# 1990
# YEAR BOOK OF
# PULMONARY DISEASE®

## The 1990 Year Book® Series

**Year Book of Anesthesia®:** Drs. Miller, Kirby, Ostheimer, Roizen, and Stoelting

**Year Book of Cardiology®:** Drs. Schlant, Collins, Engle, Frye, Kaplan, and O'Rourke

**Year Book of Critical Care Medicine®:** Drs. Rogers and Parrillo

**Year Book of Dentistry®:** Drs. Meskin, Ackerman, Kennedy, Leinfelder, Matukas, and Rovin

**Year Book of Dermatology®:** Drs. Sober and Fitzpatrick

**Year Book of Diagnostic Radiology®:** Drs. Bragg, Hendee, Keats, Kirkpatrick, Miller, Osborn, and Thompson

**Year Book of Digestive Diseases®:** Drs. Greenberger and Moody

**Year Book of Drug Therapy®:** Drs. Hollister and Lasagna

**Year Book of Emergency Medicine®:** Dr. Wagner

**Year Book of Endocrinology®:** Drs. Bagdade, Braverman, Halter, Horton, Kannan, Korenman, Molitch, Morley, Odell, Rogol, Ryan, and Sherwin

**Year Book of Family Practice®:** Drs. Rakel, Avant, Driscoll, Prichard, and Smith

**Year Book of Geriatrics and Gerontology®:** Drs. Beck, Abrass, Burton, Cummings, Makinodan, and Small

**Year Book of Hand Surgery®:** Drs. Dobyns, Chase, and Amadio

**Year Book of Hematology®:** Drs. Spivak, Bell, Ness, Quesenberry, and Wiernik

**Year Book of Infectious Diseases®:** Drs. Wolff, Barza, Keusch, Klempner, and Snydman

**Year Book of Infertility:** Drs. Mishell, Paulsen, and Lobo

**Year Book of Medicine®:** Drs. Rogers, Des Prez, Cline, Braunwald, Greenberger, Wilson, Epstein, and Malawista

**Year Book of Neonatal and Perinatal Medicine:** Drs. Klaus and Fanaroff

**Year Book of Neurology and Neurosurgery®:** Drs. Currier and Crowell

**Year Book of Nuclear Medicine®:** Drs. Hoffer, Gore, Gottschalk, Sostman, Zaret, and Zubal

**Year Book of Obstetrics and Gynecology®:** Drs. Mishell, Kirschbaum, and Morrow

**Year Book of Occupational and Environmental Medicine:** Drs. Emmett, Brooks, Harris, and Schenker

**Year Book of Oncology:** Drs. Young, Longo, Ozols, Simone, Steele, and Weichselbaum

**Year Book of Ophthalmology®:** Drs. Laibson, Adams, Augsburger, Benson, Cohen, Eagle, Flanagan, Nelson, Reinecke, Sergott, and Wilson

**Year Book of Orthopedics®:** Drs. Sledge, Poss, Cofield, Frymoyer, Griffin, Hansen, Johnson, Springfield, and Weiland

**Year Book of Otolaryngology–Head and Neck Surgery®:** Drs. Bailey and Paparella

**Year Book of Pathology and Clinical Pathology®:** Drs. Brinkhous, Dalldorf, Grisham, Langdell, and McLendon

**Year Book of Pediatrics®:** Drs. Oski and Stockman

**Year Book of Plastic, Reconstructive, and Aesthetic Surgery:** Drs. Miller, Bennett, Haynes, Hoehn, McKinney, and Whitaker

**Year Book of Podiatric Medicine and Surgery®:** Dr. Jay

**Year Book of Psychiatry and Applied Mental Health®:** Drs. Talbott, Frances, Frances, Freedman, Meltzer, Schowalter, and Yudofsky

**Year Book of Pulmonary Disease®:** Drs. Green, Ball, Loughlin, Michael, Mulshine, Peters, Terry, Tockman, and Wise

**Year Book of Speech, Language, and Hearing:** Drs. Bernthal, Hall, and Tomblin

**Year Book of Sports Medicine®:** Drs. Shephard, Eichner, Sutton, and Torg, Col. Anderson, and Mr. George

**Year Book of Surgery®:** Drs. Schwartz, Jonasson, Peacock, Shires, Spencer, and Thompson

**Year Book of Urology®:** Drs. Gillenwater and Howards

**Year Book of Vascular Surgery®:** Drs. Bergan and Yao

Editor

**Gareth M. Green, M.D.**

*Professor of Respiratory Medicine, Department of Medicine, The Johns Hopkins University School of Medicine; Professor and Chairman, Department of Environmental Health Sciences, The Johns Hopkins University School of Hygiene and Public Health, Baltimore*

Associate Editors

**Gerald M. Loughlin, M.D.**

*Associate Professor of Pediatrics; Director, Eudowood Division of Pediatric Respiratory Sciences, The Johns Hopkins University School of Medicine, Baltimore*

**John R. Michael, M.D.**

*Associate Professor of Medicine, University of Utah Health Science Center, Salt Lake City*

**James L. Mulshine, M.D.**

*Head, Biotherapy Section, National Cancer Institute–Navy Medical Oncology Branch, National Naval Medical Center, Bethesda, Maryland*

**Stephen P. Peters, M.D., Ph.D.**

*Professor of Medicine, Associate Director, Division of Pulmonary Medicine and Critical Care, Jefferson Medical College, Thomas Jefferson University, Philadelphia*

**Peter B. Terry, M.D.**

*Associate Professor of Medicine, Associate Professor of Anesthesiology and Critical Care Medicine, Associate Professor of Environmental Health Sciences, The Johns Hopkins University School of Medicine, Baltimore*

**Melvyn S. Tockman, M.D., Ph.D.**

*Associate Professor of Environmental Health Sciences, The Johns Hopkins University School of Hygiene and Public Health, Baltimore*

**Robert A. Wise, M.D.**

*Associate Professor of Medicine, The Johns Hopkins University School of Medicine, Baltimore*

1990

# The Year Book of PULMONARY DISEASE®

Editor

**Gareth M. Green, M.D.**

Associate Editors

**Gerald M. Loughlin, M.D.**
**John R. Michael, M.D.**
**James L. Mulshine, M.D.**
**Stephen P. Peters, M.D., Ph.D.**
**Peter B. Terry, M.D.**
**Melvyn S. Tockman, M.D., Ph.D.**
**Robert A. Wise, M.D.**

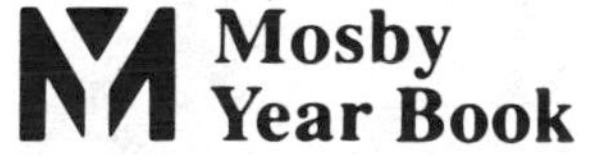


St. Louis  Baltimore  Boston  Chicago  London  Philadelphia  Sydney  Toronto

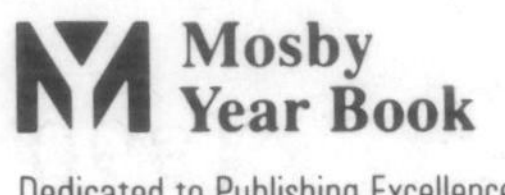


Editor-in-Chief, Year Book Publishing: Nancy Gorham
Sponsoring Editor: Gretchen C. Templeton
Manager, Medical Information Services: Edith M. Podrazik
Senior Medical Information Specialist: Terri Strorigl
Assistant Director, Manuscript Services: Frances M. Perveiler
Assistant Managing Editor, Year Book Editing Services: Wayne Larsen
Production Coordinator: Max F. Perez
Proofroom Supervisor: Barbara M. Kelly



Mosby-Year Book, Inc.
11830 Westline Industrial Drive
St. Louis, MO 63146



Editorial Office:
Mosby-Year Book, Inc.
200 North LaSalle St.
Chicago, IL 60601

International Standard Serial Number: 8756-3452
International Standard Book Number: 0-8151-3882-2

# Table of Contents

The material covered in this volume represents literature reviewed up to October 1989.

# Journals Represented

Year Book Medical Publishers subscribes to and surveys nearly 850 U.S. and foreign medical and allied health journals. From these journals, the Editors select the articles to be abstracted. Journals represented in this YEAR BOOK are listed below.

APMIS: Acta Pathologica, Microbiologica et Immunologica
Acta Paediatrica Scandinavica
Acta Radiologica
American Heart Journal
American Industrial Hygiene Association Journal
American Journal of Diseases of Children
American Journal of Epidemiology
American Journal of Gastroenterology
American Journal of Industrial Medicine
American Journal of Medicine
American Journal of Obstetrics and Gynecology
American Journal of Physiology
American Journal of Public Health
American Journal of Roentgenology
Americal Review of Respiratory Disease
Annals of Internal Medicine
Annals of Occupational Hygiene
Annals of Thoracic Surgery
Anticancer Research
Archives of Internal Medicine
Archives of Pathology and Laboratory Medicine
British Journal of Cancer
British Journal of Clinical Pharmacology
British Medical Journal
Cancer
Cancer Letters
Cancer Research
Chest
Circulation
Cleft Palate Journal
Clinical Radiology
Clinical Science
Critical Care Medicine
Early Human Development
Environmental Research
Epidemiologic Reviews
European Respiratory Journal
Experimental and Molecular Pathology
Health Physics
Immunology
Infection and Immunity
International Disability Studies Journal
Journal of Acquired Immune Deficiency Syndromes
Journal of Allergy and Clinical Immunology
Journal of the Applied Physiology
Journal of Clinical Investigation
Journal of Clinical Microbiology
Journal of Epidemiology and Community Health

Journal of Immunology
Journal of Infectious Diseases
Journal of Molecular Endocrinology
Journal of Parenteral and Enteral Nutrition
Journal of Pathology
Journal of Pediatrics
Journal of Thoracic and Cardiovascular Surgery
Journal of the American Medical Association
Journal of the Canadian Association of Radiologists
Journal of the National Cancer Institute
Lancet
Lung
Nature
New England Journal of Medicine
New Zealand Medical Journal
Pediatric Pulmonology
Pediatrics
Presse Medicale
Radiology
Respiration
Respiration Physiology
Respiratory Medicine
Scandinavian Journal of Infectious Diseases
Scandinavian Journal of Work Environment and Health
Science
Southern Medical Journal
Thorax
Toxicology and Applied Pharmacology
Western Journal of Medicine

## Standard Abbreviations

The following terms are abbreviated in this edition: acquired immunodeficiency syndrome (AIDS), the central nervous system (CNS), cerebrospinal fluid (CSF), computed tomography (CT), electrocardiography (ECG), and human immunodeficiency virus (HIV).

# Introduction

The 1990 YEAR BOOK OF PULMONARY DISEASE provides evidence of a significant shift of focus in pulmonary disease from diagnosis and treatment of patients in a medical care setting to better understanding of the genetic mechanisms regulating health and disease and to prevention of disease through control of environmental and other etiologic factors. Most gratifying is the evidence that the public is growing in its appreciation of the overwhelming significance of cigarette smoking, occupational exposures, and community air pollution in the etiology and pathogenesis of chronic pulmonary disease, respiratory infection, and lung cancer. The linkage of strategies for maintaining air quality through pollution control with the hazards of environmental tobacco smoke for nonsmokers has directed the powerful social forces of individual and collective rights to health via reduction of pollutants disseminated by others at the cigarette smoking issue. The result is no smoking in restaurants, hospitals, elevators, office buildings, airliners, and other public transportation, with a net dramatic improvement in the quality of indoor air. The growing governmental emphasis on indoor air quality and the renewal of the Clean Air Act are further evidence of significant progress in preventing pulmonary disease through control of environmental air contaminants.

The effect of the past four decades of research into and education about the role of cigarette smoking and other air pollutants in lung cancer and respiratory infection has been the beginning of a leveling off and even decline of lung cancer associated with smoking cessation among some populations. This is most encouraging news considering the decades long, epidemic rise of lung cancer mortality. Unfortunately, such is not the case yet for chronic respiratory disease: morbidity and mortality continue to rise to epidemic proportions. This dissociation between mortality curves for lung cancer and diffuse respiratory disease, both of which share similar etiologic agents, may provide a clue to the differences in their pathogenetic mechanisms.

Lung cancer mortality falls most rapidly during the first 5 years after smoking cessation, as does the incidence of respiratory symptoms of cough, phlegm, and chronic infection. This early response to smoking cessation suggests immediate and short-term effects of smoking as an agent in promotion or progression of lung cancer and immunosuppression of pulmonary infection. If, in addition, smoking affects the pathogenesis of chronic pulmonary disease by chemoattraction of inflammatory cells into the pulmonary parenchyma, one would expect early reduction of chronic respiratory disease as a response to smoking cessation as well. However, the pathologic process in chronic obstructive pulmonary disease and pulmonary fibrosis may be such that the injury is perpetuated by long-term retention of previously inhaled physicochemically toxic particulate material. It is perhaps too early to draw this conclusion, but the divergence of these two curves will be important to track in the decade of the '90s.

The second major trend illustrated by the papers collected in the 1990 YEAR BOOK OF PULMONARY DISEASE is the increasing sophistication of molecular biologic research in respiratory disease, along with the rapidly growing elucidation of the genetic mechanisms that control cell function in health and disease. Injury to the genes, as in deletion of tumor suppressor genes or activation of tumor oncogenes, appears to be critical in the multistep process of carcinogenesis, but the DNA repair process itself may be toxic to cells because of the depletion of antioxidant defenses such as NAD+. In addition, molecular genetics is spawning a new technology for monitoring environmental exposures via characterization of DNA adduct patterns, offering the promise of improved accuracy in dosimetry in occupational and community environments.

Other themes that emerge in the 1990 YEAR BOOK include the prominence of immune dysfunction in pulmonary disease, either through immunodeficiency and infection—best illustrated by the complications of HIV-1 infection—or through allergy and hypersensitivity, exemplified as always by asthma and as dramatically demonstrated by the new findings on beryllium disease. In contrast, advances in diagnosis and treatment are modest, but worth reviewing in the areas of asthma, critical care, sleep-disordered breathing, and pediatric lung disease. We particularly are proud of the exceptionally strong chapter on pediatric lung disease this year, the first full year that attention has been directed specifically to the pulmonary disease problems of neonates, infants, and developing children. Lung cancer and occupational and environmental lung disorders also receive greater attention in this volume. We hope you will both enjoy and learn from the selected articles abstracted in the 1990 YEAR BOOK OF PULMONARY DISEASE and that the commentary and editorials will be informative and thought-provoking. We encourage any commentary the readers wish to make to the editors of this volume.

**Gareth M. Green, M.D.**

# 1 Respiratory Infection

## Introduction

The area of respiratory infection continues to be dominated by the problems of infection in the immunocompromised host. Infection with HIV-1, along with its manifestations as AIDS, capture the limelight because it is new, awesome in its pathologic mechanism, and frightening by its inevitable consequences. The thought of an independent replicating microorganism capturing the genetic machinery of the very cell (CD4+ lymphocyte) that is designed for protection against the microbial world is as terrifying as the mutagenic process of cancer. In fact, the two are closely related to their focus on the genetic machinery, and the knowledge of molecular biology gained in the study of one is assisting in unraveling the secrets of the other.

We continue to be dazzled by the incredibly rapid advancement of knowledge about HIV infection gained through molecular biologic research, but the more prosaic studies of nutritional deficiencies and environmental immunosuppressants may in the long run have greater significance in reducing, preventing, and controlling respiratory infection and chronic respiratory disease on a worldwide basis. As we study the relationship of nutritional deficiencies and environmental exposures to the prevalence and pathogenesis of respiratory infection in economically emerging nations, opportunities become available to better understand the passage of our own country through the era of high mortality from respiratory infection in the 19th and early 20th centuries when tuberculosis and pneumonia were the leading causes of mortality. The development of antibiotics has had an impressive impact on that mortality, but an effective medical care system must be available to make antibiotics available to the persons afflicted with respiratory infection. Underlying susceptibility factors such as nutrition and housing require attention; immunization against potentially lethal childhood infections are a mandatory component; and economic resources to support treatment, prevention, and infrastructure must be identified and developed. Although the scope of this chapter does not cover the last feature, the work on vitamin A deficiency presents a new twist to an old tale, which, when coupled with epidemiologic studies showing the impact of vitamin A supplements on the reduction of respiratory morbidity, is extremely encouraging for worldwide prevention and control.

Another dimension of the problem of the immunocompromised host is the ability to diagnose the condition and recognize the secondary microbial invaders, which may be more lethal than the primary disease. Here, advances in molecular technology and cytotechnology, combined with traditional techniques for obtaining meaningful specimens from the lung, give new diagnostic power to the mundane and unglamorous sputum specimen.

These considerations of immunodeficiency merge with improved diagnostic technology in the clinical management of AIDS. We have included 15 articles primarily dedicated to the topic this year and several more in which AIDS is an indirect issue: for example, the role of AIDS as a reservoir for active tuberculosis and for dissemination of tuberculosis in medical settings, in prisons, and among the homeless.

Finally, the resistant problem of nosocomial infection, which remains a major cause of mortality among hospitalized patients and a source of high medical costs, receives attention primarily as another manifestation of impaired pulmonary host defense mechanisms. No major breakthroughs appear here, but we continue to chip away at an inherently stubborn problem: these infections are a limiting factor in the successful deployment of advanced medical technology such as organ transplantation and antitumor chemotherapy. The prospects for more precise control of molecularly targeted pharmacologic agents offer new vistas for medical investigators and new tools for clinicians. However, these developments will continue to challenge scientists and physicians to develop working knowledge of genetic control mechanisms of immune and defense systems and of the ways that these controls can be manipulated pharmacologically for more effective treatment of respiratory infection.

**Gareth M. Green, M.D.**

## Etiology and Pathogenesis

► In developing countries around the world, acute respiratory infection is rapidly replacing diarrheal disease as the principal cause of infant mortality. Part of the reason for this replacement is the decline of lethal diarrheal disease because of more effective dissemination of knowledge and technology for the treatment of infantile diarrhea and for the provision of sanitary services. The other part of the reason for the rise in mortality from acute respiratory illness is the persistence of nutritional deficiency, notably vitamin A and protein deficiencies, and the exposure of infants to indoor air pollutants. These latter conditions also preferentially affect the susceptibility to pulmonary infections of infants born into lower socioeconomic family status, and, along with limitations in medical care, account for the excessive morbidity and mortality from respiratory infections in the industrialized countries. Fortification of foodstuffs with vitamin A incorporated by conventional or novel techniques has made significant inroads into the prevalence of vitamin A deficiency and promises to do much more, and elimination of protein deficiency is an ongoing battle in economically deprived populations, but the control of indoor and outdoor air pollution is proving to be a more stubborn problem to resolve.

The first 3 papers of this section on the etiology and pathogenesis of respiratory infections discuss these 2 susceptibility factors. The first (Abstract 1–1) presents evidence that vitamin A deficiency alters the epithelial barrier of the respiratory mucosa, allowing increased bacterial binding to the respiratory epithelial cells. Epithelial colonization increases the quantitative dose of infectious organisms locally and in the distal lung on inhalation or aspiration of nasal pharyngeal secretions into the lower respiratory tract. Conditions that lower resistance to the contaminating bacteria, such as nitrogen oxides produced by cooking fuels—notably gas cooking—would obviously work in concert with the greater infectious dose to increase susceptibility to acute respiratory infection. G.M. Green, M.D.

**Increased Bacterial Binding to Respiratory Epithelial Cells in Vitamin A Deficiency**

Chandra RK (Mem Univ of Newfoundland, St John's)

*Br Med J* 297:834–835, Oct 1, 1988 1–1

An important risk factor for infection is malnutrition. Vitamin A deficiency is associated with a high incidence of infection, especially respiratory disease, and contributes greatly to childhood morbidity and mortality. Vitamin A plays an important part in regulating immunocompetence. The barrier function of epithelial cells in vitamin A deficiency is poorly understood. Before systemic invasion begins, bacteria must adhere to mucosal cells. The changes that occur in respiratory epithelial cells in this deficiency suggest that the ability of mucosal cells to prevent penetration by pathogenic bacteria is compromised. The binding of bacteria to nasopharyngeal epithelial cells in vitamin A-deficient children was reported.

A total of 3 groups of Indian children were studied: the first was apparently healthy, the second had mild vitamin A deficiency, and the third had eye signs of moderately severe vitamin A deficiency. A dietitian recorded 3 24-hour dietary intakes. Plasma retinol concentration was assessed, and nasopharyngeal secretions were obtained. The number of bacteria adhering to nasopharyngeal epithelial cells was significantly greater in children with vitamin A deficiency (table).

Respiratory epithelial surfaces of children with vitamin A deficiency may allow increased colonization and thus penetration of mucosa, resulting in systemic infection. If vitamin A supplements were found to correct the abnormal bacterial adherence, a cause-and-effect relationship would be established between vitamin A deficiency and this pathologic process.

▶ This simple and straightforward study was performed carefully, combining categorization of level of vitamin A deficiency by clinical signs, dietary history, and plasma retinol concentration. The association of vitamin A deficiency with general malnutrition is indicated by the correlation with body-weight-for-height standards. As shown in the table, as the vitamin A levels declined, the number of bacteria binding per epithelial cell climbed beyond 100%.

The first step in host defense is to minimize colonization to control the infectious dose. What is required to confirm the significance of the association is a study to correlate quantitative bacterial adherence with incidence and morbidity of bacterial infection, and to confirm the role of vitamin A by observing reductions in morbidity and epithelial colonization in the deficient group when provided with vitamin A supplements.—G.M. Green, M.D.

Clinical Data and Bacterial Binding to Epithelial Cells

| | Children without vitamin A deficiency (group 1) | Children with mild vitamin A deficiency (group 2) | Children with moderately severe vitamin A deficiency (group 3) |
|---|---|---|---|
| No. in group | 14 | 10 | 12 |
| Mean (SE) age (months) | 22 (3) | 24 (4) | 20 (3) |
| No. of boys:girls | 8:6 | 6:4 | 7:5 |
| Serum retinol (umol/L): | | | |
| Mean (SE) | 2·2 (0·3)* | 1·1 (0·1)* | 0·4 (0·1)* |
| Range | 1·4–3·4 | 0·7–1·4 | 0·1–0·7 |
| Mean (SE) dietary vitamin A intake (retinol equivalents) | 321 (44)* | 201 (29)* | 186 (22)* |
| No. with: | | | |
| Xerophthalmia | | 4 | 9 |
| Bitot's spots | | 2 | 6 |
| Corneal opacity | | 1 | 4 |
| Mean (SE) weight-for-height (% of standard) | 81 (4) | 77 (3) | 74 (5) |
| Mean (SE) no. of bacteria/epithelial cell | 4·8 (0·6)* | 7·9 (1·0)* | 10·3 (0·8)* |

*$P < .01$.
(Courtesy of Chandra RK: *Br Med J* 297:834–835, Oct 1, 1988.)

**Effect of Nitrogen Dioxide Exposure on Susceptibility to Influenza A Virus Infection in Healthy Adults**

Goings SAJ, Kulle TJ, Bascom R, Sauder LR, Green DJ, Hebel JR, Clements ML (Johns Hopkins Univ; Univ of Maryland)

*Am Rev Respir Dis* 139:1075–1081, May 1989 1–2

Experimental and epidemiologic studies have not resolved the existing controversy over the impact of nitrogen dioxide ($NO_2$) at ambient concentrations on pulmonary function. Previous animal studies suggested that $NO_2$ concentrations as low as 1.5 ppm adversely affect pulmonary function and increase susceptibility to respiratory virus infection. This 3-year randomized, placebo-controlled trial assessed the effect of $NO_2$ exposure on susceptibility to respiratory virus infection.

The study was done with 152 healthy, nonsmoking volunteers, aged 18 to 35, who breathed either filtered clean air or air with $NO_2$ concentrations of 2 ppm, 3 ppm, and 1 or 2 ppm in an environmentally controlled research chamber. All were seronegative to the live, attenuated, cold-adapted influenza A/Korea/l/82 (H3N2) virus administered intranasally immediately after the second exposure. Each underwent spirometric and bronchial reactivity testing at baseline and at predetermined intervals thereafter. Influenza A virus infection was defined as virus shedding, development of a fourfold rise in serum or nasal wash antibody titer, or both.

Only 1 of the 152 volunteers had a low-grade fever; none of the others had any symptoms. Pulmonary function measurements and nonspecific airway reactivity to methacholine were unchanged after $NO_2$ exposure, virus infection, or both. Only exposure to 1 or 2 ppm $NO_2$ during the third year of the study caused a higher incidence of virus infection, but the difference was statistically not significant. Therefore, these findings only suggest, but do not prove, that exposure to $NO_2$ may have a role in increasing adult susceptibility to respiratory virus infections.

▶ Evidence that oxidant air pollutants such as $NO_2$ unfavorably alter resistance to respiratory infection is substantial. The characteristics of that alteration, however, are not fully understood. Animal studies have definitely shown greater lethality for bacterial pneumonias after exposure to $NO_2$. Additional studies have demonstrated that the rate at which inhaled bacteria are killed in the lung is retarded by $NO_2$ exposure. Furthermore, animals given influenza viral infection, exposed to $NO_2$, and then challenged with a bacterial inoculum show impaired clearance of the bacteria.

Studies of human beings have been limited to epidemiologic measurements. Numerous references cited in this paper define the increased prevalence and morbidity from respiratory infection in households with elevated levels of $NO_2$ related to gas cooking and heating. Most of the papers describe these effects in children, who may be particularly affected by the $NO_2$ exposures either because of a biologic susceptibility or because they are present in the homes for virtually 100% of their lives during infancy.

The study by Goings and colleagues is particularly interesting, even with its negative results, because it is a carefully conducted exposure of healthy adult volunteers to $NO_2$ at levels up to 6 times the ambient standard for exposure. Despite slight changes in the direction of increased susceptibility, differences between control and study groups were not significant. Part of this problem may be that the test virus was sufficiently infective so that 60% or more of the nonexposed volunteers became infected. Furthermore, the use of an attenuated cold-adapted influenza A virus may have resulted in a sufficiently nonpathogenic challenge to detect any potential effect of $NO_2$. After all, children and adults in a community are infected with virulent organisms that would be expected to more readily identify a condition of impaired resistance induced by $NO_2$ exposure. So, once again, the effect of $NO_2$ on host susceptibility to respiratory infection in human beings is unresolved, although the epidemiologic evidence that this problem may be of substantial importance in children, perhaps particularly those children with less than optimal nutrition, continues to mount, gas cooking tends to be more prevalent in communities with lower socioeconomic status.

The next paper offers additional experimental evidence to explain why exposure to $NO_2$ should be considered a risk factor for respiratory infection.— G.M. Green, M.D.

---

**Nitrogen Dioxide Exposure in Vivo and Human Alveolar Macrophage Inactivation of Influenza Virus in Vitro**

Frampton MW, Smeglin AM, Roberts NJ Jr, Finkelstein JN, Morrow PE, Utell MJ (Univ of Rochester, NY)

*Environ Res* 48:179–192, April 1989 1–3

---

Respiratory infection and illness have been associated with increased indoor levels of nitrogen dioxide ($NO_2$), and animal exposure studies have related brief exposures to peak levels of $NO_2$ to increased morbidity. In the present study normal volunteers were exposed to 0.6 or 2.0 ppm of $NO_2$ during bicycle exercise. Inhalational challenges with aerosolized carbachol were carried out. Cells obtained by bronchoalveolar lavage were exposed in vitro to influenza virus.

Inhalation of $NO_2$ by normal volunteers did not significantly alter lung function or airway reactivity. Alveolar macrophages from those exposed to continuous 0.6 ppm of $NO_2$ tended to inactivate influenza virus in vitro less effectively than cells collected after exposure to air. Macrophages from all subjects whose cells were defective in inactivating virus exhibited increased production of interleukin-1 in association with $NO_2$.

Effects of pollutants on defenses in the lower respiratory tract can be assessed by examining lavaged alveolar macrophages after controlled exposure to a pollutant. In vitro challenge with influenza virus provides information on human respiratory disease without having to produce clinical infection.

▶ This very nice experimental study of human beings shows a physiologic defect in alveolar macrophages obtained from human volunteers exposed to $NO_2$

at near standard levels and provides another piece in the puzzle supporting the picture of $NO_2$ as a significant risk factor for respiratory infection. Furthermore, this study is of interest in demonstrating that less than half of the tested persons showed the positive effect and that this effect was associated with increased production of the cytokine interleukin-1. Given the individual variation in susceptibility to infection, the pathways to unraveling the relationship of $NO_2$ and susceptibility will have to be mechanistically defined to characterize, identify, and distinguish the susceptible portion of the population from the nonsusceptible, even when the susceptible population is a small fraction of the total. Mechanistic studies such as described in this paper represent a productive pathway to pursue. It is of special interest that the exposures that showed effects on viral inactivation by alveolar macrophages showed no effects on pulmonary function or airways reactivity. This is a good paper for the experimental clinical investigator to read and analyze.— G.M. Green, M.D.

► ↓ The next 4 papers elaborate on the various cellular mechanisms of host resistance to infection; Abstracts 1–5 and 1–6 define additional mechanisms by which cigarette smoke enhances susceptibility to respiratory infection by a suppressive effect on alveolar macrophages.— G.M. Green, M.D.

---

**Rapid Recovery of Lung Histology Correlates With Clearance of Influenza Virus by Specific CD8$^+$ Cytotoxic T Cells**

Mackenzie CD, Taylor PM, Askonas BA (Natl Inst for Med Research, London; Michigan State Univ)

*Immunology* 67:375–381, July 1989 1–4

---

Cytotoxic T cells protect against lethal infection by some viruses, such as influenza, and promote viral clearance from the lungs. Histologic changes in the lungs were related to viral clearance following transfer of influenza-specific cytotoxic T cell clones into infected mice. Influenza virus A/X31 and the BALB/c cytotoxic T cell clones T5/5 and T9/13 were used in the study. T cells were transferred 7 to 10 days after antigenic stimulation in vitro. Intranasal infection of mice with A/X31 produces lung tissue changes that persist for 8 to 10 days.

Transfer of the T cell clone T9/13 to infected mice led to a transiently increased loss of epithelium and much reduced epithelial abnormality by day 6, compared with untreated infected mice. Lung viral titers were significantly reduced by day 6. By day 8, virus was cleared and the lungs appeared normal. The T cell clone T5/5, which has greater cytolytic activity, led to significant recovery of lung tissue by day 4.

Adoptive transfer of cloned cytotoxic T cells may hasten the recovery of lung tissue after influenza virus infection. Histologic improvement correlates with a reduction in the level of pulmonary virus. Whether actual lysis of infected cells is responsible remains to be established.

► This paper is interesting because it shows the correlation of the course of histopathology with the timing of the immune response and the eradication of the pathogen. By providing antiviral immune cytotoxic lymphocytes at the time of inoculation of the virus, the cellular immune apparatus was able to go to work against the virus immediately rather than wait for the development of endogenous antiviral immunity, which takes 4 to 5 days. Because specific cellular immunity was provided earlier, it is not surprising that viral inactivation would occur earlier and that immunoreactive pathology would also occur earlier and resolve earlier. The provision of specific immune cytotoxic T cells early in the course of infection is perhaps analogous to the reinfection phenomenon, in which a viral inoculum confronts a specific immune system earlier in the course of the infection.

The interesting finding is the early and enhanced sloughing of the respiratory epithelium in the CD8-inoculated animals. The finding recalls the acceleration and exaggerated response of the chronic bronchitic to viral reinfection when sputum is dramatically increased early in the course of the infection. Perhaps part of this accelerated response is related to the interaction of an already specific immune cytotoxic lymphocyte system. By aggravating and accelerating epithelial destruction, specific immune cytotoxic lymphocytes could accelerate and exaggerate the secretory and symptomatic response to infection of the bronchitic.—G.M. Green, M.D.

**Phagocytosis and Killing of *Listeria monocytogenes* by Alveolar Macrophages: Smokers Versus Nonsmokers**

King TE Jr, Savici D, Campbell PA (Natl Jewish Ctr for Immunology and Respiratory Medicine, Denver; Univ of Colorado)

*J Infect Dis* 158:1309–1316, December 1988 1–5

Previous studies have demonstrated that cigarette smoking alters the presence and function of alveolar macrophages in otherwise healthy persons. However, studies of the phagocytic and bactericidal activity of alveolar macrophages in smokers and nonsmokers have yielded conflicting results. *Listeria monocytogenes* is a facultative intracellular bacterium that is widely used as a model of T cell-mediated immune response affecting macrophage function. The phagocytic and bactericidal capabilities of alveolar macrophages from normal smokers and nonsmokers against *L. monocytogenes* was investigated.

A group of 21 men and 11 women aged 21 to 71 years (mean, 44 years) had no respiratory symptoms and normal chest radiographs and pulmonary function tests. Of the 32 persons, 15 were current smokers and the others were nonsmokers or ex-smokers. All underwent bronchoalveolar lavage (BAL) to recover alveolar macrophages, which were tested for their ability to ingest *L. monocytogenes* in a previously described bactericidal assay.

There were no significant differences between smokers and nonsmokers in the alveolar macrophages' ability to phagocytose *Listeria.* However, the alveolar macrophages from nonsmokers killed *Listeria,* whereas those from smokers did not. Therefore, alveolar macrophages from healthy smokers can phagocytose, but not kill *Listeria,* suggesting a defect in the immunoregulation of alveolar macophages in smokers.

▶ It is well documented that cigarette smokers have more difficulty handling respiratory tract infection than nonsmokers. At one time this difficulty was attributed to the increased mucus and sputum in smokers and the "irritant effect" of the tobacco smoke. That intrapulmonary bactericidal activity was more critical to the defense of the lung against infection than mucociliary clearance focused attention on the effects of cigarette smoke on the alveolar macrophage as the principal resident phagocyte responsible for the intrapulmonary bactericidal activity.

This paper continues in the series of mechanistic studies that has been ongoing for the last 20 years. It uses the dependence of eradication of *Listeria monocytogenes* on the intracellular bactericidal action of the lung for control of this infection. Cigarette smoke was found to affect alveolar macrophages via intracellular destruction of *Listeria* rather than its uptake as a particle into the macrophage. This is a particularly interesting finding, because the cigarette smokers from whom the alveolar macrophages were obtained were clinically healthy but walking around with a previously unsuspected and important physiologic deficit in a key defense mechanism of the lung. How broad or significant this physiologic defect is in regard to susceptibility to a broader range of viral and bacterial potential pathogens remains to be determined.

Cigarette smoke has other effects on the human alveolar macrophage that are important to the mobilization of bronchopulmonary defense mechanisms. Human alveolar macrophages synthesize and release interleukin-1, which mobilizes inflammatory responses. As the next paper shows, release but not synthesis of interleukin-1 is inhibited by cigarette smoking in otherwise normal, healthy smokers; smoke also affected the release of prostaglandin $E_2$. This is further evidence of the chronically altered state of immunoresponsiveness of respiratory tract defense mechanisms in the cigarette smoker. Other environmental pollutants may produce similar or related effects in these cells and alter unfavorably the versatile and integrated immunodefense mechanisms of the lung, including responses to infectious challenges and possibly tumor surveillance. These are very sensitive assays of biologic effects of an important environmental pollutant. The effects do not appear to interfere with the normal state of health of the immunodefense apparatus, but impair responses to challenges from infectious or chemical exposures. Is this environmentally induced defect a significant risk for smokers?—G.M. Green, M.D.

---

**Cigarette Smoking Decreases Interleukin 1 Release by Human Alveolar Macrophages**

Brown GP, Iwamoto GK, Monick MM, Hunninghake GW (VA Hosp, Iowa City; Univ of Iowa)

*Am J Physiol* 256:C260–C264, 1989 1–6

---

Defective host defenses may have a role in the smoking-induced risk of bronchogenic carcinoma. Macrophages in particular are considered to be important antitumor effector cells. Release of interleukin-1 (IL-1) by alveolar macrophages was studied by obtaining bronchoalveolar lavage samples from 11 nonsmokers, 4 light smokers with less than 10 pack-years of exposure and 9 heavy smokers with more than 10 pack-years of exposure.

In the presence of lipopolysaccharide, macrophages from heavy smokers released significantly less IL-1 than cells from nonsmokers, and light smokers had intermediate values. Decreased release of IL-1 by cells from heavy smokers did not result from an altered dose response to lipopolysaccharide. It appeared that release, not production, of IL-1 was defective. Cells from heavy smokers also released less prostaglandin $E_2$ ($PGE_2$). Release of IL-1 was not augmented in the presence of indomethacin, which abolished the release of $PGE_2$.

Release of IL-1 from alveolar macrophages is defective in chronic heavy smokers. Release of $PGE_2$ also is impaired, and inflammatory and immune processes in the lungs may be altered as a result of these abnormalities.

---

**Alveolar Macrophages Differ From Blood Monocytes in Human IL-1β Release: Quantitation by Enzyme-Linked Immunoassay**

Wewers MD, Herzyk DJ (Ohio State Univ)

*J Immunol* 143:1635–1641, Sept 1, 1989 1–7

---

Interleukin-1 (IL-1) is an important regulatory cytokine with a variety of proinflammatory functions. One of its 2 constituent proteins, IL-1β, lacks a signal peptide or hydrophobic peptide sequence that would act to regulate protein secretion. In this study antigenic assays were used to characterize IL-1β release by alveolar macrophages. These assays overcome the problem of interference that arises with bioassays and are able to accurately measure the nonfunctional precursor of IL-1β.

A sensitive, specific enzyme-linked immunosorbent assay showed that blood monocytes from normal persons released 13 ng/$10^6$ cells of IL-1β, compared with 3.5 ng/$10^6$ for alveolar macrophages. Total production of IL-1β actually was greater for alveolar macrophages. A relative increase in intracellular IL-1β in alveolar macrophages was confirmed by Western blot analysis of cell lysates. Studies of production of tumor necrosis factor (TNF) showed that the limitation in IL-1 release was not a generalized defect. When fresh monocytes matured in vitro, they had a greater than 20-fold decrease in ability to release IL-1β, while ability to release TNF increased sixfold to eightfold.

Alveolar macrophages and blood monocytes differ in their ability to process and release IL-1β precursor protein. Regulation of IL-1β differs substantially from that of TNF-α. A better understanding of the mechanisms involved may throw light on how circulating and tissue mononuclear phagocytes respond to microbial invasion.

## Diagnosis

---

**Quantitative Bacterial Cultures of Bronchoalveolar Lavage Fluids and Protected Brush Catheter Specimens From Normal Subjects**

Kirkpatrick MB, Bass JB Jr (Univ of South Alabama, Mobile)
*Am Rev Respir Dis* 139:546–548, February 1989 1–8

Flexible bronchoscopy with the use of a protected brush catheter (PBC) is used routinely to identify pathogens in the lower respiratory tract. Quantitative bacterial cultures obtained from bronchoalveolar lavage (BAL) fluid might be able to identify lower airway pathogens. Quantitative bacterial cultures from BAL fluid were compared with those from PBC specimens obtained from 8 normal, nonsmoking volunteers who had no history of acute or chronic respiratory disease.

Before bronchoscopy, saline was aspirated through the bronchoscope channel and submitted for quantitative culture to assess the cleanliness of the bronchoscope. A PBC specimen was obtained from each person's right middle lobe. A BAL specimen was then obtained from the same location. All specimens were cultured quantitatively for aerobic and anaerobic organisms. In addition, lidocaine levels were measured in both BAL fluid and PBC specimens to determine whether lidocaine was present in concentrations high enough to inhibit bacterial growth.

Six of the 8 bronchoscope specimens taken for culture taken before bronchoscopy were sterile. Two bronchoscopes were contaminated as a result of violations of standard bronchoscope cleaning techniques. Seven of the 8 PBC specimens were sterile; 1 specimen yielded small quantities of normal oropharyngeal flora. Seven of 8 BAL fluid cultures were positive, yielding 1–4 bacterial strains per culture. Quantitation of the cultures indicated that the bacteria were oropharyngeal contaminants. Lidocaine concentrations in BAL fluids and PBC specimens were low enough not to interfere with the recovery of bacteria.

Bronchoalveolar lavage fluid is often contaminated by oropharyngeal bacterial flora, but quantitation of the recovered bacteria may allow separation of contaminant from pathogenic organisms.

▶ Thirty years ago, Lees and McNaught (1) demonstrated the sterility of the lower respiratory tract below the carina by careful quantitative culture of bronchial secretions obtained at bronchoscopy. This observation was used to hypothesize that existing bronchopulmonary defense mechanisms were capable of maintaining sterility in the peripheral lung despite the presumed contamination by inhalation or aspiration of infective material from the upper respiratory tract. The focus of consideration of defense mechanisms at that time was on the mucociliary apparatus that mechanically sweeps inhaled and aspirated material from the peripheral bronchi to the trachea and glottis where the material is swallowed, thus the term *bacterial clearance of the lung.* Later investigators, in repeating these studies, found that the topical anesthetic could inhibit the outgrowth of bacteria from contaminated specimens and threw these earlier studies into question. However, direct cultures of the lung tissue from numerous animal species have confirmed that the normal peripheral lung in most species is indeed sterile.

Numerous subsequent studies of human beings have attempted to protect the sampling process from upper respiratory tract contamination, as was done in this study. By using the protected brush catheter adapted to the flexible bronchoscope, these authors have avoided contamination by upper respiratory tract secretions in 7 of 8 patients and offer evidence of a useful and reliable technique for obtaining specimens from the lower bronchial region that represent that region without contamination from the upper respiratory tract.

Their findings raise several questions: first, the long-asked question, "How does the normal peripheral lung maintain its sterility?" and second, "What is the significance of finding mixed bacterial flora in this normally sterile region?" The first question was addressed by Green and Kass (2) and by Laurenzi (3), who used aerosol infections in quantitative culture to characterize the kinetics of the normal clearance of bacteria experimentally introduced into mouse lung. Then, Green and Kass (4), using radiotracer-labeled microorganisms, found that the inhaled organisms were killed in situ long before the tracer material was physically eliminated by the mucociliary stream. Using immunofluorescent labeling techniques, these authors then demonstrated that the microorganisms were taken up by alveolar phagocytes, accounting for the in situ bactericidal activity inferred by the radiotracer studies.

Since those studies, countless others have varied the experiments to show that many bacterial species, particularly those that become pathogenic, resist the bactericidal activity of the alveolar macrophages and either are taken up by secondarily infiltrated polymorphonuclear leukocytes or replicate in the lung to produce infection. The finding of positive cultures from the lower respiratory tract suggests a relative defect in the normal bactericidal activity of these cells such that the flora are not eradicated. The significance, then, of finding viable organisms in the distal bronchopulmonary tract may be the indication of a dysfunctional bactericidal system in the peripheral lung.

The clinical significance of positive cultures without symptomatic or radiologic lower respiratory tract findings has not been worked out, in part because of the lack of a simple technique that assures the interpretation of microbial cultures of the lower respiratory tract without contamination from above. The data in this paper indicate that the protected brush catheter technique employed to obtain bronchoalveolar lavage fluids at flexible bronchoscopy provides a suitable method of pursuing such studies in human beings.—G.M. Green, M.D.

*References*


1. Lees AW, McNaught W: *Lancet* 2:1112, 1959.
2. Green GM, Kass EH: *J Clin Invest* 43:769, 1964.
3. Laurenzi G et al: *J Clin Invest* 43:759, 1964.
4. Green GM, Kass EH: *J Exp Med* 119:167, 1964.


---

**Gram Stain and Culture of Morning and 24 h Sputum in the Diagnosis of Bacterial Exacerbation of Chronic Bronchitis: A Dogma Disputed**

Medici TC, von Graevenitz A, Shang H, Böhni E, Wall M (Univ of Zürich; Hoffmann-La Roche & Co Ltd, Basel, Switzerland)

*Eur Respir J* 1:923–928, December 1988 1–9

Exacerbation of chronic bronchitis is commonly diagnosed by Gram stain and culture of freshly expectorated morning sputum. Some investigators prefer examination of 24-hour sputum for antibiotic trials because the 24-hour sputum volume is considered a sensitive parameter of antibiotic efficacy. However, others believe that bacterial viability is lost when cultivation is delayed. To clarify this issue, the bacteriologic results from microscopic and cultural examinations of morning and 24-hour sputa were compared.

Fresh morning and 24-hour sputum aliquots were collected from 12 patients with untreated bacterial exacerbation of chronic bronchitis. Patients were assigned randomly to collect sputa on 2 consecutive days, collecting either fresh morning sputum for 3 hours in the early morning on the first day and a 24-hour sputum collection on the second day, or vice versa. The diagnosis of exacerbation of chronic bronchitis was based on worsening of clinical signs and symptoms, sputum cytology, and total bacterial count on the Gram stain.

With respect to *Haemophilus* and pneumococci, no difference was noted between bacteriologic findings in fresh morning sputum in the 24-hour sputum. *Haemophilus influenzae,* pneumococci, and neisseriae were identified more often in Gram stains than in cultures. The Gram-stained specimens of 3-hour and 24-hour sputa had similar counts of *Haemophilus*-like and *Pneumococcus*-like microorganisms. Staphylococci and gram-negative rods were seen more often in cultures than in Gram stains, suggesting bacterial overgrowth. However, the overgrowth did not interfere substantially with the growth of *Haemophilus* or pneumococci. Approximately 50% of the bacteria identified as pneumococci failed to grow in cultures.

For confirmation of bacterial exacerbation of chronic bronchitis, microscopic examination of the Gram stain is superior to cultural examination. Furthermore, Gram stains of 24-hour sputum produce comparable results to those of morning sputum.

▶ Chronic bronchitis is perhaps the best example of impaired bactericidal defensive mechanisms in the lower respiratory tract. Not all patients with symptoms of chronic bronchitis, persistent cough, and phlegm show bacterial microflora in the lower respiratory tract, indicating that these symptoms may be caused by allergens, chemicals, or other physical irritants and do not universally require microbial infection for their appearance. However, chronic bronchitic patients who have the characteristic recurrent exacerbations associated with bacterial overgrowth show persistent microbial flora between the periods of exacerbation. According to the rationale expressed in the discussion of the previous paper, the persistence of microflora suggests a chronic impairment of the normal bactericidal mechanisms of the lower respiratory tract. The bacterial species usually found are *Haemophilus influenzae* and *Stretococcus pneumoniae.* It is unlikely that the microorganisms cause the bacterial exacerbations of chronic bronchitis because they are chronically present in lower respiratory tract secretions of bronchitic patients, but it does appear that they replicate more actively during the exacerbations and that the exacerbations are ameliorated by appropriate antibacterial therapy.

The problem addressed in this paper by Medici and co-workers is how to gather specimens of lower respiratory tract secretions that reliably measure the bacterial content during these exacerbations without resorting to invasive techniques such as are employed in the previous paper. The paper examines the relative efficacy of different sputum collection techniques and examination by Gram's stain smears vs. culture. The results are instructive, but the relevant question in exacerbations of chronic bronchitis is the quantitative changes that occur in microbial flora. The predominance of *Haemophilus* and pneumococcal-like organisms is so great that many clinicians do not immediately use cultures, but routinely treat with broad-spectrum antibiotics at the onset of symptoms of exacerbation and resort to cultures only when failure to respond suggests a change or emergence of a bacterial species other than the predominant two. However, the above conclusions on the relative value of Gram's stains vs. cultures, and fresh morning vs. 24-hour sputum samples, provides useful clinical guidance.—G.M. Green, M.D.

---

**The Use of Mucolysed Induced Sputum for the Identification of Pulmonary Pathogens Associated With Human Immunodeficiency Virus Infection**

Ng VL, Gartner I, Weymouth LA, Goodman CD, Hopewell PC, Hadley WK (Univ of California, San Francisco)

*Arch Pathol Lab Med* 113:488–493, May 1989 1–10

---

Because of the projected increase in the number of new cases of AIDS in the near future, efficient and accurate microbiologic procedures are needed to diagnose *Pneumocystis carinii* pneumonia. A method for the routine diagnosis of *P. carinii* pneumonia and other pulmonary complications in patients with HIV infection is described.

Technique.—Sputum is induced by inhalation of a 3% saline aerosol solution. The induced sputa are mucolysed, concentrated by centrifugation, and stained with a rapid modified Giemsa stain. When *P. carinii* is found, the specimen is also stained for acid-fast organisms and cultures for mycobacteria and fungi. When *P. carinii* is not found, fiberoptic bronchoscopy with bronchoalveolar lavage (BAL) is performed.

During a 10-month period, 404 induced sputum specimens obtained from 358 HIV-infected patients were examined for the presence of *P. carinii.* All patients had suspected HIV-associated pulmonary disease. *Pneumocystis carinii* was found in 222 of the 404 specimens (55%). Bronchoalveolar lavage subsequently identified *P. carinii* in 50 of 118 episodes in which sputum specimens were negative for *P. carinii.* Mycobacteria were recovered from 6% of the specimens positive for *P. carinii* and from 12% of the positive bronchoscopic specimens. None of the positive sputum or bronchoscopic specimens contained potentially pathogenic fungi. Mycobacteria were detected in 23.5% of the specimens negative for *P. carinii*, and pathogenic fungi were recovered from 50% of the negative specimens.

Bronchoscopy need only be performed in patients whose induced sputum specimens do not yield *P. carinii*. Mycobacterial and fungal cultures need only be done on bronchoscopic specimens in which *P. carinii* is not detected.

▸ The resurgence of interest in obtaining efficient and accurate diagnostic procedures for lower respiratory tract infection results from the growing problem of respiratory tract infection in the immunocompromised host, especially in patients with HIV infection. The most common agent for infection in that disease is the organism *Pneumocystis carinii*, which has a peculiar predilection for replication in the presence of HIV infection. The single fortunate aspect of this predilection is that *P. carinii*, a unicellular parasite, is readily distinguished microscopically and is pathognomonic for infection. All that is necessary is to obtain a reliable sample from the lower respiratory tract by the simplest possible procedure. Twenty years ago, the customary procedure was done via open-lung biopsy of infected tissue. Then, Harrow and colleagues (1) showed, with an animal model of *P. carinii* infection, that the organism could be readily identified by bronchopulmonary lavage. These findings were subsequently confirmed in human beings, obviating the need for the invasive procedure to make the diagnosis.

About 30 years ago, Alvin Barach designed a technique of stimulating lower respiratory tract secretions to improve the sputum sample for diagnosing diseases such as bronchopulmonary carcinoma and tuberculosis. The technique was designed, and has been used for decades, to provide better cytologic testing for bronchogenic cancer. Sputum induced by hypertonic saline aerosols reliably produces fresher specimens containing cellular material from the lower respiratory tract and alveoli.

These 2 streams of investigation have now been brought together by the authors of this paper, whose data support a systematic methodology for identifying the principal pulmonary pathogens associated with HIV infection, *P. carinii*, and *Mycobacterium tuberculosis*. The high frequency of positivity for mycobacteria is a reminder of the important association of tuberculosis with human AIDS. Following this methodology would diminish the number of instances of examination by fiberoptic bronchoscopy being required.—G.M. Green, M.D.

*Reference*

1. Harrow EM et al: *Am Rev Respir Dis* 112:7, 1975.

**Transthoracic Aspiration Needle Biopsy: Value in the Diagnosis of Pulmonary Infections**

Conces DJ Jr, Clark SA, Tarver RD, Schwenk GR (Indiana Univ, Indianapolis)

*AJR* 152:31–34, January 1989 1–11

In a 5-year period, most of the 441 transthoracic needle aspiration biopsies at 1 center were performed for presumed malignancy, but 13 patients proved to have infection, and 67 biopsies were done on the indication of pulmonary infection. The results of these 80 biopsies, performed on 76 patients with an average age of 49 years, were reviewed. More than half of the patients had disorders that compromised immune defenses. Biopsies were done under fluoroscopic guidance in most instances.

Infectious organisms were found in approximately half of the specimens obtained from patients with suspected infection. In 10 cases a specific noninfectious diagnosis was made. Eighteen biopsies yielded nonspecific findings. A wide range of infections was present in the patients with biopsies for suspected malignancy. Complications included pneumothorax in 14 patients, contusion in 9, and hemoptysis in 2. Four patients with pneumothorax required a chest tube.

Transthoracic needle aspiration biopsy is a useful means of diagnosing pulmonary infections. In 80% of patients, information used in making treatment decisions was obtained. If possible, biopsy should be done before antibiotic therapy begins. For many specimens, either the stain or culture was positive, but not both; therefore, multiple studies are appropriate. The complication rate was acceptable.

▶ Of course, another approach to sampling pulmonary secretions in tissues for diagnosing pulmonary infection is aspirating secretions in tissue by transthoracic needle biopsy. This approach may be particularly useful in a localized infection, but many previous studies have shown that the approach by the luminal route of bronchoalveolar lavage is superior and avoids the complications of pneumothorax. This technique is available, however, should the tracheobronchial approach not yield diagnostic information in a situation where infection is highly suspected. Such an example is illustrated in the comparison of transtracheal aspiration and fine-needle aspiration biopsy for the diagnosis of pulmonary infection in heart transplant patients (1).—G.M. Green, M.D.

*Reference*

1. de Vivo F et al: *J Thorac Cardiovasc Surg* 96:696, 1988.

▶ ↓ In contrast to the continuing evaluation of decades-old techniques for assessing bacterial infection in the lung, advances in immunology and molecular biology have brought exciting and precise methodologies for assessing viral infection and other lung disease processes as indicated by the next 3 papers (Abstracts 1–12 through 1–14). The first demonstrates the use of pooled murine monoclonal antibodies for rapid screening of respiratory secretions for several respiratory viruses in 1 test, the second uses the exotic technique of in vitro hybridization to identify adenovirus in lung tissues from patients with adenovirus pneumonia, and the third measures levels of soluble interleukin-2 receptors to distinguish rejection from infection after lung or heart–lung transplantation.—G.M. Green, M.D.

**Evaluation of a Monoclonal Antibody Pool for Rapid Diagnosis of Respiratory Viral Infections**

Stout C, Murphy MD, Lawrence S, Julian S (Univ of Tennessee, Knoxville)
*J Clin Microbiol* 27:448–452, March 1989 1–12

Rapid diagnosis of viral respiratory diseases may promote the effective use of antiviral drugs and limit unneeded antibiotic therapy. Viral isolation can take as long as 2 weeks. The enzyme-linked immunosorbent assays are useful for demonstrating respiratory syncytial virus (RSV) but not other respiratory viruses, and fluorescent antibody staining has had varying sensitivity and specificity. A reagent of pooled murine monoclonal antibodies (MAbP) were directed against several respiratory viruses, including adenovirus, RSV, influenza viruses A and B, and parainfluenza viruses types 1, 2, and 3. The procedure consisted of a 2-step, fluorescent staining method applied to cells harvested from culture and on exfoliated nasopharyngeal or tracheal cells. Individual antiviral antibody stains served to identify specific viruses from MAbP-positive specimens.

When 241 respiratory specimens were tested to confirm cell culture, MAbP was 91% sensitive and 94% specific. A total of 376 specimens then were assessed by direct staining of exfoliated cells, and the results were compared with those of cell culture isolation. The MAbP method was 69% sensitive and 97% specific.

The MAbP method served to detect several respiratory viruses at 1 test session in a highly specific and a fairly sensitive manner. It can serve as a rapid screening technique for respiratory secretions and, as such, may be a cost-effective viral detection method. Sensitivity might be increased by testing a larger sample of adenovirus and parainfluenza virus-positive specimens.

▶ The specificity of the monoclonal antibody technique is remarkable and, of course, results from the highly specific antiviral antibody that is produced by the monoclonal technique. Thus, once the identification of viral etiology is determined by a positive reaction of the pooled antiserum, specific identification of the causative virus by direct staining of the exfoliated cells for the virus is close to 100%. Pooling of the several highly specific monoclonal antibodies greatly extends the sensitivity in the initial detection of viral etiology. This technique is not readily available in clinical laboratories, but it clearly has strong promise for the future and its development should be watched closely for appropriate application to clinical diagnosis of respiratory viral infections.—G.M. Green, M.D.

**In Situ Hybridization Studies of Adenoviral Infections of the Lung and Their Relationship to Follicular Bronchiectasis**

Hogg JC, Irving WL, Porter H, Evans M, Dunnill MS, Fleming K (John Radcliffe Hosp, Oxford, England)
*Am Rev Respir Dis* 139:1531–1535, June 1989 1–13

On the basis of serologic studies of patients with bronchiectasis and histologic examination of lobectomy specimens removed for bronchiectasis, chronic adenovirus infection may play a role in the etiology of this disorder.

A total of 20 lung samples obtained from 9 patients with chronic bronchiectasis, 14 lung samples obtained from 3 patients with adenovirus pneumonia, 1 lung sample obtained 3 months after confirmed acute adenovirus pneumonia, and 1 lung sample obtained 3 years after adenovirus pneumonia were studied. The patients with bronchiectasis had undergone resection of 1 or 2 lobes that all had the histopathologic changes of follicular bronchiectasis. The 3 patients with acute adenovirus pneumonia died of their disease. All lung samples had been fixed and stored in paraffin blocks for several years.

HepII cells were inoculated with a single adenovirus species and incubated for 24 to 36 hours. These cells were then embedded in paraffin to be used as positive controls. A commercially available biotin-labeled DNA probe was used to detect nucleic acid sequences of adenovirus in the HepII cells and in the fixed paraffin-embedded tissue blocks.

The DNA probe detected adenovirus in all HepII cells that had been specifically infected with types 3, 35, 5, 8, and 4, representing Genera B1, B2, C, D, and E, with a sensitivity of 5–10 copies per cell. The probe also detected adenovirus in the 14 lung samples obtained from patients with acute adenovirus pneumonia. However, the probe failed to identify adenovirus in the samples from patients examined 3 months and 3 years after acute adenovirus infection, and in the samples from patients with chronic follicular bronchiectasis.

The in situ hybridization technique is useful for investigating active pulmonary adenovirus infection. It could not be determined if the failure to detect adenovirus in the other lung samples resulted from the true absence of adenovirus in these blocks, or whether the virus was present in a latent form below the level of sensitivity of this technique.

▶ In situ hybridization uses a stainable labeled DNA sequence that hybridizes with viral protein-producing specific RNA to detect the evidence of viral protein-producing machinery in cells and tissues. It detects not the virus itself, but the manufacturing machinery for the virus. It is thus far more specific evidence to implicate viral etiology in chronic disease than either immunoserology or viral culture because it traces the evidence of virus infection in relation to the abnormal cells and tissues of the acute or chronic disease. The distinction between positive and negative findings in adenovirus pneumonia, either acute or postinfection, is complete, as are the 100% negative findings in follicular bronchiectasis. Although the negative findings appear to exclude chronic adenoviral infection as causative of follicular bronchiectasis because no viral-producing machinery is identified, it does not exclude the possibility that adenoviral pneumonia initiated a process that is no longer dependent on continuing viral replication. The use of this highly specific technique likely will do much to clarify the alleged role of chronic viral infection in a variety of chronic pulmonary disorders.—G.M. Green, M.D.

**Dynamic Changes in Soluble Interleukin-2 Receptor Levels After Lung or Heart–Lung Transplantation**

Lawrence EC, Holland VA, Young JB, Windsor NT, Brousseau KP, Noon GP, Whisennand HH, Debakey ME, Nelson DL (Methodist Hosp; Baylor College of Medicine, Houston; Natl Cancer Inst, NIH, Bethesda, Md)

*Am Rev Respir Dis* 140:789–796, September 1989 1–14

Accurate diagnosis of allograft rejection is a major limitation of successful lung and heart–lung transplantation. Because there is evidence that serum levels of soluble interleukin-2 receptor (IL-2R) correspond to heart–lung transplant rejection, a prospective, blind trial was designed to evaluate the dynamics of soluble levels of IL-2R after transplantation.

Twelve patients who had single-lung, double-lung, or heart–lung transplantation participated in the study. Control sera were obtained from 85 normal volunteers and 24 patients with various disorders including adult respiratory distress syndrome.

Levels of soluble IL-2R were markedly elevated during rejection episodes. Elevations up to 5,000 units/mL were present in sepsis, but levels exceeding 6,750 units/mL occurred only with rejection.

Markedly elevated levels of soluble IL-2R are associated with rejection of lung or heart–lung transplants. A low level of soluble IL-2R excludes transplant rejection. This determination may help distinguish rejection from infection after lung or heart lung transplantation. Dynamic changes in soluble IL-2R also may occur when a liver or heart transplant is rejected.

▶ A means of distinguishing among infectious, septic, and rejection episodes in post-lung or heart–lung transplant patients is needed to guide both antibiotic and immunosuppressive postoperative management. Clinical and radiologic signs are not sufficiently specific in many instances, and the finding of a more specific biologic monitor for rejection would allow for increasing immunosuppressive treatment without increasing the risks of the infection. The use of a marker of the immune response, the IL-2 soluble receptor, is an interesting approach. However, lymphocyte activation is a part of infectious diseases in those with bacterial infection and sepsis as evidenced by the findings of elevated IL-2R levels in this paper. Thus, although some distinction can be made in the levels of IL-2R in groups of patients, the overlap is sufficient to make it extremely difficult to distinguish one etiology from another in the individual patient. The approach in this paper is well worth pursuing, but additional or more specific markers will be required to provide adequate guidance in posttransplantation pulmonary disease.—G.M. Green, M.D.

## AIDS

▶ The phenomenon of pulmonary infection as a serious or lethal complication of infection with HIV-1 and its associated AIDS has stimulated a necessary resurgence of interest in immune mechanisms of resistance to infection in the lung and the effectiveness of diagnostic procedures in verifying the etiology of the complicating infecting organism. The human immunodeficiency virus enters the lymphocyte subset responsible for cell-mediated immunity by attachment to the CD4+ cellular receptor. Infection, replication, and release of fresh virus is associated with the reduction of CD4+ lymphocytes and a decline in cell-mediated immunity. Because the respiratory tract harbors potential respiratory pathogens and is open for infection to the external environment, it is commonly the first and principal organ to show the effects of the impaired immune response.

By far, the most common serious infection in the lung, for reasons that are not clearly understood, is that by the protozoan *Pneumocystis carinii,* which is normally easily suppressed but replicates in the absence of cellular immunity mediated by the CD4+ lymphocytes. The *Pneumocystis* organism is readily recognized in cytologic or pathologic material from the infected lung and is essentially pathognomonic of infection with that organism. However, this is not the only organism to infect the lung under the conditions produced by HIV-1 virus infection. Cytomegalovirus, mycobacterial organisms, and fungi are prone to spread to immunocompromised lungs in patients with AIDS who are also more vulnerable to, although less frequently infected with, the ordinary range of bacteria and viruses. The finding of *Pneumocystis* organisms, while pathognomonic for that infection, does not exclude the possibility of other simultaneously infecting pathogens, which should always be looked for in the specimens retrieved for the diagnosis of *Pneumocystis carinii* pneumonia.

Gall and associates (1) present a well-documented review of pulmonary pathology in AIDS, including a well-thought-out protocol for the sequence of studies to gather information on the etiology of symptomatic pulmonary infection with or without abnormal chest x-ray results. This sequence proceeds from the examination of induced sputum through bronchoscopy, bronchoalveolar lavage, and bronchial brushings to transbronchial biopsy and open lung biopsy with the option to terminate investigative studies at each step with the identification of the *Pneumocystis* organism. The article is worth reviewing and contains a comprehensive review of the literature. New tests still emerge from time to time to improve the evaluation of pulmonary infiltrates in immunocompromised patients.

The work by Xaubet and co-workers (2), who evaluated the use of the telescoping plug catheter in bronchoalveolar lavage, is an example. That the finding of *Pneumocystis carinii* on bronchoscopy in patients infected with HIV is virtually pathognomonic of infection, even in symptom-free patients, is indicated by Lundgren and colleagues (3), who found no evidence of *Pneumocystis carinii* in symptom-free patients with AIDS who were positive for HIV.—G.M. Green, M.D.

*References*

1. Gall AA et al: *Surgical Pathol* 1:325, 1988.
2. Xaubet A et al: *Chest* 95:130, 1989.
3. Lundgren JD et al: *Thorax* 44:68, 1989.

---

**Diagnosis of *Pneumocystis carinii* Pneumonia by Induced Sputum in a City With Moderate Incidence of AIDS**

O'Brien RF, Quinn JL, Miyahara BT, Lepoff RB, Cohn DL (Denver Gen Hosp; Univ of Colorado, Denver)
*Chest* 95:136–138, January 1989 1–15

*Pneumocystis carinii* pneumonia (PCP) remains the most common, yet treatable, life-threatening infection in patients with AIDS. Examining induced sputum from patients with AIDS has provided a noninvasive diagnosis of PCP in 10% to 76% of patients. These previous studies were done in centers with a high incidence of AIDS. To determine whether this test could be successfully implemented in a center with a lower incidence of patients with AIDS, a study was done.

In 13 months, 25 (66%) of 38 AIDS patients with PCP had positive Giemsa stains of induced sputum. Patients who had positive test results could not be identified before sputum induction on the basis of clinical severity, including increased alveolar-to-arterial gradient or serum lactic dehydrogenase (LDH) levels. Previous observations that a normal serum LDH level was found in only 5% of documented patients with PCP were subsequently confirmed.

This noninvasive technique for diagnosing PCP in patients with AIDS can significantly reduce the number of bronchoscopies done and result in a considerable cost savings. The essential components of successfully implementing this technique are the training of a skilled parasitology technologist, a careful clinical screening process that identifies patients with a high likelihood of having PCP, and standardization of the sputum induction procedure by a limited number of technicians who do the test during normal working hours.

▶ O'Brien and associates found 66% of AIDS patients with PCP to be positive by induced sputum examination. The brief paper by Leigh and co-workers (1), which reported the yield by bronchoalveolar lavage after negative induced sputum examination to be only 1 in 25, achieved a sensitivity of 95% and a negative predictive value of 96% compared with bronchial lavage. In both cases, the yield by induced sputum is well worth careful use of this technique before proceeding to more invasive procedures. However, a negative finding by induced sputum should be followed by more aggressive diagnostic procedures for the patient with suspected PCP.—G.M. Green, M.D.

*Reference*

1. Leigh TR et al: *Lancet* 2:205, July 22, 1989.

▶ ↓ The next series of papers follows 2 lines of investigation regarding *Pneumocystis carinii* pneumonia: the first set of papers explores the pathogenesis of *Pneumocystis carinii* pneumonia in HIV-1 infection; the second series evaluates additional diagnostic techniques to increase the sensitivity and accuracy of the diagnosis of *Pneumocystis carinii* pneumonia.—G.M. Green, M.D.

**Nonspecific Interstitial Pneumonitis Without Evidence of *Pneumocystis carinii* in Asymptomatic Patients Infected With Human Immunodeficiency Virus (HIV)**

Ognibene FP, Masur H, Rogers P, Travis WD, Suffredini AF, Feuerstein I, Gill VJ, Baird BF, Carrasquillo JA, Parrillo JE, Lane HC, Shelhamer JH (Clinical Ctr, Natl Cancer Inst, Natl Inst of Allergy and Infectious Diseases, NIH, Bethesda, Md)

*Ann Intern Med* 109:874–879, Dec 1, 1988 1–16

An unprecedented incidence of *Pneumocystis carinii* pneumonia has been associated with HIV infection. The reason for this is unknown. A fraction of HIV-infected patients may have subclinical *P. carinii* pneumonia and *P. carinii* cysts, and inflammatory changes may be present without obvious signs and symptoms of pneumonia. The incidence of *P. carinii* organisms, *P. carinii* pneumonia, or other pulmonary pathologic processes in HIV-infected persons without pulmonary symptoms or previous history of *P. carinii* and with normal results of chest radiography was investigated.

Twenty-four HIV-positive patients with a nonpulmonary manifestation of AIDS or an absolute CD4 lymphocyte count of $0.2 \times 10^9$ cells/L or less were studied. In addition to having no pulmonary symptoms and a normal chest radiograph, all had no history of *P. carinii* pneumonia nor of treatment with antipneumocystis prophylaxis. Pulmonary assessment was done using several techniques. Mean alveolar-arterial gradient was 1.1 mm Hg, and mean diffusion capacity was 73% of predicted. No patient had *P. carinii* or other pathogens on stains of bronchoalveolar lavage fluid, nor histologic evidence of *P. carinii* pneumonia. Transbronchial biopsy specimens revealed chronic, nonspecific interstitial pneumonia in 11 of 23 patients and no pathologic anomaly in the rest. *Pneumocystis carinii* pneumonia developed in 6 patients in the 2 to 18 months of follow-up.

In this study, HIV-infected patients without pulmonary symptoms had no detectable *Pneumocystis* organisms in bronchoalveolar lavage fluid or transbronchial biopsy specimens. However, 11 of 23 had evidence of chronic, nonspecific interstitial pneumonitis. *Pneumocystis* species in pulmonary specimens from symptomatic patients most likely indicate the cause of pulmonary dysfunction, even if only a few are observed.

▶ This study of 24 HIV-positive patients without pulmonary symptoms or radiographic changes identified functional and morphological evidence of interstitial pneumonitis in half without evidence of *Pneumocystis carinii.* In 6 of these patients, *Pneumocystis carinii* pneumonia (PCP) subsequently developed, but there was no evidence of the etiology at the time of study. It is not clear from this article whether the interstitial pneumonitis was of a different etiology or whether the disease may manifest itself histologically months before the organisms are detected in the tissue or secretions.—G.M. Green, M.D.

▶ ↓ The case for the association of interstitial infiltrates with prediagnostic *Pneumocystis* infection is supported in the next paper by Hartelius and colleagues (Abstract 1–17), and in the following paper by Smith and associates (Abstract 1–18).—G.M. Green, M.D.

**Computed Tomography of the Lungs in Acquired Immunodeficiency Syndrome: An Early Indicator of Interstitial Pneumonia**

Hartelius H, Gaub J, Ingemann Jensen L, Jensen J, Faber V (Rigshospitalet, Copenhagen; Univ of Copenhagen)

*Acta Radiol* 29:641–644, November–December 1988 1–17

The radiographic findings have been described previously in patients with AIDS who acquire opportunistic lung infections. However, all of these findings are based on conventional chest radiography. Computed tomography of the chest is routinely performed at 1 center whenever AIDS is suspected. After the chance observation that CT revealed gross interstitial infiltration in the presence of a normal chest radiographs, 26 homosexual men with end-stage HIV disease were examined using 42 CT scans and normal radiographs of the lungs. Twenty men with confirmed AIDS had 34 CT examinations, and 6 men with symptoms of AIDS had 8 examinations. Eighteen patients also underwent diagnostic fiberoptic bronchoscopy with bronchoalveolar lavage. All patients have died. The median time from the first CT scan of the lungs to death was 8.5 months.

Seventeen patients had both abnormal chest radiographs and abnormal lung scans. Bronchoscopy, or lung biopsy, or both, identified an etiologic agent in most of these patients. At some time during the study period, CT of the lungs revealed unequivocal interstitial infiltration in the presence of normal chest radiographs in 9 of these 17 patients. An etiologic diagnosis subsequently was confirmed in all 9 patients. The remaining 9 patients had symptoms suggestive of pulmonary infection, but all had normal chest radiographs and normal lung scans. None of these 9 patients were found to have current opportunistic lung infections on further diagnostic testing or on clinical grounds.

Computed tomography of the lungs appears more accurate than conventional chest radiography in identifying the presence of diffuse pulmonary pathology in AIDS patients.

▶ This paper, which shows that CT scanning can identify pulmonary infiltrates before they show up on the routine chest radiograph, supports the view in the previous papers that the lung may be infiltrated for some time before the pneumonitis shows up on the routine radiograph. It would be interesting to correlate the identification of infiltrate by CT scans with exercise-induced desaturation, as described in the previous paper; or with immunoglobulin or lymphocyte changes, described in the following papers. At any rate, these techniques for early identification of pulmonary infiltration will improve the timing of chemotherapy or chemoprophylaxis in patients with AIDS.—G.M. Green, M.D.

**Severe Exercise Hypoxaemia With Normal or Near Normal X-Rays: A Feature of *Pneumocystis carinii* Infection**

Smith DE, McLuckie A, Wyatt J, Gazzard B (St Stephens Hosp; Westminster Hosp, London)

*Lancet* 2:1049–1051, Nov 5, 1988 1–18

Cyanosis and hypoxia are well-recognized late features of *Pneumocystis carinii* pneumonia (PCP). However, some patients with symptoms suggestive of PCP have normal arterial blood gas values. Because low arterial oxygen pressure ($PaO_2$) is associated with high mortality in patients with PCP, the detection and treatment of these patients before they become hypoxic at rest may improve survival.

To determine whether PCP can be detected while still in its early phase by the degree of exercise-induced oxygen desaturation, arterial oxygen saturation was measured by continuous pulse oximetry after 10 minutes of exercise in 16 patients with biopsy-proven PCP and a low resting $PaO_2$, 24 patients with biopsy-proven PCP and a normal resting $PaO_2$, 19 patients with other chest diseases and a normal resting $PaO_2$, and 12 healthy age- and sex-matched volunteers.

In 15 (94%) of the 16 patients with PCP and a low resting $PaO_2$ and in 19 (80%) of the 24 patients with PCP and a normal resting $PaO_2$, oxygen saturation fell to 90% or less after 10 minutes of exercise. However, in only 2 (10%) of the 19 patients with other chest diseases did oxygen saturation fall to 90% or less with exercise. In none of the healthy controls did oxygen saturation fall below 90% after 10 minutes of exercise.

Desaturation to 90% or less after 10 minutes of exercise is a useful diagnostic tool in the detection of early PCP. The equipment required for measuring the oxygen desaturation response to exercise is inexpensive, is easily moved, and does not require a specialist for operation. Results are available within 10 minutes, and the equipment need not be sterilized between examinations.

▶ Smith and co-workers have shown that 94% of HIV patients with proven *Pneumocystis* infection and with reduced arterial oxygen pressures showed desaturation on exercise, as did 80% who had normal oxygen pressures at rest. This study suggests that exercise desaturation could be a useful diagnostic tool in the detection of early PCP. Although the study's patients had normal or near normal x-ray results, they did have biopsy-proven PCP. What is needed is a prospective study of HIV-1-infected populations that would serially measure exercise-induced desaturation to determine whether this measurement is predictive of *P. carinii* or detects the effects of the pneumonitis before evidence is available by examination of induced sputum. If oxygen desaturation occurs before microbiologic evidence of *P. carinii,* the serial testing of patients infected with HIV-1 might be in order with more intensive studies for *P. carinii,* or even institution of prophylaxis near the onset of exercise-induced desaturation. The paper by Stover and colleagues (1) comes close to meeting this need in finding the simple exercise test in patients with AIDS who were evaluated for PCP to have a sensitivity and negative predictive value of 100%, but a specificity of only 36%. To quote the authors, "a normal exercise test virtually eliminates *Pneumocystis* pneumonia in HIV-1 infected patients with pulmonary symptoms."—G.M. Green, M.D.

*Reference*

1. Stover DE et al: *Am Rev Respir Dis* 139:1343, 1989.

---

**Humoral and Cellular Responses to *Pneumocystis carinii,* CMV, and Herpes Simplex in Patients With AIDS and in Controls**

Hofmann B, Nielsen PB, Ødum N, Gerstoft J, Platz P, Ryder LP, Poulsen A-G, Mathiesen L, Dickmeiss E, Norrild B, Andersen HK, Faber Westergaard B, Møller Nielsen C, Holten-Andersen W, Mojon M, Nielsen JO, Svejgaard A (State Univ Hosp; Hvidovre Hosp, Copenhagen; Copenhagen Univ; Århus Univ, Århus, Denmark; Université Claude Bernard, Lyon, France)

*Scand J Infect Dis* 20:389–394, 1988 1–19

---

*Pneumocystis carinii* pneumonia (PCP) is the single most life-threatening opportunistic infection for patients with AIDS. However, some patients with AIDS do not acquire PCP, although they are exposed regularly to *P. carinii* infection in their environment. Those AIDS patients in whom PCP develops lack IgM antibodies to *P. carinii.*

The distribution of IgM, IgG, and IgA antibodies to *P. carinii* in 36 AIDS patients with or without PCP, and in a similar number of healthy controls was examined. The 36 AIDS patients, aged 19–76 years (median, 38 years), included. 15 who had PCP as confirmed with biopsy or bronchial lavage and 21 who did not.

The titers of IgG and IgA antibodies to *P. carinii* in the AIDS patients did not differ significantly from those in the controls. However, only 2 (13%) of 15 patients with PCP had IgM antibody titers of 5 or more, compared with 63% of controls and 43% of patients without PCP. The risk of acquiring PCP for patients without IgM antibodies to *P. carinii* was 5 times more than for patients who did have these antibodies. All patients had high titers of antibodies to cytomegalovirus and herpes simplex virus, but all had normal total immunoglobulin levels. None of the patients responded in lymphocyte transformation to *P. carinii,* cytomegalovirus, or herpes simplex virus antigens.

Lack of IgM antibodies may be a marker for an immunodeficiency to *P. carinii.* However, an explanation for the selective lack of IgM antibodies to *P. carinii* in AIDS patients with PCP was not found.

▶ Selective lack of IgM antibodies to *P. carinii* in patients with PCP, although unexplained, may be related to HIV-1 infection of lymphocytes and to a risk of *Pneumocystis* infection high enough to warrant chemoprophylaxis. However, a prospective study of an HIV-1-positive population without *Pneumocystis carinii* pneumonia is needed to determine whether the IgM deficiency appears as the

HIV-1 infection progresses in those patients destined for the complication of *Pneumocystis carinii* pneumonia.—G.M. Green, M.D.

▶ ↓ The next paper by Masur and associates continues the theme that risk for *Pneumocystis* infection in HIV-positive persons may be identified by changes in physiologic parameters, in this case the CD4+ lymphocyte cell count. Retrospectively studied patients with pulmonary infection or Kaposi's sarcoma had a C4/PD4 lymphocyte count of less than 200 cells/mm$^3$ within 60 days of the episode. This conclusion requires confirmation in a prospective study, but it is consistent with the IgM findings reported in the previous paper. What is unclear is whether the immunologic decline precedes and causes, or is a component of, the subsequent pulmonary infection.—G.M. Green, M.D.

**CD4 Counts as Predictors of Opportunistic Pneumonias in Human Immunodeficiency Virus (HIV) Infection**

Masur H, Ognibene FP, Yarchoan R, Shelhamer JH, Baird BF, Travis W, Suffredini AF, Deyton L, Kovacs JA, Falloon J, Davey R, Polis M, Metcalf J, Baseler M, Wesley R, Gill VJ, Fauci AS, Lane HC (Natl Inst of Allergy and Infectious Diseases; Natl Cancer Inst, NIH, Bethesda; Program Resources Inc, Frederick, Md)

*Ann Intern Med* 111:223–231, Aug 1, 1989 1–20

Opportunistic infections in patients infected by HIV result directly from depletion of CD4 cells. Further knowledge of the course of these infections might allow timely and cost-effective prophylaxis. The predictive value of circulating CD4+ lymphocyte counts was examined in 100 patients with HIV infection who had 119 episodes of pulmonary dysfunction within 2 months of CD4 lymphocyte estimation.

Circulating CD4 cell counts were less than $0.2 \times 10^9$ cells/L (200 cells/mm$^3$) before 46 of 49 episodes of *Pneumocystis* pneumonia, all 8 episodes of cytomegalovirus pneumonia, all 7 episodes of *Cryptococcus neoformans* infection, and all but 2 of 21 episodes of *Mycobacterium avium-intracellulare* infection. Counts were quite variable before episodes of nonspecific interstitial pneumonia. The percentage of CD4+ lymphocytes and the CD4+ cell count had comparable predictive value, but serum p24 antigen levels had no predictive value.

Patients infected with HIV who have a CD4 cell count less than $0.2 \times 10^9$ cells/L or fewer than 20% CD4 cells are especially likely to benefit from antipneumocystis prophylaxis.

**Phenotypical and Functional Analysis of Bronchoalveolar Lavage Lymphocytes in Patients With HIV Infection**

Agostini C, Poletti V, Zambello R, Trentin L, Siviero F, Spiga L, Gritti F, Semenzato G (Padua Univ, Padua; Bellaria Hosp; Maggiore Hosp, Bologna; Cittadella Hosp, Padua, Italy)

*Am Rev Respir Dis* 138:1609–1615, December 1988 1–21

Patients with AIDS often acquire unusual opportunistic and nonopportunistic lung infections. Patients with AIDS are characterized by a number of immunologic abnormalities that have been examined extensively in peripheral blood cells but not in cells obtained from the lung. To clarify the immunopathogenesis of infectious lung complications in patients with AIDS, Bronchoalveolar lavage lymphocytes obtained from 24 patients with clinical signs and symptoms of HIV infection were characterized using a panel of monoclonal antibodies. The bronchoalveolar lavage lymphocytes recovered from 8 healthy persons with normal lung function were used as controls.

Most bronchoalveolar lavage lymphocytes from patients with HIV infection expressed CD8 determinants. The percentage and absolute number of pulmonary CD8 cells were significantly more than those in controls, whereas lung CD4 cells were reduced in percentage but not in absolute number. An exception was noted in 4 patients with full-blown AIDS who had a significant decrease in the absolute number of CD4 cells in the bronchoalveolar lavage fluid. Consequently, all patients had a marked reversal of the ratio of CD4 to CD8 cells in the lung. Six 24 patients had a lymphocytic alveolitis, 4 of whom had full-blown AIDS. Although the number of bronchoalveolar lavage cells bearing natural killer related determinants was higher in patients with HIV, in vitro natural killer cell activity could not be demonstrated.

Because natural killer cells in the lung represent 1 of the first lines of natural resistance against infection, impaired natural killer cell activity in the lungs of HIV patients may be 1 of the mechanisms that leads to the in situ immunodeficiency state and the characteristic pulmonary complications of AIDS.

▶ This is a study of 24 HIV-1 seropositive patients who underwent bronchoalveolar lavage with phenotypic and functional characterization of the recovered lymphocytes. The principal changes were increase in CD8 cells, decrease in CD4+ lymphocytes in patients with full-blown AIDS, and no natural killer (NK) cell activity despite a normal number of NK lymphocytes. These studies point to both anatomical (decreased CD4+ cells) and functional (decreased NK cell activity) abnormalities in AIDS. This study suggests that the hypersusceptibility of AIDS patients for pulmonary infections with microorganisms controlled by lymphocyte cell-mediated immunity is related both to the CD4 cell deficiency and NK cell dysfunction.— G.M. Green, M.D.

---

**Pulmonary Involvement in Patients With HTLV-I–Associated Myelopathy: Increased Soluble IL-2 Receptors in Bronchoalveolar Lavage Fluid**

Sugimoto M, Nakashima H, Matsumoto M, Uyama E, Ando M, Araki S (Kumamoto Univ, Kumamoto, Japan)

*Am Rev Respir Dis* 139:1329–1335, June 1989 1–22

A chronic spastic myelopathy endemic in tropical regions and southwest Japan often is associated with high antibody titers in serum and CSF to human T-cell lymphotropic virus type I (HTLV-I). Because large amounts of soluble interleukin-2 receptor (IL-2R) are released by HTLV-I–positive T cell lines, soluble IL-2R may have an important role in negatively modulating IL-2–dependent immune responses. Serum and bronchoalveolar lavage fluid levels of soluble Il-2R were estimated in 18 patients who had HTLV-I–associated myelopathy (HAM); all had high antibody titers in serum and CSF against HTLV-I. Five HTLV-I carriers without myelopathy and 13 healthy persons also were studied.

Patients with HAM had significantly increased serum levels of IL-2R, and 1 of the 5 HTLV-I carriers also had an increased level. Bronchoalveolar lavage levels of IL-2R were detectable in low amounts in 4 healthy persons and 1 HTLV-I carrier, but the patients with HAM had markedly elevated levels that averaged nearly 13 times the serum levels. Levels of IL-2R in lavage fluid correlated well with the numbers of T lymphocytes and CD4+ cells in the patients with HAM. Lavage fluid lymphocytes from these patients synthesized DNA spontaneously when cultured in vitro.

It appears that in patients with HAM an increased number of T lymphocytes in the lungs is activated locally to produce soluble IL-2R. Immunologic mechanisms may be important in the development of pulmonary lesions in this setting.

▶ The last paper in this series continues the association of lymphocyte activity with immunologically mediated pulmonary disease, this time by identifying elevated lymphocyte cell product, the IL-2R lymphokine, in patients with an HTLV-I–associated myelopathy. Although this interesting observation may have significance for diagnosis of immune function in the future, it is still too early to draw firm conclusions from cytokine levels. Perhaps the time will come when we will use these tests much like blood chemistries and other biochemical tests used today.—G.M. Green, M.D.

▶ ↓ New studies done to more sensitively identify the *Pneumocystis* organism are presented in the next 2 papers. The first (Abstract 1–23) compared the use of the Giemsa stain with the methenamine silver nitrate stain for the rapid identification of the *Pneumocystis* trophozoites on bronchoalveolar lavage samples, and found the Giemsa stain both simpler and more sensitive. The other technique (Abstract 1–24) involves a monoclonal antibody that stains with an immunoperoxidase technique specific for the organism. There was a 94% agreement between the results using the monoclonal antibody and the conventional staining method. The advantage of this method is the specificity of the monoclonal antibody for the *Pneumocystis* organism. The possible advantage of a quicker identification of the organism is counterbalanced by the longer time taken to carry out the procedure.

Linnemann and co-workers (1) reported on the recovery of HIV-1 virus from 100% of the BAL fluids that they cultured from 9 patients with AIDS; the article is a needed reminder that these specimens are potentially infectious even when studied for PCP and other secondary pathogens.—G.M. Green, M.D.

*Reference*

1. Linnemann CC et al: *Chest* 96:64, 1989.

**Comparison of Methenamine Silver Nitrate and Giemsa Stain for Detection of *Pneumocystis carinii* in Bronchoalveolar Lavage Specimens From HIV Infected Patients**

Holten-Andersen W, Kolmos HJ (Hvidovre Hosp, Copenhagen)

*APMIS* 97:745–747, August 1989 1–23

*Pneumocystis carinii* is a common cause of pneumonia in patients with AIDS. Because *P. carinii* cannot be distinguished from other causes of pneumonia on clinical grounds alone, it must be demonstrated microscopically in material obtained from the lower respiratory system. The parallel use of Giemsa and methenamine silver nitrate (MSN) stains for demonstrating *P. carinii* in bronchoalveolar lavage (BAL) specimens from patients infected with HIV is reported.

During a 1-year period, 77 BAL samples were obtained from 64 HIV-infected patients admitted with pulmonary symptoms. After the BAL samples were centrifuged a drop of sediment was spread on 2 slides. One slide was stained with a 4% Giemsa solution, and 1 was stained with MSN. In the Giemsa stain trophozoites and intracystic sporozoites appear pale blue with red nuclei. In the MSN stain the cyst wall and parenthesis-like structures stain a brownish color. Each slide was scanned for 30 minutes.

*Pneumocystis carinii* was detected in 47 BAL samples (61%). Thirty-seven samples (48%) were positive with both stains, and 10 samples (13%) were positive only with the Giemsa stain. All 30 samples that were negative with the Giemsa stain also were negative with the MSN stain. Therefore, the demonstration of trophozoites in a Giemsa stained BAL sample is a more sensitive method for diagnosing *P. carinii* than the demonstration of cysts on an MSN-stained slide. Because staining with MSN takes much more time than staining with Giemsa, the latter method should be used for the initial screening for *P. carinii* in BAL samples, and the MSN stain should be reserved for the presumably few samples in which cysts are the only evidence of *P. carinii* infection.

**Use of a Monoclonal Antibody to Detect *Pneumocystis carinii* in Induced Sputum and Bronchoalveolar Lavage Fluid by Immunoperoxidase Staining**

Blumenfeld W, Kovacs JA (VA Med Ctr, San Francisco; Clinical Center, NIH, Bethesda, Md)

*Arch Pathol Lab Med* 112:1233–1236, December 1988 1–24

The diagnosis of *Pneumocystis carinii* pneumonia currently is based on morphological recognition of the organism in material removed from patients. Before the AIDS epidemic, open-lung biopsy was the diagnostic procedure of choice, but the increasing prevalence of *P. carinii* pneumonia as a major complication of AIDS has created the need for a less invasive diagnostic technique. The use of a monoclonal antibody to *P. carinii* in bronchoalveolar lavage (BAL) fluid and sputum obtained from patients with possible *P. carinii* pneumonia was examined. An immunoperoxidase antibody staining technique was used to stain the slides.

Sputum or BAL specimens obtained during 50 procedures in 44 patients with AIDS. Of 18 sputum specimens 12 (67%) contained *P. carinii* by conventional Diff-Quik staining, and of 32 BAL fluid specimens, 16 (50%) contained *P. carinii* by Diff-Quik staining. All specimens were reacted with a monoclonal antibody to *P. carinii* and visualized by an avidin-biotin horseradish peroxidase staining technique.

The monoclonal antibody clearly identified *P. carinii* in specimens prepared from either sputa or BAL fluid. All 12 specimens of induced sputum identified as positive for *P. carinii* by Diff-Quik staining also were positive by immunoperoxidase staining. For the 32 BAL specimens, agreement between Diff-Quik staining and immunoperoxidase stain was noted in 29. Two Diff-Quik-positive specimens were negative by immunoperoxidase staining, and 1 Diff-Quik-negative specimen was positive by immunoperoxidase staining. Overall agreement between the results of conventional Diff-Quik staining and immunoperoxidase staining was 94%. These discrepancies were attributed to the random distribution of *P. carinii* on smears.

Use of a monoclonal antibody specific for *P. carinii* with immunoperoxidase staining accurately identifies the presence by *P. carinii* in sputum and BAL specimens.

---

**Serum Lactate Dehydrogenase Activity in Patients With AIDS and *Pneumocystis carinii* Pneumonia: An Adjunct to Diagnosis**

Kagawa FT, Kirsch CM, Yenokida GG, Levine ML (Santa Clara Valley Med Ctr, San Jose, Calif)

*Chest* 94:1031–1033, November 1988 1–25

---

The value of lactic dehydrogenase activity as a marker for *Pneumocystis carinii* pneumonia (PCP) was examined in patients with AIDS or AIDS-related complex by estimating lactic dehydrogenase levels in 30 adults with AIDS and PCP. Patients with AIDS or AIDS-related complex and non-*Pneumocystis* pneumonia and patients with pneumococcal pneumonia and bacteremia served as controls.

Lactic dehydrogenase levels were elevated in patients with AIDS and PCP compared with those in both control groups. None of the study patients had normal values of lactic dehydrogenase. Alveolar-arterial oxygen tension difference values were significantly elevated in both patients with AIDS and PCP and patients with pneumococcal pneumonia. Lymphocyte counts were lower in patients with AIDS or AIDS-related complex than in those with pneumococcal pneumonia alone.

Elevated lactic dehydrogenase levels in patients with AIDS and PCP appear to be caused by PCP-related lung injury. Estimation of lactic dehydrogenase can be a useful adjunct in the diagnosis of PCP in patients with AIDS. Levels of lactate dehydrogenase appear to correlate with the defect in oxygen transfer.

▶ Yet another test to distinguish *Pneumocystis* from pneumonias of other etiologies is measurement of the serum lactate dehydrogenase level, which is elevated in *Pneumocystis* pneumonia but not in patients with pneumococcal pneumonia. The differences in alveolar arterial oxygen tension may identify the pneumonic process with either etiology, but the finding of elevated levels of lactate dehydrogenase in patients with *Pneumocystis* pneumonia is a useful piece of substantiating information. However, the techniques for retrieving and identifying the *Pneumocystis* organism in induced sputum is a more direct approach. The level of lactic dehydrogenase might be included along with counts of immunoglobulin M and CD4+ lymphocytes in attempting to identify the etiology of pneumonitis in AIDS patient. The reference by Singer (1) adds the finding of elevated angiotension-converting enzyme levels in *Pneumocystis carinii* pneumonia, as in sarcoidosis. G.M. Green, M.D.

*Reference*

1. Singer F et al: *Chest* 95:803, 1989.

---

**Acute Respiratory Failure Secondary to *Pneumocystis carinii* Pneumonia in the Acquired Immunodeficiency Syndrome: A Potential Role for Systemic Corticosteroids**

Montaner JSG, Russell JA, Lawson L, Ruedy J (Univ of British Columbia, Vancouver)

*Chest* 95:881–884, April 1989 1–26

---

The prognosis for patients with HIV infection and *Pneumocystis carinii* pneumonia (PCP) has been improved with the use of specific antimicrobials. However, when acute respiratory failure develops, the mortality rate of PCP is more than 80%. Because the use of corticosteroids in the treatment of acute respiratory failure in AIDS-related PCP is controversial, the incidence and mortality of acute respiratory failure in AIDS-related PCP was determined retrospectively, the impact of systemic corticosteroid administration on outcome was evaluated.

During a 6-year period, 127 patients with AIDS-related PCP were identified, 27 (21%) of whom had acute respiratory failure and required ventilatory support. Three patients who refused ventilatory support soon died without receiving corticosteroids. Eighteen of the remaining 24 patients received corticosteroids intravenously in addition to conventional antimicrobial therapy. Three of 24 patients, 2 women and 1 man, had contracted HIV infection through blood transfusion. None was an intravenous drug abuser.

The overall mortality for patients with acute respiratory failure secondary to AIDS-related PCP was 50%. Adjunctive corticosteroid therapy was responsible for a reduction in mortality; 7 (39%) of 18 corticosteroid-treated patients and 5 (84%) of those not treated with corticosteroids died. Survivors also were younger and were identified earlier than nonsurvivors. All survivors were discharged from the hospital after a mean stay of 20 days. Known AIDS, previous episodes of PCP, and arterial blood gas values at the onset of acute respiratory failure did not appear to affect outcome.

If begun early, treatment with adjunctive corticosteroids appears to improve the survival rate of patients with ARF secondary to AIDS-related PCP. Prospective studies are under way to confirm these findings.

▶ The possible benefit of early adjunctive corticosteroid therapy in acute respiratory failure secondary to *Pneumocystis carinii* pneumonia in AIDS patients is consistent with the value of corticosteroid use for other manifestations of AIDS. One might anticipate that further immunosuppression by corticosteroids in patients already severely immunosuppressed would result in a worse outcome. However, the exudative process of ARDS is a greater risk, and as in other settings, corticosteroids given in short courses for acute inflammatory disorders can be given safely, from the immunosuppression point of view, when effective antimicrobial therapy is available. The series of patients reported is very small and, as indicated by the author, requires a randomized prospective study to confirm the findings. Friedman and colleague (1) report 36% survival in a prospective study, but the use of steroids was not randomly controlled.—G.M. Green, M.D.

*Reference*

1. Friedman Y et al: *Chest* 96:862, 1989.

---

**Empirical Treatment Without Bronchoscopy for *Pneumocystis carinii* Pneumonia in the Acquired Immunodeficiency Syndrome**

Miller RF, Millar AB, Weller IVD, Semple SJG (Middlesex Hosp, London)
*Thorax* 44:559–564, July 1989 1–27

---

It has been suggested that patients with suspected *Pneumocystis carinii* pneumonia who are seropositive for HIV-1 or who are at high risk should undergo fiberoptic bronchoscopy and bronchoalveolar lavage with or without transbronchial biopsy, for definitive diagnosis before treatment is started. An empirical approach to treating *P. carinii* pneumonia was used in a prospective study of 73 men with antibodies to HIV-1 and respiratory problems. At presentation, 49 patients were thought to have histories, physical findings, chest radiographs, and arterial blood gas tensions typical of *Pneumocystis* pneumonia; empirical treatment was started immediately. Twenty-four patients thought to have features not typical of *Pneumocystis* pneumonia were referred for bronchoscopy. Of 45 evaluable patients in the first group, 42 had *Pneumocystis* pneumonia, which was diagnosed at bronchoscopy in 40. In the second group, a specific diagnosis was made by bronchoscopy in 21 patients, 7 of whom had *Pneumocystis* pneumonia.

This empirical approach to treatment for patients with typical signs and symptoms of *Pneumocystis* pneumonia led to the correct treatment of 95% of patients. Adopting an empirical approach would have led to a misdiagnosis of AIDS in 1 patient. Bronchoscopies would have been avoided in 64% of the patients; the specificity for the diagnosis of *Pneumocystis* pneumonia was 85% and the sensitivity was 85%.

▶ It is interesting that the clinical measures of *Pneumocystis* pneumonia in AIDS patients are becoming sufficiently well characterized that empirical treatment without bronchoscopy is correct for 95% of the patients so identified. The argument for using empirical treatment is to avoid bronchoscopy and bronchoalveolar lavage. However, as reported in the previous paper by Montaner and associates, the effective use of induced sputum in the identification of the *Pneumocystis* organism in a high proportion of cases blunts the rationale of this somewhat blind approach. In addition, the use of improved staining techniques increases the sensitivity of this diagnostic procedure. There may be a case for empirical treatment on clinical grounds while awaiting the scheduling and accomplishment of bronchoscopy or induced sputum, but it seems that the laboratory techniques are sufficiently simple, available, and effective that the rationale for the treatment can be verified simply and quickly.—G.M. Green, M.D.

**Aerosolized Pentamidine as Second Line Therapy in Patients With AIDS and *Pneumocystis carinii* Pneumonia**

Montgomery AB, Debs RJ, Luce JM, Corkery KJ, Turner J, Hopewell PC (Univ of California, San Francisco)

*Chest* 95:747–750, April 1989 1–28

Pilot studies indicate that aerosolized pentamidine is an effective and relatively safe approach to first episodes of *Pneumocystis carinii* pneumonia (PCP) in patients with AIDS. This treatment was used in 10 patients for whom standard treatment was hazardous. The patients had previous or concurrent severe adverse reactions or contraindications to trimethoprim-sulfamethoxazole or parenteral pentamidine therapy. A dosage of 600 mg of pentamidine in 6 mL of sterile water was aerosolized and administered for 25 minutes once a day for an average of 10.5 days.

All of the patients improved substantially and achieved an oxygen pressure of more than 70 mm Hg or an arterial saturation of more than 94% on room air. Temperature became normal and the chest radiograph appearances improved. Six patients coughed and required pretreatment with aerosolized metaproterenol. None had clinical bronchospasm or any other adverse reactions during treatment.

Aerosolized pentamidine is an effective and safe approach to treating PCP in AIDS patients who cannot receive standard treatment. Hospitalization is not necessary.

▶ The effectiveness of aerosolized pentamidine is heartening for patients who have difficulty with the standard treatment regimens. The usual problem with such therapy is obtaining sufficiently high concentrations in the region of infection to be effective. The problem is that aerosols tend not to be drawn into the areas of pneumonia because of the poor ventilation attributable to the alveolar-filling infiltrate. If this technique is effective, then it suggests that the drug is diffused through the lung and penetrates the inflammatory lesion to act against the organism. For these reasons, the aerosolized approach should be used with caution for patients with extensive infiltrative lesions who are quite sick. There may be a rationale for its more extensive use in chemoprophylaxis where alveolar ventilation is preserved to transport the aerosol to the periphery. O'Doherty and colleagues (1) compare different nebulizers for their efficiency in pentamidine administration. Sarti (2) expands on the use of aerosolized pentamidine.—G.M. Green, M.D.

*References*

1. O'Doherty MJ et al: *Lancet* 2:1283, Dec 3, 1988.
2. Sarti GM: *Postgrad Med* 86:54, 1989.

---

**Successful Prophylaxis of *Pneumocystis carinii* Pneumonia With Trimethoprim-Sulfamethoxazole in AIDS Patients With Previous Allergic Reactions**

Shafer RW, Seitzman PA, Tapper ML (Lenox Hill Hosp, New York)
*J AIDS* 2:389–393, August 1989 1–29

---

*Pneumocystis carinii* pneumonia is the most common infection in patients with AIDS. Attempts to prevent recurrences of this infection with oral trimethoprim-sulfamethoxazole (TMP-SMX) have been limited by the high incidence of side effects.

Thirty-four homosexual patients with AIDS were treated for *P. carinii* pneumonia between April 1984 and November 1985. All 31 survivors were treated with oral TMP-SMX prophylaxis immediately after completion of intravenous therapy, despite prior occurrence of hypersensitivity reactions to the intravenous drug in 21 patients. Subsequent reactions to oral TMP-SMX required discontinuation of the drug in only 4 patients. None of the patients who continued TMP-SMX prophylaxis developed recurrent *Pneumocystis* pneumonia.

In this series oral TMP-SMX was effective in preventing recurrent *Pneumocystis* pneumonia in patients with AIDS. Hypersensitivity reactions during treatment with TMP-SMX may not be a contraindication to continuation of therapy and subsequent oral prophylaxis.

▶ This approach toward reducing morbidity and mortality from *Pneumocystis* pneumonia in AIDS patients is a promising application of the principles of chemoprophylaxis so effectively used in other pulmonary disorders such as tuberculosis. This paper demonstrates that, even in patients with previous side effects from treatment with TMP-SMX, the same drugs can be given for prophylaxis. Perhaps more promising is the potential for aerosolized drugs such as pentamidine to reduce the incidence and control the prevalence and early lethality of *Pneumocystis* pneumonia in this population. This approach is being evaluated and probably will be reported in next year's YEAR BOOK.—G.M. Green, M.D.

## Nosocomial Infection

**Tracheal Tube Biofilm as a Source of Bacterial Colonization of the Lung**
Inglis TJJ, Millar MR, Jones JG, Robinson DA (Univ of Leeds, England)
*J Clin Microbiol* 27:2014–2018, September 1989 1–30

Nosocomial pneumonia is an important cause of morbidity and mortality among patients in intensive care units. Previous studies have shown that nosocomial pneumonia is preceded by colonization of the lower respiratory tract. Tracheal intubation is a known risk factor for pneumonia, but an association between tracheal intubation and colonization of the lung has not been demonstrated. This study was conducted to investigate biofilm formation in tracheal tubes and the potential interaction between luminal biofilm and ventilator gas flow.

The amount of luminal biofilm was measured in 40 tracheal tubes with internal diameters of 7.5–9.5 mm, which had been used in adult patients from 2 hours to 10 days. The tubes were marked at 1-cm intervals from the lower end and were cut into 20 1-cm lengths without disturbing the biofilm. All visible biofilm was examined under the electron microscope. Qualitative and quantitative cultures were performed on 45 tracheal tubes that had been used from 12 hours to 26 days. Seventy-eight heat and moisture exchanger filter units removed from ventilator circuits were studied for the presence of bacteria. Flow studies also were performed.

In 30 of the 40 tubes examined, the dry weight of the biofilm was 50 mg or greater. Electron microscopy confirmed the presence of bacteria in the biofilm. Quantitative cultures demonstrated bacterial counts of up to 10 million/cm of tube length. Bacteria were also isolated from the patient side of 18 of the 78 heat and moisture exchanger–microbiologic filter units. Flow studies showed how particles that detach from the tracheal tube biofilm may be projected as far as 45 cm from the tracheal tube tip.

These findings suggest that, after contamination of a tracheal tube's biofilm with a ventilated patient's own gastrointestinal tract flora, production of a cloud of contaminated particles from the luminal biofilm surface provides the mechanism for initial and repeated lung colonization.

▶ This is a practical goal-oriented study that has collected data to support a logical hypothesis for the mechanism of pathogenesis of nosocomial pneumonia in intubated patients. The investigators have quantified the development of secretion-like biofilm on tracheal tubes withdrawn from patients after 2–10 days, have quantified the bacterial content of the biofilm, and have demonstrated that the biofilm can be entrained by the inflow of ventilator air with bacterial particles projected up to 45 cm beyond the tracheal tube. To prove that this is the pathway by which the lower respiratory tract becomes colonized with oropharyngeal flora with subsequent outgrowth as nosocomial pneumonia, a study must demonstrate a reduction in lower respiratory tract colonization and nosocomial pneumonia under conditions by which the biofilm is prevented or bacterial contamination of the biofilm is eliminated. We will look forward to such technology, which might involve the creation of special services or materials in tracheal intubation tubes.—G.M. Green, M.D.

---

**Nosocomial Pneumonia in Patients Receiving Continuous Mechanical Ventilation: Prospective Analysis of 52 Episodes With Use of a Protected Specimen Brush and Quantitative Culture Techniques**

Fagon J-Y, Chastre J, Domart Y, Trouillet J-L, Pierre J, Darne C, Gibert C (Hôpital Bichat, Paris)

*Am Rev Respir Dis* 139:877–884, April 1989 1–31

---

The incidence of nosocomial bacterial pneumonia in critically ill patients undergoing continuous mechanical ventilation remains high. The diagnosis of pneumonia in these patients is difficult because serious underlying disease may mask pneumonia, and because clinical assessment cannot distinguish between bacterial colonization of the tracheobronchial tree and nosocomial pneumonia. In this study, uncontaminated airway secretions were obtained directly from the involved area in the lower respiratory tract, using fiberoptic bronchoscopy with a protected specimen brush (PSB).

Fiberoptic bronchoscopic examinations were performed in 567 patients who were undergoing mechanical ventilation for more than 72 hours during the 41-month study, and in whom pneumonia was suspected because of the presence of a new pulmonary infiltrate and purulent tracheal secretions. The diagnosis of ventilator-associated (V-A) pneumonia was retained only if the PSB specimen yielded more than $10^3$ colony-forming units of at least 1 microorganism per milliliter.

Of the 567 patients, 49 (9%) had 52 episodes of V-A pneumonia. The actuarial risk of V-A pneumonia during the first 30 days of mechanical ventilation was 6.5% at 10 days, 19% at 20 days, and 28% at 30 days. No patient with negative cultures of PSB specimens was subsequently found to have had pneumonia. Patients with pneumonia had a greater average age and a higher incidence of serious underlying illness, but no other significant differences were found.

Isolated microorganisms included 51 gram-negative and 33 gram-positive bacteria. *Pseudomonas aeruginosa* was involved in 31% of the pneumonias and *Staphylococcus aureus* in 33% of the pneumonias; 21 episodes were caused by more than 1 pathogen. The overall mortality in patients without pneumonia was 29%, compared with a 71% overall mortality in patients with pneumonia. Only 13% of patients with pneumonia caused by *Pseudomonas* or *Acinetobacter* species survived, compared with 45% of patients who had pneumonia caused by other bacteria.

▶ This paper makes 2 points: first, that the PSB and quantitative culture techniques used with the fiberoptic bronchoscope can distinguish V-A bacterial pneumonia from other causes of pulmonary infiltration; and second, that the risk of V-A pneumonia rises progressively with the duration of mechanical ventilation. The overall mortality among patients with pneumonia was 2.5 times that among patients without pneumonia, but it is quite likely that the former acquired pneumonia in part because of impaired defenses related to a more severe status of illness. The value of the vigorous pursuit of a bacterial diagnosis is indicated by the finding that no patient with negative cultures was subsequently found to have had pneumonia.—G.M. Green, M.D.

---

**Diagnosis of Nosocomial Bacterial Pneumonia in Intubated Patients Undergoing Ventilation: Comparison of the Usefulness of Bronchoalveolar Lavage and the Protected Specimen Brush**

Chastre J, Fagon J-Y, Soler P, Bornet M, Domart Y, Trouillet J-L, Gibert C, Hance AJ (Hôpital Bichat, Paris)

*Am J Med* 85:499–506, October 1988 1–32

---

Nosocomial bacterial pneumonia is a common, life-threatening complication in intubated patients undergoing mechanical ventilation. Because the clinical signs of pneumonia also may occur in the presence of other pathologic processes, intubated patients suspected of nosocomial pneumonia require further investigation. The diagnostic usefulness was compared of specimens obtained by bronchoalveolar lavage (BAL) and by the protected specimen brush (PSB).

Specimens were obtained by PSB and BAL from 21 patients who had received mechanical ventilation for 3–35 days and were suspected of having nosocomial pneumonia. All specimens were processed for quantitative bacterial and fungal culture by standard methodology. Total cell counts were performed on an aliquot of resuspended original BAL fluid. Differential cell counts were made on at least 500 cells. In addition, 300 cells were examined at high-power magnification; the percentage of cells containing intracellular microorganisms and the average number of extracellular organisms per oil-immersion field were determined.

The diagnosis of bacterial pneumonia was confirmed clinically in 5 of 21 patients. Specimens obtained with the PSB were positive in all 5 patients with bacterial pneumonia and negative in all 13 patients without this infection. Results were not available until 24–48 hours after bronchoscopy. The remaining 3 patients died with no pathologic evidence of pneumonia at autopsy.

Quantification of intracellular organisms in cells recovered by BAL also was useful in the diagnosis of pneumonia. In all 5 patients with confirmed bacterial pneumonia, more than 25% of cells recovered by BAL contained intracellular organisms, whereas less than 1% of cells recovered from 9 of 13 patients without bacterial pneumonia contained intracellular bacteria. These results were immediately available. However, quantitative culture of BAL fluid revealed bacterial growth in all but 1 patient and thus was useless for identifying infected patients.

The quantitative culture of specimens recovered by PSB and of intracellular organisms in cells recovered by BAL are both useful techniques for confirming bacterial pneumonia in intubated patients who require mechanical ventilation, as the techniques yield complementary information.

▶ This paper confirms the utility of PSB in the diagnosis of bacterial pneumonia in mechanically ventilated patients, and adds the observation that a finding of intracellular bacteria in cells obtained at BAL provides immediate information for the diagnosis of nosocomial bacterial pneumonia in intubated patients. The quantitative culture of alveolar lavage fluid, however, did not provide useful information. It would seem, therefore, that the addition of the BAL procedure to the culture of bronchial secretions obtained by PSB is not worth the added small risk of the lavage procedure unless immediate information is required for treatment purposes.—G.M. Green, M.D.

▶ ↓ The next paper, by Papazian and colleagues, shows that blind distal bronchial sampling of tracheobronchial secretions without a fiberscope produces identical results with samples obtained by fiberoptic protected brush biopsy in 94% of the specimens where paired samples were obtained by both techniques. It would appear, then, that a good sampling of tracheobronchial secretions, whether by blind distal bronchial sampling or fiberoptic protected brush biopsy, is the most reliable guide to the etiology of nosocomial pneumonia; that fiberoptic bronchoscopy adds little to the case in which a positive sample is obtained by blind distal bronchial sampling; and that bronchoalveolar lavage adds little definitive information.—G.M. Green, M.D.

---

**Comparison of Two Methods of Bacteriologic Sampling of the Lower Respiratory Tract: A Study in Ventilated Patients With Nosocomial Bronchopneumonia**

Papazian L, Martin C, Albanese J, Saux P, Charrel J, Gouin F (Hôpital Sainte-Marguerite, Marseille, France)

*Crit Care Med* 17:461–464, May 1989 1–33

---

The bacterial diagnosis of pulmonary infections in mechanically ventilated or tracheostomized patients who are being cared for in the intensive care unit is a difficult problem. Recent studies have shown good correlation between fiberoptic protected brush biopsy (FPBB) and blind distal bronchial sampling (DBS) of tracheobronchial secretions without a fiberscope. A prospective study was conducted to compare the 2 sampling techniques.

The study population consisted of 28 men and 5 women aged 16–88 years, who had been treated with mechanical ventilation for a mean of 20 days and who had bilateral or predominantly right lung infiltrates on chest radiographs suggestive of bronchopneumonia. The mean delay between admission to the intensive care unit and bacteriologic sampling was 11.4 days. A total of 47 paired specimens were obtained by both DBS and FPBB; 9 patients underwent repeated sampling. Distal bronchial sampling and FPBB were always performed within 24 hours.

Identical results were obtained in 44 of the 47 paired samples. The remaining 3 pairs showed contradictory results. A single microorganism was isolated in 23 pairs; 2 organisms were isolated in 4 pairs; and 3 organisms, in 1 pair of samples. No bacteria were detected in the remaining 16 pairs of samples. In 5 patients, identical organisms were found simultaneously in blood cultures, in cultures obtained by DBS, and in cultures obtained by FPBB. The simultaneous samples obtained from all 9 patients who underwent repeated sampling were identical. These findings support those of earlier studies indicating that FPBB is not more efficient than DBS in the bacteriologic assessment of lower respiratory tract infections in mechanically ventilated patients.

► ↓ With the preceding papers, it would seem that a strategy might be developed to diminish the incidence of life threatening nosocomial pneumonia in intubated and ventilated patients, and that a more vigorous effort to develop such preventive protocols is in order. An effective protocol would begin by adopting methods of preventing the development of a biofilm on the inner lining of the tracheal tube, to inhibit bacterial colonization in the biofilm, to monitor the course of colonization of tracheobronchial secretions through periodic blind distal bronchial sampling and quantitative bacteriology, and to suppress bacterial overgrowth from contaminated and colonized lower respiratory tract secretions, when identified. The following article by Mandelli and co-workers confirms that reliance on antibiotic prophylaxis fails to reduce significantly the incidence of nosocomial pneumonia in the early stages of intubation. Therefore, a more complex strategy needs to be developed to control this serious and often life-threatening complication of the intensive care setting in the modern acute care hospital.—G.M. Green, M.D.

---

**Prevention of Pneumonia in an Intensive Care Unit: A Randomized Multicenter Clinical Trial**

Mandelli M, Mosconi P, Langer M, Cigada M, Intensive Care Unit Group of Infection Control (Istituto Ricerche Farmacologiche "Mario Negri"; Ospedale Maggiore, Milan, Italy)

*Crit Care Med* 17:501–505, June 1989 1–34

---

A recently completed trial showed that more than 50% of all acquired pneumonias appeared within 4 days of admission to an intensive care unit (ICU). This type of early pneumonia was classified as early-onset pneumonia (EOP). It was hypothesized that EOP pneumonia is caused by the aspiration of oropharyngeal contents at the acute onset of the illness that precipitates the ICU admission. Thus, EOP may represent an indication for antibiotic prophylaxis, as such massive aspiration is a single event of limited duration and is different from the continuous microaspirations occurring in long-term intubated or tracheostomized patients. A randomized, multicenter clinical trial was conducted to assess the effect of antibiotic prophylaxis in the prevention of EOP.

During a 4-month study period, 1,319 patients in 23 ICUs were enrolled in the study. Of these patients, 181 were treated with cefoxitin; 196, with penicillin G; and 193 received no antibiotic prophylaxis. The remaining patients were excluded for a variety of reasons. Prophylaxis was initiated as soon as possible after ICU admission, but not later than 24 hours. No other antibiotics were administered during the first 48 hours of admission.

Early-onset pneumonia was diagnosed in 11 of 181 cefoxitin-treated patients, in 12 of 196 penicillin-treated patients, and in 14 of 193 controls. The 15.3% reduction in EOP incidence was statistically nonsignificant. During hospitalization, 21 cefoxitin-treated patients, 27 penicillin-treated patients, and 30 control patients died. These data confirm that acquisition of EOP is a risk factor for death in ICU patients, but antibiotic prophylaxis does not prevent it.

## Tuberculosis

▶ ↓ A resurgence of interest in tuberculosis is taking place, largely because of the growth of immigrant populations and susceptibles associated with the spread of HIV infection among intravenous drug users and homosexual populations (1). Infection with HIV, by causing a reduction in lymphocyte-mediated cellular immune mechanisms on which immunity to tuberculosis rests, is producing an expanding reservoir of mycobacterial infection that acts as a source for spread of infection to non-HIV-infected persons in close quarters such as prisons, nursing homes, and shelters. The importance of the expanding reservoir of susceptibles and infecteds is the subject of 7 of the following 11 articles on tuberculosis. One article deals with a new diagnostic technique, and the final 3 articles deal with treatment.—G.M. Green, M.D.

*Reference*

1. Rieder HL et al: *JAMA* 262:385, 1989.

**A Prospective Study of the Risk of Tuberculosis Among Intravenous Drug Users With Human Immunodeficiency Virus Infection**

Selwyn PA, Hartel D, Lewis VA, Schoenbaum EE, Vermund SH, Klein RS, Walker AT, Friedland GH (Montefiore Med Ctr—Albert Einstein College of Medicine, New York)

*N Engl J Med* 320:545–550, March 2, 1989 1–35

Epidemiologic data from the United States suggest a significant association of tuberculosis with AIDS, but few prospective trials have been done. A 2-year prospective study of tuberculosis in 520 intravenous drug users in a New York City methadone maintenance program was performed. Of these, 217 patients were seropositive for HIV at the outset. Ten other patients had seroconversion by the end of the 2 years.

Skin testing with purified protein derivative (PPD) was positive at baseline in 23% of seropositive and 20% of seronegative patients. Rates of conversion on retesting after a mean of 22 months were 11% and 13%, respectively, in the seropositive and seronegative groups. Active tuberculosis developed in 4% of the seropositive patients, but in none of those who were seronegative. Seven of 8 patients with active disease had had previously positive PPD tests. The case rate was 8 per 100 person-years in patients with a previous positive PPD test and 0.3 in those with negative tests.

These findings suggest that tuberculosis in HIV-infected persons most often results from reactivation of latent infection. Aggressive chemoprophylaxis is warranted in HIV-infected patients with a positive PPD test. Household members and health care workers may be at secondary risk of contracting tuberculosis from seropositive patients.

▶ This study of the relationship among HIV seropositivity, PPD reactivity, and active tuberculosis in a population of drugs users in a methadone maintenance program is instructive in demonstrating the relationships among prior tuberculous infection, HIV infection, and active tuberculosis. Although 42% of this population was seropositive for HIV infection, the prevalence of PPD skin test positivity was equivalent at 23% and 20% among seropositive and seronegative patients, respectively, and the rate of skin test conversion 2 years later was the same, at 12% in both groups. However, only the HIV seropositive patients (4%) had active tuberculosis; none of the seronegative did. The findings strongly support that the activity of tuberculosis in this population is related to the reactivation of infection as immune competency declines with HIV infection, and that the strategy of chemoprophylaxis for skin-positive and HIV-seropositive patients is sound and to be pursued vigorously.

The high rates of PPD skin test conversion over the short 2-year period of follow-up graphically illustrate the risk of infection with tubercle bacilli in this population and reinforce the need to control tuberculous infectivity through chemoprophylaxis. The drug-using population must clearly be a focus for programs of tuberculosis control in the community.—G.M. Green, M.D.

---

**Increasing Incidence of Tuberculosis in a Prison Inmate Population: Association With HIV Infection**

Braun MM, Truman BI, Maguire B, DiFerdinando GT Jr, Wormser G, Broaddus R, Morse DL (New York State Dept of Health; New York State Dept of Correctional Services, Albany; New York Med College, Valhalla)

*JAMA* 261:393–397, Jan 20, 1989 1–36

Several previous studies have indicated that patients with AIDS frequently have tuberculosis (TB). Matching TB and AIDS registries in 24 states and 4 localities revealed that 645 (4.2%) of 15,181 patients with AIDS also had TB. Matching TB and AIDS registries for the New York State prison system revealed that 22 (6.9%) of 319 inmates with AIDS also had TB. Because TB poses special problems in correctional facilities, a comparison of 59 inmates with TB and 59 matched control inmates without TB was done to examine the role of AIDS in the development of TB. All 118 patients examined were seropositive for HIV.

According to univariate analysis, TB was associated with street drug use, positive Mantoux test results at entry into the New York State prison system, and New York City residence at the time of arrest. Birth outside the United States, spending 1 year or more in local jails before entry into the New York State prison system, leukopenia at entry, and Quetelet's index of thinness at entry were not associated with TB.

In most patients, TB was thought to result from reactivation of latent TB infection. However, phage typing of 16 *Mycobacterium tuberculosis* cultures suggested the possibility of inmate-to-inmate transmission in at least 1 cluster of 3 cases. Therefore, TB control measures need to be reinforced in the prison setting to counter the increased risk created by HIV infection.

▶ This paper quotes a remarkably similar prevalence of 4% of patients with AIDS also having tuberculosis; a slightly higher finding of 6.9% occurred in a population of prison inmates with AIDS. Again, the occurrence of active tuberculosis was associated with previous skin test positivity for tuberculosis at the time of entry into the prison population, supporting the view that active tuberculous infection in HIV-seropositive persons is associated more with reactivation of latent tuberculous infection than with new infection. Because prisons, like methadone treatment centers, bring this high-risk group under medical surveillance, they provide an appropriate focus for active tuberculosis control programs in the community. That 4% to 7% of persons with AIDS also had active tuberculosis is an astounding contrast with the 0.01% in the general population.—G.M. Green, M.D.

---

**Tuberculosis and Acquired Immunodeficiency Syndrome: Florida**

Rieder HL, Cauthen GM, Bloch AB, Cole CH, Holtzman D, Snider DE Jr, Bigler WJ, Witte JJ (Ctrs for Disease Control, Atlanta; Dept of Health and Rehabilitative Services, Tallahassee, Fla)

*Arch Intern Med* 149:1268–1273, June 1989 1–37

---

Between 1975 and 1984 tuberculosis rates in the United States decreased from 15.9 to 9.4 per 100,000 population, an average decline of 5.7% per year. However, in 1986 the number of reported instances of tuberculosis increased. The exact reasons for this increase are not known, but available data indicate that the current epidemic of HIV infection and AIDS accounts for part of the change in tuberculosis morbidity. Possibly, latent subclinical infection with *Mycobacterium tuberculosis* progress is more frequently to clinically active tuberculosis in patients with HIV infection because of their immunodeficient status. This records-based investigation was done to analyze the extent of overlap of tuberculosis and AIDS among different populations residing in Florida.

Between January 1, 1981, and October 31, 1986, the state of Florida reported 8,455 instances of tuberculosis, and 1,858 instances of AIDS. Of the patients with AIDS, 159 (8.6%) also had tuberculosis; of the patients with tuberculosis, 154 (1.8%) also had AIDS. Tuberculosis was diagnosed more than 1 month before AIDS was in 50% of patients, within 1 month after the diagnosis of AIDS in 30% of patients, and more than 1 month after AIDS was diagnosed in 20% of patients. Those with both diagnoses were more likely to be Haitian, non-Haitian black, or Hispanic than patients with AIDS only. They were also more likely to be younger, male, Haitian, non-Haitian black, Hispanic, or to have extrapulmonary tuberculosis, negative tuberculin skin test, or noncavitary chest radiographs than patients with tuberculosis only.

Patients with AIDS may be at increased risk of contracting clinically active tuberculosis. Patients with both AIDS and tuberculosis differ from those with AIDS only and those with tuberculosis only in a number of important demographic and clinical characteristics.

▶ This study confirms the findings of the previous paper (Abstract 1–36) in identifying an 8.6% prevalence rate of tuberculosis in persons with AIDS, in associating ethnicity and race as well as age and sex with susceptibility, and in finding a greater tendency to extrapulmonary, noncavitary, and tuberculin-negative disease in the tuberculous population with AIDS. The latter finding is consistent with impaired cellular immune mechanisms characteristic of HIV infection. An 8% tuberculous infection rate clearly warrants a targeted and aggressive chemoprophylaxis program in this population, especially considering the reduced effectiveness of their immune mechanisms in controlling and containing the mycobacterial infection.—G.M. Green, M.D.

### The Slowing of the Decline in Tuberculosis Notifications and HIV Infection

Davies PDO (Sefton Gen Hosp, Liverpool, England)

*Respir Med* 83:321–322, July 1989 1–38

In England and Wales the number of reported instances of tuberculosis steadily declined by approximately 10% per year from the 1960s to 1984. In the early 1970s, this decline was somewhat slowed as a result of an influx of immigrants from the Indian subcontinent. In 1985 the tuberculosis rate declined by only 3%, and in 1986 a small increase in the tuberculosis rate was noted. For the same 2 years, the tuberculosis rate in the United States increased 2% per year, mainly because of an increase in the rate in the 20–40 years age group in areas where positivity for HIV is prevalent.

Analysis of age-specific tuberculosis rates in England and Wales for the

5-year period between 1982 and 1986 revealed that tuberculosis rates for men aged 15–34 years declined from 16.2 to 10.8 per 100,000 population. For men aged 35–54 years rates declined from 18.6 to 13.3 per 100,000 population. Rates for the other age and sex groups also declined during that period, except that rates for women aged 35 years or more remained almost static.

When rates of tuberculosis for each age and sex group were expressed as a percentage of the total number of reported instances for a particular year, rates for women aged 55 and older increased from 12.4% to 14.6% of the total number of reported instances during the 5-year period. For men of the same age group rates increased from 22.5% to 24.1% for the same period. Therefore, the slowing in the decline of tuberculosis rates appears to be almost entirely caused by a slow rate of decline among women aged 55 and older. Thus, it is unlikely that the slowed decline in tuberculosis rates in England and Wales is associated with HIV infection. Rather, the increase in tuberculosis rates among older persons appear to result from endogenous breakdown of infection incurred during World War II.

▶ Strong demographic factors other than AIDS govern the rate of active tuberculosis and the changes in those rates over time. Tuberculosis is disseminated under conditions of crowding, socioeconomic decline, and social disruption, as in wartime. The cohort of the population experiencing such conditions progresses through the age structure, retaining a heightened susceptibility to reactivated infection that is related to age. The careful analysis in this study clearly illustrates the difference in age distribution of active tuberculosis resulting in a slowing of the decline in notifications of tuberculosis. In the United States, this appears to result from HIV and AIDS in young males; in England and Wales, it results from an increase in rates among populations aged more than 55, especially women, which is a population that experienced wartime conditions as children.—G.M. Green, M.D.

---

**The Epidemiology of Disseminated Nontuberculous Mycobacterial Infection in the Acquired Immunodeficiency Syndrome (AIDS)**

Horsburgh CR Jr, Selik RM (Ctr for Infectious Diseases, Atlanta)

*Am Rev Respir Dis* 139:4–7, January 1989 1–39

---

Before onset of the AIDS epidemic, only 78 patients with disseminated nontuberculous mycobacterial infection (DNTM) had been reported, with disseminated *Mycobacterium avium* complex reported in only 37 patients. However, disseminated *M. avium* complex has become a frequent opportunistic infection in patients with AIDS. To assess the risk factors for DNTM in AIDS patients, records of the Centers for Disease Control collected from 1981 to 1987 were analyzed.

A total of 2,269 cases of DNTM in patients with AIDS were reported, 96% of which were caused by *M. aqvium* complex. The diagnosis of DNTM was made at the same time as diagnosis of AIDS in 1,198 patients and after the diagnosis of AIDS in 1,071 patients. Diagnosis was made at autopsy in 375 patients. Those AIDS patients with Kaposi's sarcoma had DNTM less often than other AIDS patients. Hispanic persons had a lower frequency of DNTM than black or non-Hispanic white persons. The means of acquiring HIV infection and the patient's sex did not affect DNTM rates significantly. Rates of disseminated *M. avium* varied by geographic region. The AIDS patients with DNTM were not more impaired immunologically than AIDS patients with other opportunistic infections. Life-table analysis demonstrated that AIDS patients with DNTM survived for a median of 7.4 months, whereas AIDS patients without DNTM survived for a median of 13.3 months.

It is probable that DNTM is acquired by unpreventable environmental exposure to food and water and is not sexually transmitted. Because DNTM contributes to patient mortality, it merits diagnosis and therapy; however, effective therapies often are not available.

▶ The impairment of lymphocyte-mediated cellular immunity is a generalized phenomenon that heightens the susceptibility of persons with AIDS to a variety of organisms that otherwise would be noninfective or of extremely low infectivity. This paper is an important reminder that the background of impaired immune-based resistance that characterizes AIDS mandates an alert and broad based infection surveillance program in this population. The study is also a reminder that the increased risk found in AIDS patients is related not only to activation of endogenous infection with *Mycobacterium* tuberculosis, *Pneumocystis carinii*, or other carried organism, but also to environmentally acquired infections such as *Mycobacterium avium*, *Legionella pneumophila*, and other organisms transmitted through food, air, and water.—G.M. Green, M.D.

---

**Endobronchial Tuberculosis in the Acquired Immunodeficiency Syndrome**
Wasser LS, Shaw GW, Talavera W (Beth Israel Med Ctr, New York)
*Chest* 94:1240–1244, December 1988 1–40

---

The incidence of tuberculosis (TB) has been increasing coincident with the increase in the incidences of AIDS and AIDS-related complex. With the development of effective antituberculosis chemotherapy, TB of the tracheobronchial tree has become a rare. Endobronchial TB was diagnosed in 3 patients with AIDS and AIDS-related complex, a finding not reported previously.

The patients included a 34-year-old man with AIDS-related complex and a history of oropharyngeal candidiasis, a 30-year-old man with a history of *Pneumocystis carinii* pneumonia and AIDS, and a 32-year-old Hispanic woman with a previous history of *P. carinii* pneumonia and AIDS. Diagnosis at the time of hospital admission was problematic, resulting in a significant delay in the initiation of antituberculosis chemotherapy. All 3 patients had nonspecific symptoms of fever and cough, but none had the classic findings of dyspnea, wheezing, or hemoptysis suggestive of an endobronchial process. Each patient was given empiric antimicrobial agents for at least 1 week before undergoing fiberoptic bronchoscopy. Smears of sputum were nondiagnostic. Chest radiographs revealed mediastinal and hilar adenopathy in 2 patients and a lower lobe consolidation in the third. All 3 had small, ipsilateral pleural effusions consistent with a variety of infectious or neoplastic processes commonly noted in AIDS patients.

Bronchoscopic findings were similar in all 3 patients, including white or pink exophytic masses obstructing the airways, mimicking bronchogenic carcinoma. Two patients had areas of classic primary tuberculosis. In all 3 patients cultures of bronchial washing specimens grew fully sensitive *Mycobacterium tuberculosis*. All 3 patients had improvement clinically and radiographically after receiving antituberculosis chemotherapy.

In view of the frequent occurrence of TB in patients with AIDS and AIDS-related complex, involvement of the tracheobronchial tree should be suspected in patients with endobronchial lesions. To avoid a delay in diagnosis, bronchial washings should be examined for the presence of acid-gast bacilli as soon as possible.

▶ The immunologic impairment associated with AIDS may alter the presentation and pathogenesis of tuberculosis, in this case manifesting endobronchial spread of the tuberculous infection. This form of the disease may not be suspected because of the absence of the typical chest radiologic infiltrates. At the same time, this disease is highly contagious because of the ease with which viable bacilli enter the airstream in large numbers, generating extremely infectious aerosols that may spread throughout clinics, hospital rooms, or air conditioning systems to infect other persons at some distance. Thus, the best preventive is a high index of suspicion for tuberculous infection, even in unusual forms, in patients known to have AIDS.

Adopting an aggressive diagnostic stance will not only benefit the individual patient but help to contain the spread of infection to others. In turn, the medical team should be always alert to maintaining respiratory precautions in AIDS patients; although HIV-1 is not disseminated by the airborne route, secondary infecting organisms such as tubercle bacilli are highly contagious by infectious aerosols. The AIDS population, because of its high incidence rate for active tuberculosis (4% to 8%), is a potential hazard for spreading tuberculosis in the health care team.—G.M. Green, M.D.

---

**Bronchopulmonary Cross-Colonization and Infection Related to Mycobacterial Contamination of Suction Valves of Bronchoscopes**

Wheeler PW, Lancaster D, Kaiser AB (St Thomas Hosp, Nashville, Tenn; Vanderbilt Univ)

*J Infect Dis* 159:954–958, May 1989 1–41

---

Although glutaraldehyde seems to be an effective bactericidal and mycobactericidal agent in bronchoscopy, direct exposure of organisms for an adequate period is critical. Three episodes of mycobacterial contamination of bronchoscopy specimens and 1 pulmonary infection related to inadequate disinfection of the bronchoscope suction valve were detected at 1 center. Preparation of the instruments used involved both povidone-iodine and 2% glutaraldehyde solution, the latter being forced repeatedly through the valve.

*Mycobacterium avium* was isolated from bronchial washings of 2 patients on the same day. Several weeks later 4 patients had *M. tuberculosis* cultured from bronchial washings, and 1 of them became infected. Despite adoption of a commercial endoscope washer, a third episode of cross-contamination ensued. The suction valve on the proximal end of the scope seemed a likely source of contamination. The valves of intact bronchoscopes were preferentially contaminated by *M. fortuitum,* and isolated valves remained contaminated despite a 30-minute exposure to 2% glutaraldehyde solution. Most of 14 hospitals surveyed did not use a more intensive disinfection regimen than was in use at this center.

Because of the time needed to isolate mycobacterial organisms, there is a considerable chance of overlooking outbreaks of cross-contamination or even infection. Presently, valves are steam-autoclaved after cleaning, and disinfection with glutaraldehyde continues for at least 30 minutes at room temperature. No further episodes have occurred in the past 2 years, and the suction valves have continued to function well.

▶ Technologic advancements may be associated with infective hazards; in this case, a standard protocol for disinfecting bronchoscopes was found to be inadequate for reliably eliminating mycobacterial organisms. Caveat emptor!—G.M. Green, M.D.

---

**Differentiation of Sarcoidosis From Tuberculosis Using an Enzyme-Linked Immunosorbent Assay for the Detection of Antibodies Against *Mycobacterium tuberculosis***

Levy H, Feldman C, Wadee AA, Rabson AR (Hillbrow Hosp; South African Inst for Med Research; Univ of the Witwatersrand, Johannesburg, South Africa)

*Chest* 94:1254–1255, December 1988 1–42

---

Because sarcoid granulomas are not pathognomonic and cannot be distinguished from other types of granulomas, sarcoidosis presently is diagnosed only by long-term observation of patients. Differentiation between sarcoidosis and tuberculosis (TB) is often difficult clinically, particularly in the presence of positive results of purified protein derivative skin testing. An enzyme-linked immunosorbent assay (ELISA) using an adsorbed fraction of mycobacterial sonicates as an antigen was analyzed for its ability to differentiate between TB and sarcoidosis in 11 patients with active sarcoidosis, 7 patients with untreated sputum-positive TB, and 7 normal volunteers. Ten patients with sarcoidosis had at least 1 clinical or laboratory feature of active sarcoidosis; 7 were being treated with oral corticosteroids. Serum samples from each participant were subjected to ELISA.

Statistical analysis of ELISA results revealed a highly significant difference between ELISA findings for normal volunteers and for patients with sarcoidosis, and ELISA findings in patients with TB. The ELISA findings for patients with sarcoidosis did not differ from those in normal volunteers.

A rapid, relatively inexpensive, reproducible immunoassay ELISA differentiates sarcoidosis from TB with a high degree of certainty.

▶ The abstract says it all, and Figure 1 of the original paper is dramatic. The availability of a simple blood test to identify circulating antibody to mycobacterial antigen should be of significant assistance in attributing granulomatous disease either to the infectious organism, if the test result is positive, or to a sarcoid process, if the result is negative. Pursuit of positive cultures obviously is required when the test is positive.—G.M. Green, M.D.

▶ ↓ Tuberculous pleurisy is an immunoinflammatory response of pleural tissues to mycobacterial antigen released into the pleural space of a sensitized host. Tuberculous pleurisy also may result from the formation of exudative granulomata on the pleural surface or in subpleural tissue. Corticosteroids are well known for their anti-inflammatory activity and are effective in suppressing effusion in serosal surfaces. Their effectiveness in accelerating the subsidence of clinical symptoms and pleural effusion is logical and to be expected.

The risk of corticosteroid treatment is the associated immunosuppression that lowers resistance to infection and may impair the resolution of infection unless an alternative to immune control is available. Isoniazid and, especially, rifampin provide the bactericidal capability that can compensate for steroid-induced immunosuppression and achieve a bacteriologic response even in the presence of corticosteroids. When it is important to control the inflammatory response, corticosteroids seem to be effective and are safe in an infectious process so long as potent and effective antimicrobial therapy is available.—G.M. Green, M.D.

---

**Corticosteroids in the Treatment of Tuberculous Pleurisy: A Double-Blind, Placebo-Controlled, Randomized Study**

Lee C-H, Wang W-J, Lan R-S, Tsai Y-H, Chiang Y-C (Chang Gung Mem Hosp, Taipei, Taiwan)

*Chest* 94:1256–1259, December 1988 1–43

---

Tuberculous pleurisy has long been treated with a combined regimen of corticosteroids and antimicrobial agents, but most clinical trials of this approach were performed before the modern chemotherapy for tuberculosis had been developed fully. Since then, the efficacy of a combined regimen of multidrug antituberculosis chemotherapy and corticosteroids in the treatment of tuberculous pleurisy has not been reassessed.

A prospective, double-blind, randomized clinical trial was carried out in 40 patients diagnosed with tuberculous pleurisy, 21 of whom were assigned randomly to receive prednisolone and 19 of whom received placebo. All patients underwent an antituberculosis regimen comprised of isoniazid, rifampin, and ethambutol. The 2 groups were identical with respect to age, sex, time from onset of symptoms to diagnosis, and initial amount of pleural effusion.

Clinical signs and symptoms, including fever, chest pain, and dyspnea, subsided after an average of 2.4 days in the prednisolone-treated group and after an average of 9.2 days in the placebo-treated group. Radiographic evidence of clearing of the lungs occurred after an average of 54.5 days in the group given prednisolone and after an average of 123.2 days in those given placebo. The differences were statistically significant. Pleural adhesions developed in 1 steroid-treated patient (4.8%) and 3 placebo-treated patients (15.8%), but the difference did not reach statistical significance. Transient moon face, lower limb edema, and epigastric pain developed in 1 patient after prednisolone administration, but these side effects resolved after the steroid dosage was tapered.

Corticosteroid administration in conjunction with antituberculosis chemotherapy hastens the resolution of clinical symptoms and radiographic findings in tuberculous pleurisy.

▶ ↓ The potency of modern antibiotic combined regimens, particularly those that include rifampin, is indicated in the following paper (Abstract 1–44), which provides effective management of active tuberculosis with thrice-weekly treatment with a combination of streptomycin, isoniazid, rifampin, and pyrazinamide for 4 months in intially smear-negative cases, and 6 months for initially smear-positive disease.—G.M. Green, M.D.

---

**A Controlled Trial of 3-Month, 4-Month, and 6-Month Regimens of Chemotherapy for Sputum Smear-Negative Pulmonary Tuberculosis: Results at 5 Years**

Hong Kong Chest Service/Tuberculosis Research Centre, Madras/British Med Research Council (Hong Kong; Madras, India; London; Girling DJ, Brompton Hosp, London)

*Am Rev Respir Dis* 139:871–876, April 1989 1–44

---

Many patients worldwide are diagnosed with pulmonary tuberculosis on the basis of clinical and radiographic findings alone. A study from Hong Kong showed that, in patients with at least 1 of 5 initial sputum cultures positive, 2- and 3-month daily regimens of streptomycin, isoniazid, rifampin, and pyrazinamide were followed by relapse rates of 16% and 7%, respectively. The corresponding relapse rates for patients with all their initial cultures negative were only 1% and 2%, respectively. A study was done to determine whether, in patients with smear-negative pulmonary tuberculosis, 3- or 4-month regimens of streptomycin, isoniazid, rifampin, and pyrazinamide given daily or 3 times a week would be effective, or whether chemotherapy should be continued for 6 months, especially for culture-positive patients.

A total of 1,710 Chinese patients with radiologically active pulmonary tuberculosis with sputum negative for acid-fast bacilli on at least 4 initial examinations were studied for 5 years. Five hundred ninety-two (35%) of these patients had at least 1 initial sputum culture positive for *Mycobacterium tuberculosis.* By random assignment, these patients were given streptomycin, isoniazid, rifampin, and pyrazinamide daily for 4 months or 3 times weekly for 4 or 6 months. The remaining 1,118 patients also were randomly assigned to the same treatment arms. The 5-year relapse rates for the patients on the 4-month regimen were 2% in patients with drug-susceptible cultures initially; 8% in patients with cultures resistant to isoniazid or streptomycin, or both, but susceptible to rifampin initially; and 4% in patients with all negative cultures initially. For patients on the 3-month regimen, the combined relapse rate in those with all cultures initially negative was 7%.

Patients in the Hong Kong Government Chest Service diagnosed as having active but smear-negative pulmonary tuberculosis are treated with the 4-month thrice weekly regimen. Patients with smear-positive disease have isoniazid and rifampin continued 3 times a week for up to 3 months.

▶ ↓ The final paper by Dutt, Moers, and Stead provides similar results from this country in smear- and culture-negative tuberculosis with 4-month treatment with only isoniazid and rifampin. Close follow-up is important to provide additional months of chemotherapy for the very small percentage with relapses. The advent of rifampin has had a significant impact on the approach to treatment and control of tuberculosis.—G.M. Green, M.D.

---

**Smear- and Culture-Negative Pulmonary Tuberculosis: Four-Month Short-Course Chemotherapy**

Dutt AK, Moers D, Stead WW (Arkansas Dept of Health, Little Rock)

*Am Rev Respir Dis* 139:867–870, April 1989 1–45

---

It seems reasonable that culture-negative tuberculosis requires less treatment for a cure. In 1980 a 4-month course of treatment with isoniazid and rifampin was used in 414 patients with a positive tuberculin reaction and abnormal chest radiograph but negative bacteriologic studies. At least 3 negative smears and cultures were required. Pulmonary infiltration often was extensive, and 30 patients had suggestive cavitary changes. Significant medical disorders were present in 16% of patients.

Twenty-eight percent of patients had a clinical or radiographic response, or both, to treatment. Side effects occurred in about 5% of treated patients. The incidence of toxic hepatitis was 0.9%. The rate of relapse during a median follow-up of 44 months was 1.2%. Relapsers received the same drugs for 9 months longer.

Four months of chemotherapy in patients suspected of having tuberculosis despite negative bacteriologic findings is as effective as 9 months of treatment in smear- and culture- positive patients. The rate of toxic hepatitis was low despite the average patient age of 60 years.

# 2 Asthma and Selected Immunologically Mediated Lung Diseases

## Introduction

This chapter of the YEAR BOOK OF PULMONARY DISEASE has been organized into sections concerning clinical syndromes and associations, pathogenesis, and therapy, similar to previous editions. Many of the articles abstracted and discussed serve mainly to update the reader about well-established concepts that are familiar to many persons, but a few topics might be completely novel for at least some readers.

In the section titled Clinical Syndromes and Associations, we discuss not only rather traditional topics such as environmental causes of asthma, smoking and bronchial reactivity, hypersensitivity pneumonitis, and the clinical usefulness of wheezing, but also relationships between asthma and dilated cardiomyopathy, a possibly dangerous β agonist, an effective approach to the diagnosis of sinusitis, and "gustatory rhinitis." In the section Pathogenesis, not only are immunoglobulin E and airway hyperreactivity (and its associations with viral infections, ozone exposure, day-to-day variability in disease expression, and inflammatory changes in the airway) discussed, but also lessons for the airways from congestive heart failure, interleukin-2 and tumor necrosis factor, the pathogenesis of clubbing, and vasoactive intestinal polypeptide and platelet-activating factor. In the section Therapy, traditional discussions of β-agonists and corticosteroids (including a 10-year morphological study of patients on inhaled steroids) are complemented by articles discussing air cleaning devices; self-management of asthma; new, nonsedating antihistamines; and the chronic fatigue syndrome. We hope readers find at least some of these articles interesting and informative.

Finally, when we began to edit this chapter on the YEAR BOOK OF PULMONARY DISEASE 5 years ago, we began our discussion of the first article by saying, "No event is more devastating to a family than the death of a child . . ." as a prelude to a discussion of deaths from asthma (1986 YEAR BOOK OF PULMONARY DISEASE, p 76). During the past year we had the misfortune to experience just such a tragedy in a different context. This section of the YEAR BOOK is dedicated to your memory, Craig.

**Stephen P. Peters, M.D., Ph.D.**

## Clinical Syndromes

### Diagnosis

▶ ↓ As clinicians and teachers, we often tell our students (whether or not we believe it) that, except for an accurate and detailed medical history, a carefully performed physical examination, rather than exotic invasive tests, will provide us with the most useful information. The first 2 articles (Abstracts 2–1 and 2–2) suggest exceptions to this statement.—S.P. Peters, M.D., Ph.D.

---

**Wheezing on Maximal Forced Exhalation in the Diagnosis of Atypical Asthma: Lack of Sensitivity and Specificity**

King DK, Thompson BT, Johnson DC (Massachusetts Gen Hosp, Boston)

*Ann Intern Med* 110:451–455, March 15, 1989 2–1

---

Some patients with "atypical asthma" may have normal baseline spirometry and not report wheezing. Patients with other respiratory, cardiac, or psychiatric conditions may have symptoms that mimic asthma. To obtain an accurate diagnosis, methacholine challenge testing has been used when asthma is suspected. The finding of wheezing on maximal forced exhalation was assessed for its sensitivity and specificity in predicting asthma in patients without abnormal spirometry.

Forty-four patients referred for methacholine challenge testing had technically acceptable results. Before the test, all were evaluated for the presence of a wheeze—a continuous sound with a musical quality—during maximal forced exhalation. The most common symptoms were cough and dyspnea.

Physician observers heard wheezing in 8 of 14 patients with positive results of the methacholine challenge test. Wheezing was absent from 11 of 30 patients with negative test results. Thus in this patient group, wheezing lacked both sensitivity and specificity as a predictor of the results of methacholine challenge testing, whether the cutoff 20% fall in baseline forced expiratory volume in 1 second ($PC_{20}$) was 16, 8, or 4 mg/mL. Wheezing does seem to occur with regularity, however, in those with $PC_{20}$ values of less than 3 mg/mL.

▶ The finding in this article that wheezing on forced exhalation is neither sensitive nor specific in the diagnosis of asthma (or its surrogate, bronchial hyperreactivity) is not surprising. It is somewhat disappointing, however. Its lack of sensitivity could be overlooked (wheezing occurred in 8 of 14 patients with positive results of methacholine testing at a concentration of 8 mg/mL or less, and in 5 of 7 patients with a positive test result at less than 4 mg/mL), but the high number of "false positives" makes its use unwarranted. (Wheezing occurred in 13 of 27 patients with no response to methacholine at 16 mg/mL, a negative test). However, patient selection may have played an important role in these results. Only patients without wheezing on quiet breathing and with normal or near normal spirometry were selected. A more useful and realistic patient population to study would have been patients without wheezing on quiet breathing regardless of their spirometry because this is the setting in which such a test (as part of a routine physical examination before pulmonary function testing) would be employed.—S.P. Peters, M.D., Ph.D.

**Flexible Fiberoptic Rhinoscopy in the Diagnosis of Sinusitis**

Castellanos J, Axelrod D (Mt Carmel Mercy Hosp, Detroit)

*J Allergy Clin Immunol* 83:91–94, January 1989 2–2

Sinus infection is an important and treatable cause of headache. The role of flexible fiberoptic rhinoscopy in the diagnosis of sinus infections was evaluated in 246 patients with undiagnosed headache after an unrewarding neurologic evaluation. The patients were also examined by routine sinus radiographs.

Sinusitis was diagnosed by rhinoscopy in 98 patients (group I) and by both rhinoscopy and radiographs in 84 (group II), whereas the remaining 64 patients had neither radiographic or rhinoscopic evidence of sinusitis (group III). Antibiotics were effective in relieving headache for 94% of group I, 75% of group II, and 5% of group III patients. Patients with radiographic findings of sinusitis were older, had symptoms longer, and were afflicted by chronic sinusitis more often than patients with rhinoscopic findings. The disease Rhinoscopy may have been found earlier with rhinoscopy than with radiography.

Flexible fiberoptic rhinoscopy is useful in the office diagnosis of sinusitis. It is inexpensive and well tolerated by patients, and may provide a treatable diagnosis before the onset of chronic sinus changes.

▶ This article is interesting from a number of points of view. Regardless of these authors' practice circumstances (private practice, medical school faculty, or other), it demonstrates that useful clinical information can be obtained in the ordinary course of patient care without an inordinate amount of time, expense, or high technology. A number of findings in this study deserve mention. First, that 74% of patients with headache and a negative neurologic evaluation had rhinoscopic (with or without radiologic) evidence of sinusitis is surprisingly high. It would be interesting to know whether any aspects of the history or routine evaluation of these patients had a high positive predictive value for the diagnosis of sinusitis. Second, the authors appear to have become rather proficient at rhinoscopy as their technique missed not a single case of sinusitis diagnosed with sinus radiographs. Third, 85% of the total group of patients with abnormal rhinoscopy (groups I and II) responded to a 2-week course of antibiotics, but 64% of all patients responded to antibiotic treatment. Our goal in medicine is to establish a specific diagnosis, then prescribe a specific, effective therapy. The authors appear to have done that for these patients with a normal neurologic evaluation, headache, and rhinoscopic evidence of sinusitis. For those physicians without ready access to rhinoscopy, a trial of antibiotic therapy in the entire patient population might be in order.

A cost-benefit analysis of rhinoscopy with treatment of patients with positive rhinoscopic findings vs. empiric treatment of patients would be interesting, particularly if clues to the diagnosis of sinus disease could be obtained from routine history, physical examination, and laboratory studies to increase the chances of success with antibiotic therapy from its already rather high figure of 64%. The question posed is whether rhinoscopy of all 246 patients is justified to increase the likelihood of success with antibiotic therapy from 64% (all patients) to 85% (patients with sinusitis by rhinoscopy).—S.P. Peters, M.D., Ph.D.

## Environmental Factors

### Community Outbreaks of Asthma Associated With Inhalation of Soybean Dust

Antó JM, Sunyer J, Rodriguez-Roisin R, Suarez-Cervera M, Vazquez L (Univ of Barcelona; Institut Nacional de Meteorologia, Barcelona, Spain)
*N Engl J Med* 320:1097–1102, Apr 27, 1989 2–3

Since 1981 there have been 26 outbreaks of asthma in Barcelona in geographic relation to the harbor. An attempt was made to relate outbreaks occurring in 1985 and 1986 to the products unloaded at the harbor after asthma was coincidentally related to unloading of soybeans in 1987.

All 13 asthma-epidemic days during the 2-year study coincided with unloading of soybeans from ships in the harbor. On epidemic days, high-pressure areas and mild winds favored the movement of air to the city. Particles of starch and episperm cells were recovered from air samplers in the city and had characteristics identical to those of soybean particles. One of the harbor silos into which soybeans were unloaded lacked bag filters, allowing the release of soybean dust into the air. Soybean dust is a cause of epidemic asthma.

▶ Outbreaks of asthma associated with soybean unloading have been reported not only in Barcelona, but also in Valencia (1) and in Cartagena (2). The authors of the above article have done a first-rate job, not only in pointing out this association, but also in establishing the facts necessary for a cause and effect to be assumed. They have reported that airborne concentrations of soybean dust antigens and soybean chemical markers were higher on days in which epidemics occurred in comparison with days in which no outbreaks were reported (3), and that patients with epidemic asthma had serum immunoglobulin E antibody to soybean antigens in a much larger percentage of cases (74.4%) than did matched controls (4.6%) (4). The patients identified in these studies could prove valuable for investigating other aspects of extrinsic asthma, such as the natural history of this disorder, and perhaps physiologic and cellular changes associated with exposure. It will be interesting to see whether these authors or others are in a position to perform additional studies.—S.P. Peters, M.D., Ph.D.

*References*

1. Alvarez-Dardet C, Belda J, Peña M, et al: Letter. *N Engl J Med* 321:1127–1128, 1989.

2. Hernando L, Navarro C, Marquez M, et al: Asthma epidemics and soybean in Cartagena (Spain). *Lancet* 1:502, 1989.
3. Antó JM, Sunyer J, Grimalt J, et al: Letter. *N Engl J Med* 321:1128, 1989.
4. Sunyer J, Antó JM, Rodrigo M-J, et al: Case-control study of serum immunoglobulin-E antibodies reactive with soybean in epidemic asthma. *Lancet* 1:179–182, 1989.

**Gustatory Rhinitis: A Syndrome of Food-Induced Rhinorrhea**

Raphael G, Hauptschein Raphael M, Kaliner M (Natl Inst of Allergy and Infectious Diseases, Bethesda, Md)

*J Allergy Clin Immunol* 83:110–115, January 1989 2–4

Gustatory rhinitis occurs in some persons after eating certain foods. The syndrome is characterized by profuse watery rhinorrhea, generally without the sneezing, congestion, or pruritus common to allergic rhinitis. Twelve persons who had reported episodes of food-related rhinitis underwent food and nasal challenges to examine the underlying mechanisms responsible for this reaction.

The foods that frequently produce gustatory rhinitis include hot and spicy items (e.g., hot chili peppers, horseradish, tabasco sauce, and mustard). In 1 protocol, persons had a control nasal challenge with normal saline, then ate a bland, control food followed by a positive food. In the second protocol, the positive food challenge was repeated after treatment of the nasal mucosa with 100 μg of atropine (0.3 mL).

All persons had bilateral rhinorrhea after the positive food challenge. Facial flushing developed in about half of them. Total protein and albumin concentration were increased with ingestion of hot foods, but the ratio of albumin to total protein remained unchanged. Atropine prevented rhinorrhea after the positive food challenge, indicating a specific response to muscarinic blockade. Because histamine levels were not elevated at any time, gustatory rhinitis does not appear to involve mast cell degranulation. Sensitive persons can either avoid the offending spicy foods or be treated prophylactically with topical atropine.

▶ As the authors point out, this syndrome appears to involve neither a change in vascular permeability (because the ratio of albumin to total protein remained constant in nasal washings after challenge with a provocative food) nor mast cells (because symptoms differ from allergic rhinitis, the syndrome is inhibited by atropine, and an increase in histamine was not detected in nasal washings). They conclude, "Thus, for people with a passion for spicy foods, there may soon be an effective therapy that will allow them to eat to their heart's (and nose's) content . . . topical nasal atropine [applied] prophylactically (once it becomes available)."—S.P. Peters, M.D., Ph.D.

**Bronchial Provocation Tests Before and After Cessation of Smoking**

Israel RH, Ossip-Klein DJ, Poe RH, Black P, Gerrity E, Greenblatt DW, Rathbun S, Celebic A (Univ of Rochester, NY)

*Respiration* 54:247–254, April 1988 2–5

Some smokers may cough because of airway hyperreactivity. A prospective study was conducted to evaluate changes in airway reactivity and respiratory symptoms in symptomatic smokers before and after cessation of smoking. The study included 34 adults who wished to stop smoking after having smoked at least 10 cigarettes a day for 4 years or longer. All reported a chronic cough, with or without breathlessness on exertion.

The 6-month study was completed by 13 persons; 6 or 18 of the 34 persons had airway hyperreactivity at entry to the study, depending on the criterion used ($PD_{20}FEV_1$ or $PD_{35}S_{Gaw}$). All 13 persons who remained abstinent stopped coughing. However, there was no significant change in airway reactivity on testing with carbachol challenge after 6 months.

Some smokers do have increased airway reactivity, but loss of cough when smoking ends is not related obviously to altered airway responsiveness.

▶ The conclusion of this article, that cough in smokers usually is related to factors other than bronchial hyperresponsiveness is undoubtedly correct. However, if the relationship among smoking, airway hyperreactivity, and cough is to be explored, the population of smokers enrolled in this study was not optimal for examining these interrelationships. Only 6 of the 34 persons recruited for this study had airway hyperreactivity using the authors' more stringent criterion of $PD_{20}FEV_1$ at 150 breath units or less of carbachol. Therefore, only 6 persons would have the potential for cough to be related to airway hyperreactivity that might be ameliorated by smoking cessation. Only 2 of these 6 completed the 6 months of smoking cessation: 1 had a significant decrease in airway reactivity and 1 had no significant change in airway reactivity. Remaining unanswered by this study, therefore, is whether airway hyperreactivity is decreased by smoking cessation in patients who smoke, cough, and have airway hyperreactivity. That only 38% of persons abstained throughout the 6-month study is discouraging and consistent with previous data.—S.P. Peters, M.D., Ph.D.

**Reactive Airways Dysfunction Syndrome Presenting as a Reversible Restrictive Defect**

Gilbert R, Auchincloss JH Jr (State Univ of New York Health Science Ctr, Syracuse, NY)

*Lung* 167:55–61, 1989 2–6

In 1985, 10 patients who contracted an asthma-like disease after 1 high-level exposure to an irritating vapor, fume, or smoke were reported. The name *reactive airways dysfunction syndrome* was proposed to describe this illness. An additional patient experienced exertional dyspnea after a single high-level exposure to dust or mold in a silo.

Man, 25, had a severe cough and dyspnea while working in a silo. Previously he was a healthy farm worker. He had noticed a thick layer of white moldlike material covering the silage but no silage gas. While he was working the material was disturbed, and the air became dusty. That night his cough, dyspnea, and fever developed; 3 days later he was hospitalized. He recovered from this acute episode, but his dyspnea and fatigue became chronic, and he was referred for further assessment. Pulmonary function testing 18 months after exposure demonstrated small lung volumes and a normal ratio of the forced expiratory volume in 1 second to the forced vital capacity. This restrictive defect significantly improved with bronchodilator treatment, and changed to a mixed obstructive and restrictive defect with methacholine challenge.

This man probably had reactive airways dysfunction syndrome manifested by a restrictive instead of an obstructive defect. The syndrome most likely is caused by airway constriction at the bronchiole or alveolar duct level.

---

**Longitudinal Study of Alveolitis in Hypersensitivity Pneumonitis Patients: An Immunologic Evaluation**

Trentin L, Marcer G, Chilosi M, Sci MC, Zambello R, Agostini C, Masciarelli M, Bizzotto R, Gemignani C, Cipriani A, Di Vittorio G, Semenzato G (Padua Univ, Padua; Univ of Verona, Italy)

*J Allergy Clin Immunol* 82:577–585, October 1988 2–7

---

There are few longitudinal data on the immunologic competence of mononuclear cells that infiltrate the lung in hypersensitivity pneumonitis (HP). A study was conducted to clarify the natural history of HP alveolitis in 18 symptomatic nonsmoking patients with the disorder. Eleven patients continued to be exposed to specific antigens at work, and 7 were not so exposed despite continuing to live in an agricultural environment; 12 patients had never been treated.

Both the exposed (W+) and unexposed (W−) patients had significant lymphocytic alveolitis (Fig 2–1). The W+ patients had a persistent increase in bronchoalveolar lavage lymphocytes during follow-up. Alveolar macrophages were relatively low (although normal) in both groups of patients. The exposed group had an ongoing increase in CD8+ cells and reversal of the ratio of CD4 to CD8 and, in some patients, a persistent increase in natural killer cells. The W− group showed recovery of CD4+ cells, a decrease in CD8+ cells, and an increase to normal of the CD4:CD8 ratio 6 months after initial study. It appears that the extent of exposure to causative antigens and the duration of exposure can influence the immunologic status of the lungs in patients with HP.

▶ Exposure of the lung to organic dusts can result in an immunologically mediated lung disease we refer to as hypersensitivity pneumonitis (1). Although the

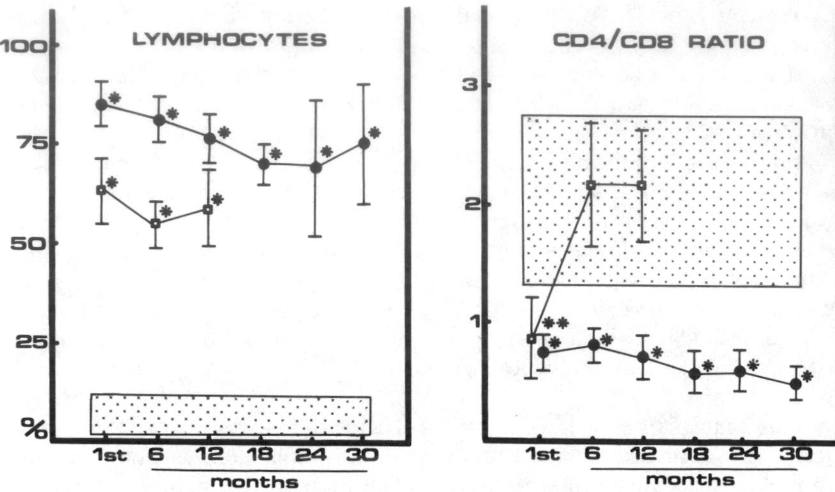


**Fig 2–1.**—Data regarding the percentage of lymphocytes and CD4/CD8 ratios in W+ *(circles)* and W− *(squares)* patients at the time of the first evaluation and during the follow-up; mean ± SEM. *Shaded areas* represent normal ranges. Statistical significance between patients with HP and controls: $^{*}P < .001$; $^{**}P < .005$. (Courtesy of Trentin L, Marcer G, Chilosi M, et al: *J Allergy Clin Immunol* 82:577–585, October 1988.)

typical physiologic abnormality present is a restrictive ventilatory defect with a defect in the diffusing capacity, an additional element of airway obstruction also may be present. Patients with hypersensitivity pneumonitis demonstrate an infiltration of the lung with lymphocytes (many of which can be recovered by bronchoalveolar lavage), a condition termed *lymphocytic alveolitis.* The patient described in the article by Gilbert and Auchincloss (Abstract 2–6) appeared to have hypersensitivity pneumonitis. Unusual about this patient was his marked response to an aerosolized bronchodilator; however, his diffusing capacity was reported to be normal, a finding unexpected in hypersensitivity pneumonitis but characteristic of asthma. It is unclear whether this patient had any of the typical immunologic abnormalities in patients with hypersensitivity pneumonitis, including a lymphocytic alveolitis as determined by bronchoalveolar lavage. Two points raised by the author should be mentioned. First, making the diagnosis of a "restrictive ventilatory defect" requires measurement of lung volumes and demonstration of a decrease in total lung capacity. Restriction can be suspected strongly from classic findings of spirometry, but patient occasionally will be misclassified using this criterion alone.

Trentin and colleagues (Abstract 2–7) did the appropriate test to document that their patient had restriction as determined by measurement of total lung capacity. They also report a sensitivity of 93% and a specificity of 82% when using spirometry alone to diagnose restriction. Second, patients with restrictive physiology occasionally will respond to a bronchodilator. Who should be suspected and tested? Any patient in whom some aspect of the history, physical examination, or screening pulmonary function tests appears inconsistent might be a good candidate for testing after treatment with a bronchodilator. More specific, patients with restriction and a normal diffusing capacity, like the patient described, might also be good candidates for testing. Finally, what about the "reactive airways dysfunction syndrome?" (2) The 10 subjects originally reported had respiratory symptoms and bronchial hyperreactivity after "high level" exposure to an irritant. Seven of the 10 subjects had obstructive lung disease, and 3 had normal pulmonary function; 6 subjects were smokers. Without knowledge of pulmonary function in these patients before irritant exposure, whether the 3 patients with normal pulmonary function ever had objective evidence of asthma, and the natural history of this disorder, it is hard to put this syndrome into any useful classification or prognostic scheme.

The second article abstracted above provides information concerning the lymphocytic alveolitis in patients with hypersensitivity pneumonitis during a 30-month follow-up. The lymphocytic alveolitis persisted for at least 12 months, even in patients who were no longer exposed to the inciting antigen. Only those subjects who continued to be exposed, however, demonstrated an increase in $CD8^+$ (suppressor) T lymphocytes and a persistent reversal of the CD4/CD8 ratio. The significance of the ongoing alveolitis and the increase in $CD8^+$ cells and reversal of the CD4/CD8 ratio is unknown, but the persistence of these abnormalities is disturbing.—S.P. Peters, M.D., Ph.D.

*References*


1. Lopez M, Salvaggio JE: Hypersensitivity pneumonitis, in Murray JF, Nadel JA (eds): *Textbook of Respiratory Medicine*. Philadelphia, WB Saunders, 1988, pp 1606–1616.
2. Brooks SM, Weiss MA, Bernstein IL: Reactive airways dysfunction syndrome (RADS). Persistent asthma syndrome after high level irritant exposures. *Chest* 88:376–384, 1985.


## Disease Associations

### Idiopathic Dilated Cardiomyopathy and Atopic Disease: Epidemiologic Evidence for an Association With Asthma

Coughlin SS, Szklo M, Baughman K, Pearson TA (Johns Hopkins Univ, Baltimore; Mary Imogene Bassett Research Inst, Cooperstown, NY)

*Am Heart J* 118:768–774, October 1989 2–8

Evidence from recent in vitro trials suggests that immediate hypersensitivity or other autoimmune mechanisms may play a role in the initiation or progression of idiopathic dilated cardiomyopathy (DCM). Patients with newly diagnosed DCM were selected from 4 Baltimore hospitals to further explore the relationship of hypersensitivity responses and autoimmunity in general to this disease. In all, 190 patients and neighborhood controls were interviewed. The groups were matched by sex and 5-year age intervals. Matched and unmatched estimates of the relative odds and conditional logistic regression methods were used to compare the 2 groups.

A significant, independent association between idiopathic DCM and a history of asthma was noted. This association was most marked among patients aged less than 55 years, 31% of whom reported a history of asthma. This finding is consistent with previous evidence suggesting that hypersensitivity mechanisms may have a role in the etiology of idiopathic

DCM. An alternative explanation is a treatment effect associated with asthma.

▶ This is a provocative article. In addition to the association of idiopathic DCM with asthma (particularly in patients aged less than 55 years), a statistically significant dose-response relationship with increasing number of atopic diseases reported and a protective effect of antihistamine use were noted. All these factors (younger age group, dose-response relationship with increasing number of atopic diseases, apparent protection by antihistamine use) suggest that mechanisms involving immediate hypersensitivity and the mast cell, rather than autoimmune mechanisms, are operating in this disorder.

The heart has been reported to be involved pathologically in as many as 80% of the cases of systemic anaphylaxis (with massive mast cell activation) (1), but we normally consider most of the severe cardiovascular manifestations of anaphylaxis to be secondary to profound vascular collapse caused by vasodilation and an increase in vascular permeability, rather than by primary myocardial dysfunction. However, an increase in adventitial mast cells in a patient with coronary artery spasm has been reported, and it has been suggested that the cells might have played an etiologic role in this person (2). If mast cell degranulation can lead to cardiac dysfunction acutely, it would not be unreasonable to assume that low-level activation of mast cells over a prolonged period could also produce organ dysfunction. Such dysfunction could result from a disruption of normal cardiac architecture, perhaps with an element of fibrosis. In fact, one of the more topical areas for discussion and investigation concerning mast cell function has been the role of mast cells in abnormal fibrosis (3). Further information concerning this association will be of interest.—S.P. Peters, M.D., Ph.D.

*References*


1. Delage C, Mullick FG, Irey NS: Myocardial lesions in anaphylaxis. *Arch Pathol Lab Med* 95:185–189, 1973.
2. Forman MB, Oates JA, Robertson D, et al: Increased adventitial mast cells in a patient with coronary artery spasm. *N Engl J Med* 313:1138–1141, 1985.
3. Claman HN: Mast cells, T cells, and abnormal fibrosis. *Immunol Today* 6:192–195, 1985.


## Mortality in Asthma

### International Trends in Asthma Mortality: 1970 to 1985

Jackson R, Sears MR, Beaglehole R, Rea HH (Univ of Auckland; Univ of Otago, Dunedin; Green Lane Hosp, Auckland, New Zealand)

*Chest* 94:914–919, November 1988 2–9

During the past 25 years, 2 epidemics of asthma deaths were reported. The second, in the late 1970s, was apparently limited to New Zealand. Recent data on deaths from asthma were examined to determine whether the New Zealand experience was an example of a worldwide increase in asthma mortality.

Health statistics were available from 14 countries for the period 1970

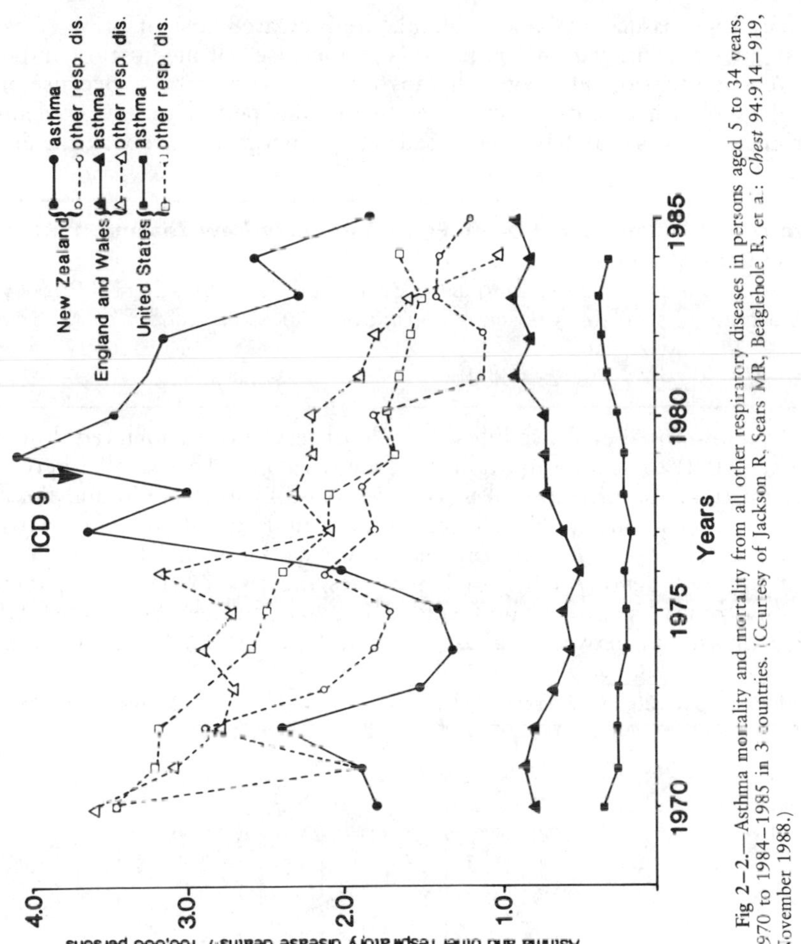


Fig 2–2.—Asthma mortality and mortality from all other respiratory diseases in persons aged 5 to 34 years, 1970 to 1984–1985 in 3 countries. (Courtesy of Jackson R, Sears MR, Beaglehole R, et al.: *Chest* 94:914–919, November 1988.)

to 1984–1985. Those studied included persons aged between 5 and 34 years. New Zealand had the highest mortalities during this period, whereas the lowest rates occurred in the United States, The Netherlands, France, and Finland. In New Zealand the death rate from asthma rose from 1.3 to 4.1 per 100,000 between 1975 and 1979, then fell abruptly to 1.85 per 100,000 by 1985. Except for Finland and Switzerland, a gradual increase has been noted since the mid-1970s. When deaths from asthma were compared with deaths from all other respiratory diseases, it became clear that in New Zealand asthma mortality was not associated with reciprocal trends in deaths for other respiratory diseases (Fig 2–2).

Changes in the International Classification of Disease coding rules or improved accuracy in diagnosing death from asthma were eliminated as causes of an apparent, but not real, increase in asthma mortality. Standardized asthma prevalence studies using accurate mortality data should clarify these issues. In New Zealand, the increased cost of primary care may have encouraged asthma patients to increase self-medication and delay corticosteroid and oxygen therapy during severe attacks. Because prescribed pharmaceuticals were free during the period of the epidemic, bronchodilators may have been used when emergency care was required.

---

**Prescribed Fenoterol and Death From Asthma in New Zealand, 1981–83: Case-Control Study**

Crane J, Pearce N, Flatt A, Burgess C, Jackson R, Kwong T, Ball M, Beasley R (Wellington School of Medicine, Wellington; Auckland School of Medicine, Auckland, New Zealand)

*Lancet* 1:917–922, Apr 29, 1989 2–10

---

Circumstantial evidence links the sale of fenoterol by metered dose inhaler (MDI) to asthma mortality in New Zealand. The parallel between the introduction of fenoterol in New Zealand in April 1976 and the beginning of a second epidemic of asthma mortality during the late 1970s is striking (Fig 2–3). A case-control study was conducted to test the hypothesis that fenoterol by MDI increases the risk of death in patients with asthma. The case group included 117 patients aged 5–45 years who died of asthma between August 1981 and July 1983. For each case, 4

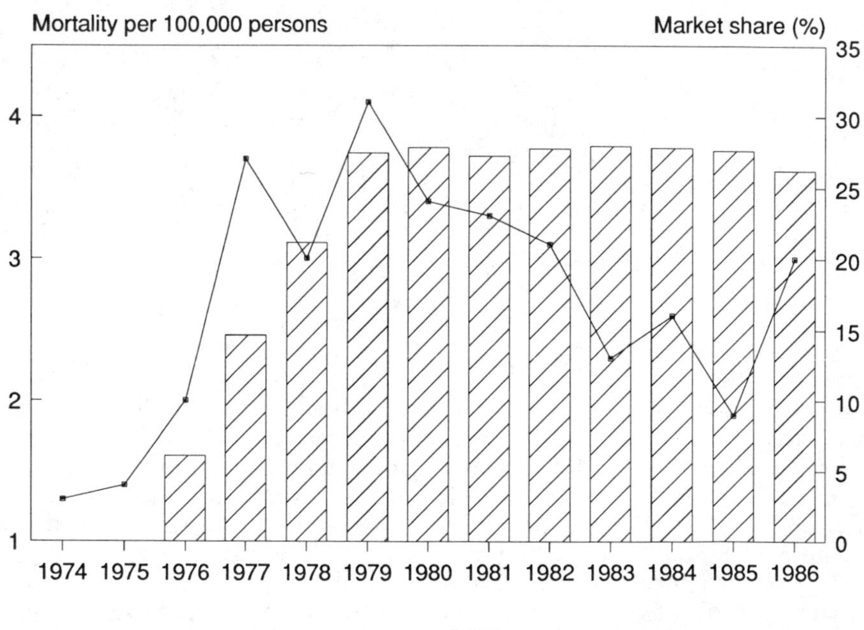


**Fig 2–3.**—Fenoterol market share of inhaled doses of β agonists (excluding nebulized presentations), after introduction in April 1976, and New Zealand asthma mortality per 100,000 persons per year (aged 5–34 years), 1974–1986. (Courtesy of Crane J, Pearce N, Flatt A, et al: *Lancet* 1:917–922, Apr 29, 1989.)

controls, matched for age and ethnic group, were selected from asthma admissions to hospitals to which the patients would have been admitted had they survived.

The relative risk of asthma death in patients prescribed fenoterol by MDI was 1.55 (95% confidence interval, 1.04–2.33) compared with those not prescribed fenoterol by MDI. This risk was increased strikingly as more restrictive definitions of asthma severity were used. The fenoterol MDI relative risk was 2.21 for patients prescribed 3 or more categories of asthma drugs, 2.19 for patients admitted to hospitals for asthma during the previous 12 months, and 6.45 for patients prescribed oral corticosteroids at the time of death or admission. More so, for the group of patients with the most severe asthma, such as those admitted during the previous year and prescribed oral corticosteroids, the fenoterol MDI relative risk was 13.29. No other asthma treatment commonly used in New Zealand increased the risk of asthma death. These findings are consistent with the hypothesis that fenoterol by MDI increases the risk of asthma death, particularly in patients with severe asthma.

▶ Several previous volumes of the YEAR BOOK OF PULMONARY DISEASE (1986, pp 76–77; 1987, pp 63–64; 1988, pp 98–99) have discussed various aspects of mortality in asthma. We reported in 1988 that the increase in asthma mortality in the United States (and other countries) led to the establishment of an Asthma Mortality Task Force with representation from the Respiratory Division of the National Heart, Lung, and Blood Institute. The first of 2 articles abstracted above (Jackson et al, Abstract 2–9) places the increase in asthma mortality observed in the United States into an international perspective. Asthma mortality may have increased in the United States during the late 1970s and early 1980s, but this increase pales in comparison with that observed in New Zealand. The second article abstracted (Crane et al, Abstract 2–10) provides strong evidence from a case-control study to suggest that fenoterol use was associated with mortality, particularly among patients with more severe disease (those requiring oral corticosteroids). The relative increased risk of 13.29 among patients who used fenoterol and both required hospital admission during the previous year and were prescribed oral corticosteroids is striking.

A number of hypotheses have been suggested to explain this apparent excess mortality. Fenoterol is administered by metered dose inhaler at a dose of 200 μg/puff, whereas albuterol, another commonly used β-agonist, is dispensed at a dose of 100 μg/puff. Therefore, both efficacy and side effects might be more significant with fenoterol than with other β-agonists. Cardiac side effects, particularly those involving various arrythmias, could increase mortality. Concerning a bronchodilator with increased efficacy, it is hypothesized that a particularly efficacious bronchodilator might cause patients not to recognize potentially dangerous exacerbations and delay in seeking medical attention. That increasing the efficacy of a bronchodilator might lead to an increase in asthma mortality is disturbing because very long lasting (and presumably more efficacious) β-agonists are now undergoing clinical trials in preparation for their release.—S.P. Peters, M.D., Ph.D.

**Psychological Defenses and Coping Styles in Patients Following a Life-Threatening Attack of Asthma**

Yellowlees PM, Ruffin RE (Flinders Med Ctr, Bedford Park, Australia)

*Chest* 95:1298–1303, June 1989 2–11

Psychological risk factors are prominent in patients with severe asthma who subsequently died of their disease. A detailed analysis was made of the psychiatric disorders and the coping styles of 25 patients who sustained a near-miss asthma death (NMAD). All 25 underwent a comprehensive psychiatric evaluation an average of 13 months (range, 1–58 months) after an NMAD. The mean age was 35.7 years.

Ten patients had psychiatric disorders at the time of assessment, including anxiety disorders in 9 and major depression in 1. Whereas the patients as a whole had high levels of denial, they appeared to respond psychologically to the NMAD by either decompensating psychiatrically and having symptoms of anxiety, or further increasing their levels of denial. Patients who decompensated psychiatrically after the NMAD had significantly higher levels of psychiatric illness in their families and in their personal histories and had a reduced perception of their quality of life when compared with patients who increased their levels of denial after the NMAD. The effects of the NMAD on patients and their families ranged from mutual anger and anxiety, although anger was often repressed, to mutual overinvolvement and overdependence.

The presence of high levels of denial of asthma and a history of psychiatric illness are factors that may increase the likelihood of death from asthma. These factors have clinical implications in the management of NMAD patients.

▶ This article contains virtually no good news and poses some vexing questions. Are patients who are mentally ill more likely to die from asthma than other patients? (Probably, particularly if their asthma is severe.) Is it likely that psychiatric disturbances will develop in patients who have almost died from their disease? (It is not an unreasonable hypothesis.) The high incidence of anxiety is understandable, but a very high level of denial, particularly in a patient with a psychiatric disorder, could be catastrophic.—S.P. Peters, M.D., Ph.D.

## Pathogenesis

### Airway Hyperreactivity

#### *Associations and Pharmacologic Alteration*

**Rhinovirus Upper Respiratory Infection Increases Airway Hyperreactivity and Late Asthmatic Reactions**

Lemanske RF Jr, Dick EC, Swenson CA, Vrtis RF, Busse WW (Univ of Wisconsin)

*J Clin Invest* 83:1–10, January 1989 2–12

Viral upper respiratory infections provoke wheezing in many patients with asthma. However, the effect of these illnesses on the airway response to inhaled antigen is not established. The effect of an experimental rhinovirus (RV) illness on airway reactivity and response to antigen was assessed in 10 ragweed allergic rhinitis adults. The series included 2 women and 8 men whose average age was 30.6 years.

Preinfection tests were done to determine airway reactivity to histamine and ragweed antigen. Patients also were assessed for late asthmatic reactions (LARs) to antigen. One month after baseline tests, patients were inoculated with live RV16 intranasally. Infection was established in all patients by rhinovirus recovery in nasal washings and respiratory symptoms. During the acute RV illness, a significant increase was noted in airway reactivity to both histamine and ragweed antigen. Only 1 patient had an LAR after antigen challenge and before RV inoculation; during the acute RV illness 8 patients had an LAR. The development of LARs was independent of alterations in airway reactivity and the intensity of the immediate antigen response.

An RV respiratory tract illness not only enhances airway reactivity but also predisposes the allergic patient to the development of LARs. This may be an important factor in virus-induced bronchial hyperresponsiveness.

▶ This article is interesting and potentially important. That viral infections can lead to an increase in bronchial reactivity and clinical asthma, as well as to an exacerbation of preexisting asthma, is consistent with the clinical observations of many physicians. Therefore, that an experimentally induced viral infection was associated with a modest increase in bronchial reactivity to histamine and to specific antigen to which the subjects were sensitive is not surprising. (That different investigators have had different results when performing similar studies is not particularly disturbing because it is reasonable to hypothesize that both viruses and subjects may differ in their abilities to induce and develop bronchial hyperresponsiveness, respectively.) Rather surprising and important is that 7 of the 10 subjects had a new late reaction after antigen challenge during the acute viral illness. According to currently accepted hypotheses, these are the conditions (the presence of bronchial hyperreactivity with the ability to develop late asthmatic reactions) in which a positive feedback loop can be established to produce the clinical condition we call asthma.—S.P. Peters, M.D., Ph.D.

---

**Ozone-Induced Changes in Pulmonary Function and Bronchial Responsiveness in Asthmatics**

Kreit JW, Gross KB, Moore TB, Lorenzen TJ, D'Arcy J, Eschenbacher WL (Univ of Michigan; Gen Motors Research Labs, Warren, Mich)

*J Appl Physiol* 66:217–222, January 1989 2–13

---

Ozone causes alterations in lung volumes in normal human beings. Forced vital capacity (FVC), inspiratory capacity, and total lung capacity are all decreased, whereas airway resistance is increased. The effects of

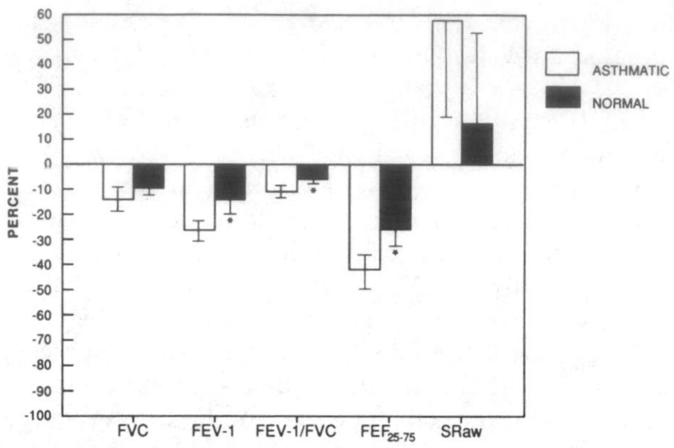


**Fig 2–4.**—Contrast test results. *Bars* represent difference (mean ± SE) between mean percent change (baseline to postexposure) in ozone and filtered purified air. *sRaw,* specific airway resistance. *Significant difference between normal and asthmatic research subjects, $P < .05$. (Courtesy of Kreit JW, Gross KB, Moore TB, et al: *J Appl Physiol* 66:217–222, January 1989.)

ozone exposure on pulmonary function and bronchial responsiveness were compared in healthy and asthmatic persons aged 18 to 35 years. Nine had relatively mild asthma, and 9 were normal. Each person was exposed, in random order, to filtered purified air and 0.4 ppm of ozone and performed intermittent, moderate exercise. Asthmatic patients discontinued taking medications during the study. All participants underwent a complete series of pulmonary function tests and answered a questionnaire regarding subjective symptoms after exposure to filtered purified air and ozone.

Exposure to ozone was associated, in both groups, with significant decreases in forced expired volume in 1 second ($FEV_1$), percent $FEV_1$, forced expired flow at 25% to 75% FVC, and inspiratory capacity. Only asthmatic persons had a significant increase in specific airway resistance (Fig 2–4). Both asthmatic persons and healthy persons had similar increases in symptoms (urge to cough, shortness of breath, and chest discomfort) and proportional increase in bronchial responsiveness to methacholine after ozone exposure. The decrease in FVC did not differ significantly between the 2 groups, indicating that, although greater airway obstruction develops in asthmatic patients than in healthy persons, their lung volume changes are similar. Thus the mechanism by which ozone alters lung volume appears not to be influenced by underlying bronchial hyperresponsiveness. Unlike previous reports that ozone had no significant effects on asthmatic patients, the study used a higher effective dose of ozone (0.4 ppm for 2 hours) and required asthmatic patients to be medication free during the study period.

▶ In summary, ozone produced equivalent decreases in lung volumes and increases in bronchial responsiveness in healthy and asthmatic patients, but a greater degree of airway obstruction in asthmatic patients than in healthy controls. These observations fit our (or at least my) preconceived notions rather well.—S.P. Peters, M.D., Ph.D.

**Nonspecific Bronchial Reactivity and Its Relationship to the Clinical Expression of Asthma: A Longitudinal Study**

Josephs LK, Gregg I, Mullee MA, Holgate ST (Univ of Southampton, England)

*Am Rev Respir Dis* 140:350–357, August 1989 2–14

The contribution of nonspecific bronchial reactivity to the daily manifestations of asthma is not known. This relationship was examined in a longitudinal investigation of 8 children and 12 adults. Reactivity to methacholine was measured every 2–3 weeks for 12–18 months. The dose that caused a 20% drop in forced expiratory volume in 1 second ($PD_{20}$) was derived. All patients kept a daily record of symptoms and treatment. Peak expiratory flow (PEF) was measured twice a day.

A significant association was noted between patients' overall reactivity and their average daily variation in morning PEF and diurnal variation in PEF. However, in examining the temporal relationship between reactivity and asthma within patients, individual $PD_{20}$ measures were inconsistently associated with concurrent asthma severity. Changes in $PD_{20}$ generally reflected simultaneous trends in symptoms or PEF in only 6 patients. Exacerbations of asthma occurred in several patients in the absence of bronchial hyperreactivity.

The relationship between nonspecific bronchial hyperreactivity and asthma is complex. This functional abnormality is only 1 mechanism contributing to the clinical expression of asthma. Because of the difficulty of interpreting measures of reactivity caused by the interaction of so many variables, the value of bronchial challenge for follow up of individual patients is questionable.

▶ This article makes 2 important points. First, although an increase in bronchial responsiveness may be a "hallmark" of the asthmatic diathesis, changes in bronchial responsiveness are not clearly related to day-to-day changes in pulmonary function and symptoms in many asthmatic patients. Second, bronchial reactivity is correlated in a general way, however, with overall severity of asthma and diurnal and day-to-day variability in peak flow rates. Such a correlation in bronchial responsiveness and variability in peak flow measurements was noted in an article abstacted last year (1989 YEAR BOOK OF PULMONARY DISEASE, pp 94–96). Such an increase in variability, as well as an increase in symptoms or a decrease in peak flow rate, should alert the physician that more intensive treatment of a patient's asthma might be in order. Of course, to demonstrate that a patient has an increase in variability, the patient must monitor his peak flow twice a day. Many physicians (and patients) are finding such home monitoring to be quite useful.—S.P. Peters, M.D., Ph.D.

*Lessons From Congestive Heart Failure*

**Protective Effect of Inhaled Furosemide on Allergen-Induced Early and Late Asthmatic Reactions**

Bianco S, Pieroni MG, Refini RM, Rottoli L, Sestini P (Univ of Siena, Italy)

*N Engl J Med* 321:1069–1073, Oct 19, 1989 2–15

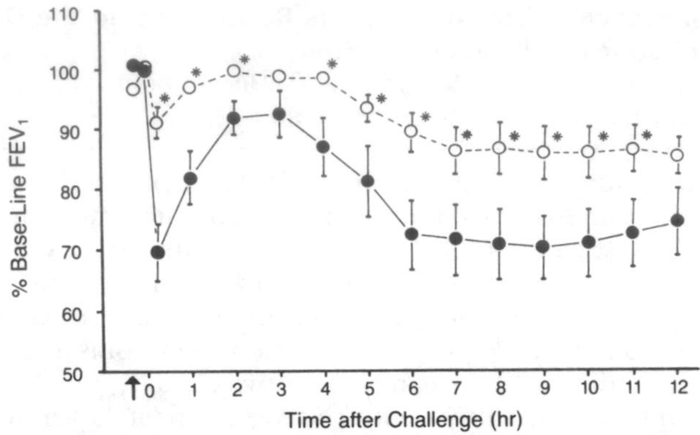


Fig 2–5.—Changes in $FEV_1$ after specific allergen challenge. Values are mean (±SE) percentages of the posttreatment value (time zero) after inhalation of placebo *(solid circles)* and furosemide *(open circles)*. The mean baseline values *(arrow)* were 4.15 L before placebo and 4.1 L before furosemide. Each asterisk denotes a significant difference between placebo and furosemide values ($P < .05$ by paired t-test). (Courtesy of Bianco S, Pieroni MG, Refini RM, et al: *N Engl J Med* 321:1069–1073, Oct 19, 1989.)

Alterations in the osmolarity and ion composition of the bronchial periciliary fluid might be important in the bronchial response to physical stimuli. A double-blind, placebo-controlled, randomized, crossover trial was done to assess the effect of inhaled furosemide on the immediate and late phases of the asthmatic response to specific allergen challenge in 11 patients with mild allergic asthma. All patients had both early and late asthmatic reactions to a specific inhaled allergen in a preliminary challenge.

After placebo was administered, the maximal changes from baseline were a 35% decrease in the forced expiratory volume in 1 second ($FEV_1$) and a 288% increase in specific airway resistance between 0 and 30 minutes after inhaling the allergen (Fig 2–5). These factors were decreased by 35% and increased by 301%, respectively, between 4 and 12 hours. After furosemide was administered all patients had a markedly attenuated early response to inhaled allergens. All but 1 patient had an attenuated late response. The maximal changes in $FEV_1$ and specific airway resistance were a decrease of 11% and an increase of 61%, respectively, between 0 and 30 minutes and a decrease of 20% and an increase of 178%, respectively, between 4 and 12 hours. No significant differences were noted in the bronchoconstrictor response to inhaled methacholine after furosemide or placebo administration.

Pretreatment with a single inhaled dose of furosemide can significantly inhibit early and later responses induced by challenge with a specific allergen. This protection was probably not caused by a direct bronchodilator effect of furosemide. A furosemide-sensitive mechanism in the airways was involved in the pathogenesis of allergic asthma responses. It is uncertain whether inhaled furosemide is useful in the treatment of allergic asthma.

▶ Pathophysiologic alterations associated with bronchial asthma are said to include smooth muscle contraction, hypersecretion of mucus, an alteration in vascular permeability, an increase in nonspecific bronchial reactivity, and inflammation. Of these, investigations of changes in vascular permeability have perhaps proven the most difficult to perform. Whether asthmatic patients have altered lung permeability at baseline (before challenge or while asymptomatic), challenge with various agents, including antigen and several mediators of immediate hypersensitivity, has been shown to produce an increase in lung permeability (1, 2). The article abstracted above demonstrates that the loop diuretic furosemide, first-line therapy for patients with congestive heart failure, inhibits both early and late asthmatic reactions after antigen challenge. No effect was seen on bronchial reactivity. The mechanism or mechanisms by which this protective effect occurred is unknown; however, the authors speculate that it might involve an inhibition of chloride ion secretion and thereby alter the osmotic or ionic environment of epithelial cells, or both. It should be noted that a rather large dose of furosemide was administered (40 mg by nebulization), so the effects of furosemide might be nonspecific. However, the results are intriguing.

Alterations in vascular permeability have the potential to modulate a number of factors we consider important in asthma (e.g., recruitment of inflammatory cells and mediators, through physical factors, by increasing the metabolism of locally produced substances, etc.). The following article (Abstract 2–16) explores one effect of altering the microenvironment of the airways, not by increasing vascular permeability, which results in a protein-rich exudate, but by increasing hydrostatic pressure, which results in a relatively protein-poor exudation of fluid.—S.P. Peters, M.D., Ph.D.

*References*

1. Rees PJ, Shelton D, Chan TB, et al: Effects of histamine on lung permeability in normal and asthmatic subjects. *Thorax* 40:603–606, 1985.
2. Persson CGA: Plasma exudation and asthma. *Lung* 166:1–23, 1988.

---

**Bronchial Hyperresponsiveness to Methacholine in Patients With Impaired Left Ventricular Function**

Cabanes LR, Weber SN, Matran R, Regnard J, Richard MO, DeGeorges ME, Lockhart A (Université René Descartes, Hôpital Cochin, Paris)

*N Engl J Med* 320:1317–1322, May 18, 1989 2–16

---

Nocturnal attacks of wheezy dyspnea are common in patients with impaired left ventricular function. In these patients, nonallergic bronchial hyperresponsiveness may result from structural changes in the bronchi. To test this hypothesis, the bronchial response to methacholine was studied in 23 patients with chronic impairment of left ventricular function secondary to coronary artery disease or dilated cardiomyopathy.

Twenty-one patients had marked bronchial hyperresponsiveness to methacholine. The mean dose of methacholine that elicited a 20% decrease in the forced expiratory volume in 1 second ($FEV_1$) was 421 μg. This is the same magnitude of bronchial hyperresponsiveness seen in patients with symptomatic asthma. In contrast, 9 of 10 patients with coronary disease but normal left ventricular function had no bronchial response to methacholine. The methacholine-induced bronchial obstruction was partially corrected (43%) by the administration of the bronchodilator albuterol. Pretreatment with α-adrenergic agonist methoxamine (a potent vasoconstrictor) prevented or attenuated the methacholine-induced decrease in $FEV_1$ in 12 patients. This protective effect of methoxamine was blocked by the administration of the α-adrenergic antagonist phentolamine to all 6 patients studied.

Most patients with impaired left ventricular function have marked bronchial hyperresponsiveness to cholinergic agonists, which may contribute to the wheezy dyspnea commonly observed in these patients. The bronchoconstriction may be mediated at least in part by dilatation of the bronchial vessels.

► The clinical importance of "cardiac asthma" has been recognized for at least 150 years. Hope wrote in 1835 that "an immense proportion of asthmas—and of the most dangerous and distressing cases, result from disease of the heart. . . ." (1) However, not all investigators who have measured bronchial reactivity in patients with impaired left ventricular have obtained results comparable to those reported here. Eichacker and colleagues (2) observed bronchial hyperreactivity in only 2 of 9 patients with impaired left ventricular function. Clues to a possible explanation for this discrepancy might come from hypotheses that have been advanced to explain bronchial hyperreactivity in patients with congestive heart failure. It is thought that pulmonary and bronchial venous hypertension could inhibit egress of blood from the bronchial system and result in congestion and edema of the airways.

In the article abstracted below (Abstract 2–17), James and associates have reported that the airway wall area of patients with asthma is increased (thickened) in comparison with controls because of an increase in the area of the epithelium, muscle, and submucosa. They also calculated that the muscle shortening required to produce airway closure was considerably less in asthmatic patients than in controls. That is, the same degree of muscle shortening in asthmatic patients and controls would lead to a much larger increase in airway resistance in asthmatic patients, with only a negligible difference in resting airway resistance in these 2 groups (see Fig 2–6). If the assumptions and calculations preformed by James and co-workers are correct, then airway thickening by whatever mechanism (inflammation as in asthmatic patients, or edema and congestion as in patients with congestive heart failure) would result in an exaggerated airway closure and increase in resistance, if airway smooth muscle were stimulated to contract. The extent to which patients with congestive heart failure have bronchial congestion and edema likely varies from patient to patient, and even in the same patient over time in response to worsening cardiac function and the extent and type of treatment administered. Therefore, individual variability in bronchial responsiveness to methacholine in patients with congestive heart failure is not unreasonable. It would be interesting to correlate bronchial reactivity with more direct measures of airway wall thickness, or at least with hemodynamic parameters, in patients with cardiac dysfunction.—S.P. Peters, M.D., Ph.D.

*References*

1. Hope J: *A Treatise on the Diseases of the Heart and Great Vessels*, ed 2. London, W Kidd, 1835, pp 345–364.
2. Eichacker PQ, Seidelman MJ, Rothstein MS, et al: *Chest* 93:336–338, 1988.

---

**The Mechanics of Airway Narrowing in Asthma**

James AL, Paré PD, Hogg JC (Univ of British Columbia; St. Paul's Hosp, Vancouver, BC)

*Am Rev Respir Dis* 139:242–246, 1989 2–17

---

A consistent feature of patients with asthma is the exaggerated airways narrowing in response to nonspecific stimuli. The internal perimeter and wall area of the airway remain constant at different lung volumes and with different degrees of airway smooth muscle shortening despite substantial changes in luminal area. This finding was used in the measurement and reconstruction of the relaxed dimensions of airways and in calculating the degree of muscle shortening required to occlude the airway lumen. The airways in postmortem specimens of lung obtained from 18 patients who had asthma were compared with the airways from 23 pa-

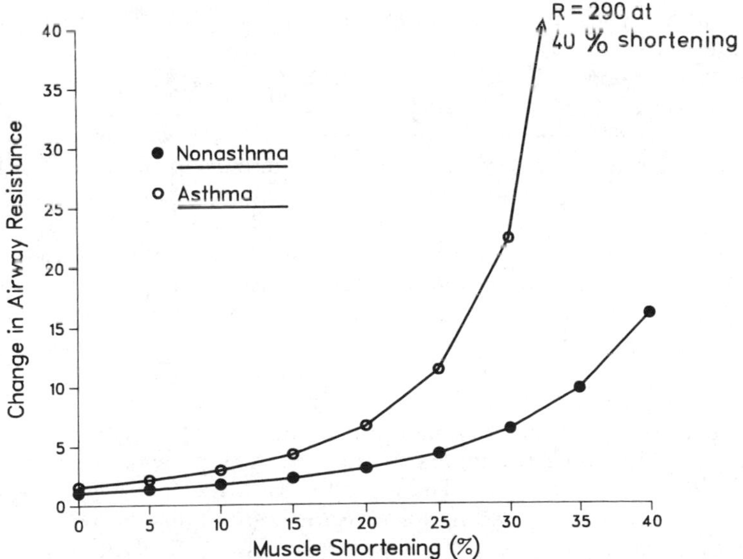


Fig 2–6.—The changes in relative resistance of cartilaginous airways (Pi < 10 mm) calculated using the mean dimensions measured in nonasthmatic and asthmatic research subjects. The baseline resistance of the nonasthmatic airway is arbitrarily set as 1.0. (Courtesy of James AL, Paré PD, Hogg JC: *Am Rev Respir Dis* 139:242–246, 1989.)

tients who had died and who were not asthmatic. To trace the internal and external perimeter of the airway and to calculate the submucosal and mucosal thicknesses, each airway was projected onto a digitizing board of microcomputer.

In asthmatic patients the wall area relative to the relaxed external area was greater in both membranous and cartilaginous airways than in non-asthmatic persons. In addition, calculated muscle shortening required to cause airway closure was less in the asthmatic patients than in the non-asthmatic persons. In nonasthmatic persons, smooth muscle shortening of 40% resulted in approximately a 15-fold increase in resistance in the airway, whereas the same degree of muscle shortening caused approximately a 290-fold increase in resistance in the airway of asthmatic patients (Fig 2–6). By using the calculations in this study, the baseline airway resistance was only slightly increased by the thickening of the airway walls observed in the asthmatic patients. As muscle shortening increases, however, its effect on airway resistance is greatly exaggerated by the wall thickening observed in asthmatic patients. This explains why less muscle shortening is required to close the airways of the asthmatic patient.

Changes produced by the chronic inflammatory process in asthmatic patients can lead to excessive airway narrowing without excessive smooth muscle contraction. Therefore, the treatment for asthma should focus on reversing these inflammatory changes in the airway wall and lumen as well as on the relaxation of the airway smooth muscle.

IMMUNOGLOBULIN E

---

### Association of Asthma With Serum IgE Levels and Skin-Test Reactivity to Allergens

Burrows B, Martinez FD, Halonen M, Barbee RA, Cline MG (Univ of Arizona)
*N Engl J Med* 320:271–277, Feb 2, 1989 2–18

---

Extrinsic asthma appears to be the predominant form of the disease in children and young adults. Intrinsic asthma is considered more common in older patients. However, the relationship between age in the general population and both allergy skin-test reactivity and serum IgE levels has not been considered. Both tend to decline with advancing age. The relationship between reported asthma and atopy and the serum IgE level was investigated in a general population of 2,657, taking into account their close interrelationship and variations with age and sex.

Regardless of atopy or age group, the prevalence of asthma was closely related to the serum immunoglobulin E (IgE) level standardized for age and sex. No asthma was noted in the 177 persons with the lowest IgE levels for their age and sex. The log odds ratio rose linearly with the serum IgE level after controlling for possible confounding variables and degree of reactivity to skin tests (Fig 2–7). However, allergic rhinitis appeared to be associated with skin-test reactions to common aeroallergens independently of the serum IgE level.

Asthma is almost always associated with some type of IgE-related reac-

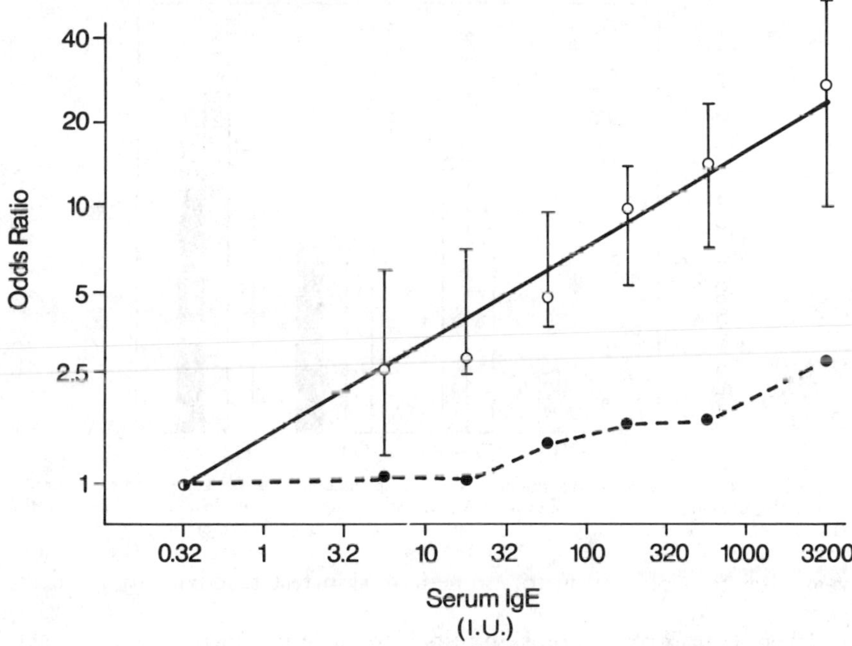


**Fig 2–7.**—Odds ratio (log scale) of having asthma *(open circles)* at 7 levels of the total serum IgE concentration after correction for age, sex, smoking habits, and skin-test index in a logistic analysis. The *solid line*, the risk of asthma, is a weighted, least-squares linear regression model fitted to the odds ratios at each log IgE level. The *vertical lines* are 95% confidence levels around the regression for each odds ratio corresponding to a given log IgE level. The *dashed line* represents the odds ratios of having rhinitis at the same 7 levels of serum IgE, after correction for the same confounders. (Courtesy of Burrows B, Martinez FD, Halonen M, et al: *N Engl J Med* 320:271–277, Feb 2, 1989.)

tion and thus has an allergic basis. These results challenge the commonly held belief in basic differences between extrinsic and intrinsic forms of asthma.

---

**Transfer of Allergen-Specific IgE-Mediated Hypersensitivity With Allogeneic Bone Marrow Transplantation**

Agosti JM, Sprenger JD, Lum LG, Witherspoon RP, Fisher LD, Storb R, Henderson WR Jr (Univ of Washington; Fred Hutchinson Cancer Research Ctr, Seattle)

*N Engl J Med* 319:1623–1628, Dec. 22, 1988 2–19

---

Several case reports suggest that immunoglobulin E (IgE)-mediated hypersensivity in a donor can be transferred by bone marrow transplantation to a previously nonreactive recipient. In a prospective study, 12 patients aged 14–47 years, undergoing allogeneic bone marrow transplantation for treatment of hematologic cancer, and their donors were studied to determine whether allergen-specific IgE-mediated hypersensitivity can be transferred by bone marrow transplantation. The donor-recipient pairs were evaluated before and at 30 days, 100 days, and more than 1

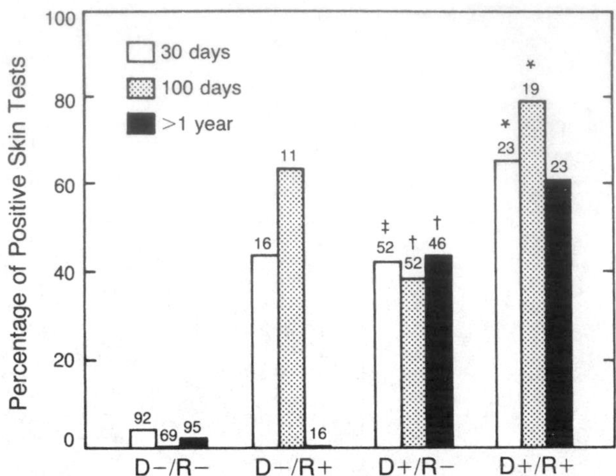


**Fig 2–8.**—Percentages of positive skin tests after transplantation categorized according to the results of pretransplantation skin tests. (Courtesy of Agosti JM, Sprenger JD, Lum LG, et al: *N Engl J Med* 319:1623–1628, Dec 22, 1988.)

year after transplantation for immediate skin test reactivity to 17 allergens.

When pretransplantation skin tests were negative for the same allergen in both donor and recipient, only 6 of 256 tests were positive for the recipient after transplantation. When pretransplantation skin tests were positive for the donors and negative for the recipients, 20 of 46 posttransplantation skin tests were positive for 8 of the 11 recipients who survived for more than 1 year after transplantation (Fig 2–8). When the donor's test was negative and the recipient's test was positive, approximately 50% of the skin tests remained positive 30 days and 100 days after transplantation, but none remained positive for more than 1 year after transplantation. Radioallergosorbent testing confirmed the long-term transfer of donor-derived mite-specific IgE in 2 recipients. Seven recipients either acquired or had exacerbation of allergic rhinitis, 2 recipients acquired asthma, and 2 has urticaria after transplantation.

Allergen-specific IgE-mediated hypersensitivity is adoptively transferred by bone marrow transplantation from donor to recipient by B cells with allergen-specific memory. These data suggest that acquisition of allergic disease may be common in recipients of bone marrow from atopic donors.

▶ The findings in the first of 2 articles abstracted above (Burrows et al, Abstract 2–18) are somewhat puzzling. One might have predicted that asthma, atopy (positive skin tests to various allergens), rhinitis, and serum IgE level would all be related to one another in some general, nonspecific manner. That rhinitis had little relationship with IgE (after controlling for positive skin tests or atopy) whereas asthma had a markedly positive association fits no overall conceptual model of these diseases that I am familiar with. That all patients with asthma had at least some quantity of IgE, or as the authors suggest, "asthma is almost always associated with some type of IgE-related reaction, and therefore has an allergic base," is also a surprise and will prove to be a controversial contention. Inherent in this and any similar study were a number of limitations, including that a questionnaire was used to determine whether patients had the diseases of interest, and that only associations and not causation can be established by such an approach. However, we should attempt to verify these results and devise hypotheses based on the authors' assertions to more rigorously test them.

Concerning the second article abstracted above (Agosti et al, Abstract 2–19), the finding that allergen-specific immediate hypersensitivity, like other immunologic reactions, can be transferred via allogeneic bone marrow transplantation is not surprising. The relatively high efficiency of transfer (20 of 46 skin tests, or 43%), and that the 5 subjects without either allergic rhinitis or asthma had one or both of these disorders after transplantation in surprising, however. Atopic disease should be considered as a likely complication of bone marrow transplantation when the donor is atopic.—S P. Peters, M.D., Ph.D.

CLUES TO THE PATHOGENESIS?

**Cellular Events in the Bronchi in Mild Asthma and After Bronchial Provocation**

Beasley R, Roche WR, Roberts JA, Holgate ST (Southampton Univ Gen Hosp, Southampton, England)

*Am Rev Respir Dis* 139:806–817, March 1989 2–20

Because of the importance of better understanding the cellular basis of asthma, a detailed cellular and ultrastructural examination was made of bronchial biopsy specimens and bronchial lavage fluid from allergic asthmatic patients to determine the nature and degree of the inflammatory processes. Eight atopic asthmatic patients with a mean $PC_{20}$ histamine of 0.90 mg/mL and 4 nonasthmatic controls underwent fiberoptic bronchoscopy. All asthmatic patients required either no treatment or inhaled albuterol alone and were clinically stable 2 weeks before bronchoscopy. Followed by endobronchial biopsy of subcarinae, a single 50-mL bronchial wash was undertaken. In the asthmatic patients 18 hours after bronchial provocation with allergen or methacholine, these procedures were repeated. All 12 then underwent bronchial reactivity testing wtih inhaled histamine. The pathologist interpreting the specimens was not aware of the clinical and physiologic data.

A significantly greater number of epithelial cells was shed by the asthmatic patients in the lavage fluid than in the nonasthmatics with values of 7.23 vs. 1.48 $\times$ $10^4$/mL. A statistically significant inverse correlation between the lavage epithelial cell count and bronchial reactivity was noted. In the asthmatic patients, there was extensive deposition of collagen beneath the epithelial basement membrane, mast cell degranulation, and mucosal infiltration by eosinophils, which exhibited morphological evidence of activation (Fig 2–9). These findings were not observed in the

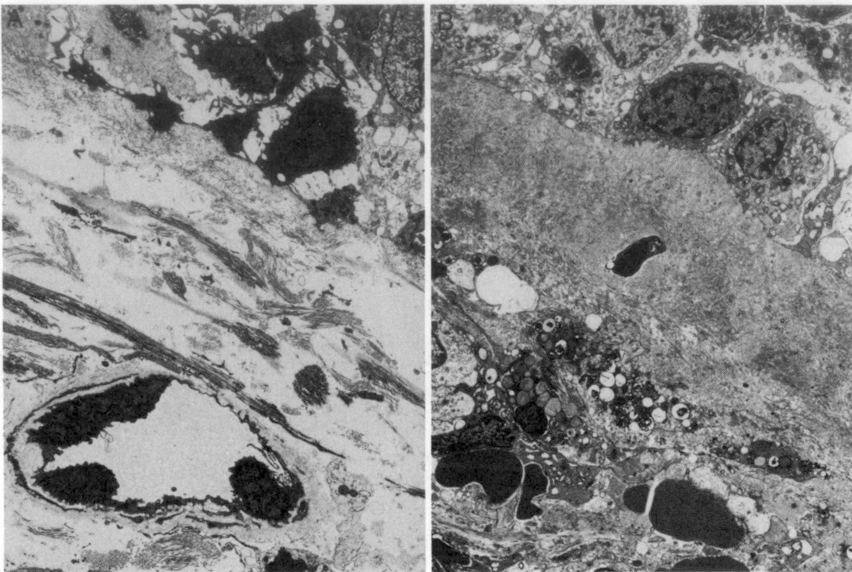

**Fig 2–9.**—Bronchial biopsy specimens (control, **left**; asthma, **right**) showing increased subepithelial collagen and numerous eosinophils in the asthmatic patient. There is marked variation in the appearance of the eosinophil granules. (Uranyl acetate-lead citrate stain; transmission electron microscopy; original magnification, ×5,000.) (Courtesy of Beasley R, Roche WR, Roberts JA, et al: *Am Rev Respir Dis* 139:806–817, March 1989.)

controls. Also, eosinophils, monocytes, and platelets were found in contact with the vascular endothelium, with emigration of eosinophils and monocytes in the asthmatic patients. These changes were observed irrespective of bronchial challenge with allergen.

Allergic asthma is accompanied by extensive inflammatory changes in the airways, even in mild clinical and subclinical disease. The findings stress the severity of the underlying disorder in what are considered mild cases of asthma.

▶ In the 1986 YEAR BOOK OF PULMONARY DISEASE (pp 99–100) we discussed an article by Laitinen and colleagues (1) in which it was reported that airway epithelial damage is common in asthmatic patients, even those with mild disease. Those results were of interest, not only because of the results per se, but also because they involved bronchoscopic biopsies of volunteers, a procedure that involves a finite amount of risk of morbidity. In both the article abstracted above and one by Jeffery and associates (2), our European colleagues have performed additional histologic and ultrastructural studies of the airways of asthmatic patients vs. controls by performing bronchoscopic, endobronchial biopsies and correlated these findings with measurements of bronchial reactivity. In these studies, epithelial damage with shedding of epithelial cells, thickening of the basement epithelial membrane (perhaps with subepithelial collagen deposition), and "inflammation" were observed. In both studies, bronchial reactivity correlated with epithelial damage (positively with epithelial loss [r = 0.67,

$P < .001$] or negatively with shed epithelial cell count after airway lavage [r = −0.64, $P$ = .03]). The type of inflammatory changes observed, however, differed in these 2 studies. Beasley and co-workers (above) observed mast cell degranulation and mucosal infiltration with eosinophils, whereas Jeffery and colleagues observed intraepithelial lymphocytes as the major inflammatory cell present. These findings correlate, in a general way, with the hypotheses advanced by these 2 groups concerning the importance of various cells in the pathogenesis of asthma. More subtle changes in other cells, including monocytes and platelets, also were noted occasionally. The extent of these inflammatory changes is surprising, even if we do not have a clear view of the role played by each of these cellular elements.—S.P. Peters, M.D., Ph.D.

*References*

1. Laitinen LA, Heino M, Laitinen A, et al: Damage of the airway epithelium and bronchial reactivity in patients with asthma. *Am Rev Respir Dis* 131:599–606, 1985.
2. Jeffery PK, Wardlaw AJ, Nelson FC, et al: Bronchial biopsies in asthma. An ultrastructural, quantitative study and correlation with hyperreactivity. *Am Rev Respir Dis* 140:1745–1753, 1989.

---

**Absence of Immunoreactive Vasoactive Intestinal Polypeptide in Tissue From the Lungs of Patients With Asthma**

Ollerenshaw S, Jarvis D, Woolcock A, Sullivan C, Scheibner T (Univ of Sydney; Royal Prince Alfred Hosp, Sydney, Australia)

*N Engl J Med* 320:1244–1248, May 11, 1989 2–21

---

Vasoactive intestinal polypeptide (VIP) is a neuropeptide present in nerve fibers of normal human lungs. Because it acts as a bronchial smooth-muscle relaxant, a reduction in VIP activity may contribute to the pathophysiology of asthma. To assess the distribution of nerve fibers immunoreactive to VIP in asthma, lung tissue was obtained at autopsy or lobectomy from 5 patients with asthma and 9 other patients without asthma. The avidinbiotin-peroxidase complex technique was used to stain tissue for immunoreactivity to VIP. At least 80 tissue sections from each patient were examined, with airway diameters ranging from 100 μm to 1.2 cm.

Immunoreactivity to VIP was found in more than 92% of lung tissue sections from patients without asthma. The immunoreactive nerve fibers were branching networks in the smooth muscle of bronchi and bronchioles, ranging from 200 μm to 1.2 cm in diameter. These fibers containing VIP were present even in areas of moderate inflammation. In contrast, no VIP was seen in any of the 468 evaluable sections obtained from patients with asthma (table). Immunostaining for substance P was undertaken as a control for the nonspecific destruction of neuropeptides. Abundant amounts of substance P were seen within nerves in tissues from the lungs of all patients.

Asthma is associated with a loss of immunoreactivity to VIP that may

Detection of Immunoreactivity to VIP in Sections From the Lungs of Patients with Asthma and Patients Without Asthma

| Subject No. | Asthma | No. of Sections | Diameter of Airway |
|---|---|---|---|
| | | *total/no. with VIP* | *range* |
| 1 | Yes | 82/0 | 200 μm–1.2 cm |
| 2 | Yes | 115/0 | 150 μm–1.0 cm |
| 3 | Yes | 80/0 | 200 μm–1.2 cm |
| 4 | No | 80/76 | 150 μm–1.1 cm |
| 5 | No | 114/107 | 200 μm–1.0 cm |
| 6 | No | 81/81 | 200 μm–1.0 cm |
| 7 | No | 90/85 | 100 μm–0.9 cm |
| 8 | Yes | 102/0 | 300 μm–0.8 cm |
| 9 | Yes | 89/0 | 250 μm–0.95 cm |
| 10 | No | 91/91 | 200 μm–0.75 cm |
| 11 | No | 89/82 | 400 μm–0.8 cm |
| 12 | No | 87/85 | 200 μm–0.8 cm |
| 13 | No | 97/97 | 200 μm–1.0 cm |
| 14 | No | 113/104 | 300 μm–1.2 cm |

(Courtesy of Ollerenshaw S, Jarvis D, Woolcock A, et al: *N Engl J Med* 320:1244–1248, May 11, 1989.)

diminish neurogenically mediated bronchodilation. Whether this loss is a cause or a result of asthma is unclear.

▶ The word *unequivocal* rarely can be used to describe a biologic phenomenon. Well, these data are unequivocal. The question is whether they are also artifactual. We have discussed neuropeptides and their possible role in asthma in several previous editions of the YEAR BOOK OF PULMONARY DISEASE (1987, pp 79–81; 1988, pp 107–108; 1989, pp 76–78). In a thoughtful letter to the editor that followed the publication of the abstracted article, Peter Barnes discussed a number of issues concerning the absence of VIP in lung tissue from patients with asthma (1). First, he argued against the hypothesis that asthma is caused by a primary deficiency in VIP-associated neurons because these neurons appear important in other organs besides the lung (i.e., the gastrointestinal tract and large blood vessels [pulmonary arteries]) and these organs appear to function normally in asthmatic patients; and because the nonadrenergic, noncholinergic, nervous system in the lung appears to function normally in patients with *mild* asthma. (The patients in whom an absence of VIP was noted had *severe* asthma.) Second, he questioned whether the observed finding might result from degradation of VIP by proteases from inflammatory cells such as mast cells, which are common in asthmatic airways and are potent sources of proteolytic enzymes such as tryptase, which has been shown to degrade VIP. The authors of the article agreed to a certain extent with Dr. Barnes and postulated that the absence of VIP appears to be a secondary phenomenon. We agree.—S.P. Peters, M.D., Ph.D.

*Reference*

1. Barnes PJ: Letter. *N Engl J Med* 321:1128–1129, 1989.

**Characterization of Serum Platelet-Activating Factor (PAF) Acetylhydrolase: Correlation Between Deficiency of Serum PAF Acetylhydrolase and Respiratory Symptoms in Asthmatic Children**

Miwa M, Miyake T, Yamanaka T, Sugatani J, Suzuki Y, Sakata S, Araki Y, Matsumoto M (Univ of Shizuoka, Oshika; Univ of Tokyo; Kansai Med School, Osaka; Shizuoka Red Cross Blood Ctr, Shizuoka, Japan)

*J Clin Invest* 82:1983–1991, December 1988 2–22

Because the accumulation of platelet-activating factor (PAF) in body fluids and tissues can be toxic, the level of acetylhydrolase, a PAF-inactivating factor, is quite important. This acid-labile factor is found in serum from both rabbits and human beings. A reproducible method for determining human serum PAF acetylhydrolase activity was developed, based on the production of [$^{14}$C]-acetate produced from 1-O-alkyl-2-[$^{14}$C]-acetyl-*sn*-glycero-3-phosphocholine on precipitation with TCA.

Of 816 healthy Japanese adults, 32 had serum PAF acetylhydrolase deficiency. Sensitivity to PAF and metabolism of PAF in platelets from the deficient persons were nearly the same as in normal persons. The deficiency appeared to be transmitted in an autosomal recessive manner in 5 families. The likelihood of deficiency was significantly greater in families with moderate or severe asthmatic symptoms than in control families. Deficiency of serum PAF acetylhydrolase could be a factor leading to severe respiratory symptoms in asthmatic children.

▶ The function of platelet activating factor is unknown. It might act as an intracellular messenger, as an autocoid acting in the immediate environment of its secretion, or as a general mediator of inflammation. It has been suggested that PAF could be an important mediator in asthma because of its ability to serve as a neutrophil and eosinophil chemoattractant and activator, and because of its ability to increase bronchial reactivity (1987 YEAR BOOK OF PULMONARY DISEASE, pp 72–75), although considerable doubt has emerged concerning the ability of PAF to modify bronchial reactivity in human beings in any meaningful way. The most important method for metabolizing PAF and "detoxifying" it appears to be through an acetylhydrolase activity. The authors of the article abstracted reported finding a deficiency of serum PAF acetylhydrolase activity in 32 of 816 healthy Japanese adults and 8 of 211 healthy children. There was a *statistical* tendency for persons with the lowest acetylhydrolase activity to have more severe asthmatic symptoms, but there was almost complete overlap of acetylhydrolase activities between various groups of persons with asthma and controls. That many subjects with a low level of acetylhydrolase activity were "healthy" suggests either that other important mechanisms exist for the metabolism of PAF or that PAF does not play an important proinflammatory role in most persons.—S.P. Peters, M.D., Ph.D.

## Miscellaneous Topics

### Interleukin-2-Induced Tumor Necrosis Factor-Alpha (TNF-α) Gene Expression in Human Alveolar Macrophages and Blood Monocytes

Strieter RM, Remick DG, Lynch JP III, Spengler RN, Kunkel SL (Univ of Michigan)

*Am Rev Respir Dis* 139:335–342, February 1989 2–23

Tumor necrosis factor-alpha (TNF-α) is a mediator of various chronic inflammatory processes, the production of which by some cells is stimulated by interleukin-2 (IL-2). Receptors for IL-2 are present on both human alveolar macrophages (AMØ) and blood monocytes (PBM). To determine whether IL-2 can stimulate expression of TNF-α from these cells, mononuclear cells purified from peripheral blood and bronchoalveolar lavage cells obtained from 11 healthy male volunteers were tested.

Blood monocytes produced 5 times their basal levels of bioactive TNF-α after stimulation by IL-2; lipopolysaccharide (LPS) stimulation resulted in a 21-fold increase in levels of TNF-α from these cells. The production of bioactive TNF-α of AMØ was doubled after incubation with IL-2, compared with sixfold increases resulting from incubation with LPS. The doses of IL-2 used to produce these effects generate lymphocyte-activated killer cells in vitro. In situ hybridization and Northern blot analyses demonstrated that IL-2 resulted in increased TNF messenger RNA accumulations by both cell types. The accumulation of TNF mRNA was delayed by 3–6 hours when induced by TNF-α compared with LPS.

These data indicate that IL-2 stimulates gene expression of TNF-α by human alveolar macrophages and blood monocytes, suggesting that IL-2 may be a mediator of lung disorders involving lymphocyte-macrophage interactions.

▶ No area of modern biology has advanced as rapidly, thanks in large part to new techniques of molecular biology, as that having to do with interleukins. These lymphokines and cytokines are involved in cell differentiation, maturation, and intercellular communication (reviewed in Strober and James [1]). Many of these substances, which were known only as biologic principles, have been purified and the genes cloned, all during the past 5 years. One of the most interesting of these is cachectin or TNF-α. This 157 amino acid peptide, purified and characterized because of its role as a mediator of cachexia and tumor necrosis, respectively (and determined thereafter to be the same molecule), has recently been suggested to be an important mediator of shock and tissue injury associated with sepsis and the adult respiratory distress syndrome (2). This material can induce shock, promote neutrophil adherence to endothelial cells, stimulate the synthesis of IL-1 from mononuclear cells, and perhaps increase vascular permeability.

More significant active or passive immunization of animals against TNF-α has provided protection against endotoxic shock (reviewed in Tracey et al). The article abstracted above demonstrates that IL-2, as well as the bacterial product lipopolysaccharide, can induce macrophages and monocytes to synthesize and release TNF-α. This provides yet another potential link between lymphocytes (which synthesize IL-2) and mononuclear cells. The methods used, in situ hybridization and Northern analysis to quantitate messenger RNA levels and gene expression, are state of the art and typical of the techniques in common use in many cell biology laboratories today.—S.P. Peters, M.D., Ph.D.

*References*

1. Strober W, James SP: The interleukins. *Pediatr Res* 24:549–557, 1988.
2. Tracey KJ, Lowry SF, Cerami A: Cachectin/TNF-α in septic shock and septic adult respiratory distress syndrome. *Am Rev Respir Dis* 138:1377–1379, 1988.

---

**The Pathology of Clubbing: Vascular Changes in the Nail Bed**
Currie AE, Gallagher PJ (Southampton Univ Gen Hosp, Southampton, England)
*Br J Dis Chest* 82:382–385, October 1988 2–24

---

Little is known of the pathogenesis or microscopic pathology of clubbing. Reports of clubbing associated with aneurysms or arteriovenous fistulas of the arm support the view that vascular changes are important; however, no attempt has been made to quantify these changes in the nail bed. For 13 patients with clubbing and 13 with normal hands, postmortem angiograms were prepared of both normal and clubbed hands and the size of the vascular bed in the terminal parts of each finger was estimated. Histologic examination also was done.

In most cases technically satisfactory angiograms were obtained and contrast was visible in vessels as small as 100 μm. No differences in the overall anatomical pattern of arteries between clubbed and control cases were found. No bony abnormalities were detected, and there was no evidence of periostitis. A wide range in the total lengths of blood vessels within the terminal parts of each digit was observed, but no differences between the 2 groups were found. Histologically, the connective tissue of the nail bed was almost entirely composed of mature collagen and no obvious qualitative differences between the 2 groups was found. No recent fibrosis or scarring in any of the clubbed fingers or toes was evident. No abnormal deposits of mucopolysaccharide and no evidence of abnormal bone formation were found.

No difference between normal and clubbed digits was found in the number or length of small blood vessels in the terminal segments. There is no associated hyperplasia of the vascular bed, and such increase in blood flow must be the result of vasodilatation. Clubbing probably is the consequence of an increased blood flow in the terminal parts of the fingers, which in turn leads to fluid accumulation in the otherwise normal connective tissue of the nail bed.

▶ This article has nothing to do with either bronchial asthma or immunologically mediated lung diseases. However, it does address an important sign in pulmonary medicine, clubbing, and suggests that the vasculature in clubbed digits is anatomically normal. Any increase in blood flow, therefore, is presumed to result from vasodilation. It has been suggested that the abnormal anatomy is caused by abnormal fluid accumulation in an otherwise normal connective tissue bed.—S.P. Peters, M.D., Ph.D.

## Therapy

### Behavioral and Environmental Considerations

**Recommendations for the Use of Residential Air-Cleaning Devices in the Treatment of Allergic Respiratory Diseases**

Nelson HS, Hirsch SR, Ohman JL Jr, Platts-Mills TAE, Reed CE, Solomon WR
(Natl Jewish Ctr for Immunology and Respiratory Medicine, Denver)
*J Allergy Clin Immunol* 82:661–669, October 1988 2–25

In February 1987 an ad hoc committee met at the request of the Food and Drug Administration and several manufacturers to consider whether standards could be recommended for room air cleaning devices. The types and performance characteristics of available domestic air-cleaning devices, available data on concentrations of allergens in the indoor air, and data from studies examining the health effects of the use of indoor air-cleaning devices were discussed.

The 2 broad categories of air cleaners include those with mechanical filtering, including high efficiency particular air (HEPA) filters, and those that use electrical attraction including electrostatic precipitators. Neither removes gases or odors; charcoal or certain chemical crystals can remove these to some extent through adsorption. Charged media filters combine both properties of mechanical and electronic filters. Air conditioning, while technically not a method of air cleaning, is an efficient way of reducing pollen and mold spores and decreasing the number of dust mites indoors.

Allergens are found in the indoor air and the quantity is related to the rate of introduction of that allergen from outdoors. Some homes may contain significant quantities of nonallergenic indoor air pollutants, such as cigarette smoke and adsorbed radon decay products.

Results of double-blind studies indicate that the addition of a central air cleaner to an air conditioning system can produce a small, often clinically significant further reduction in pollen load and symptoms compared with the major effect of the air conditioning system itself. Results of limited, double-blind studies indicate that free-standing room air cleaners failed to achieve any significant reduction in symptoms or improvement in peak flow rate in persons sensitive to house dust. Some decrease in symptoms or medication use has been shown consistently when cleaned air has been incorporated into a laminar flow device directing the air over the head of the sleeping persons.

Inadequate data on the clinical relevance of indoor ambient allergen levels and the effect of air cleaning devices on these levels prevents any firm recommendations. However, the use of air cleaning devices in the absence of other forms of environmental control is questionable.

▶ Allergic patients often ask their physicians about benefits that might be expected from using residential air-cleaning devices. As the authors of this article point out, lack of data concerning both the concentrations of indoor allergens and pollutants and the health effects of indoor air-cleaning devices preclude firm recommendations about the usefulness of these devices. However, 2 things appear noteworthy. First, high-efficiency mechanical and electronic units both produce a high degree of air purification, but use of these devices in the absence of other measures to avoid environmental insults (removal of a pet or a dust mite-infested sofa to which a person is allergic, for example) is not likely to be helpful. Second, air conditioning units, although not strictly an air-cleaning unit, may produce benefits through multiple mechanisms, including reducing exposure to outdoor pollutants and pollens and decreasing humidity (and therefore inhibiting growth of fungi and dust mites).—S.P. Peters, M.D., Ph.D.

---

**Prolongation of Simple and Choice Reaction Times in a Double-Blind Comparison of Twice-Daily Hydroxyzine Versus Terfenadine**

Goetz DW, Jacobson JM, Murnane JE, Reid MJ, Repperger DW, Goodyear C, Martin ME (Lackland Air Force Base, San Antonio; Wright-Patterson Air Force Base, Dayton, Ohio)

*J Allergy Clin Immunol* 84:316–322, September 1989 2–26

Traditional $H_1$ antihistamines sometimes produce side effects that interfere with a patient's work. Newer, nonsedating antihistamines are an attractive alternative for such patients with allergy. A double-blind, placebo-controlled, crossover trial was done to assess the differential effect of these antihistamines on reaction times and subjective symptoms in 16 healthy, asymptomatic adults.

Terfenadine, 60 mg twice daily, and hydroxyzine, 25 mg twice daily, were compared. Simple and choice reaction times were measured with a computer based, eye–hand, reaction-time testing device. Reaction times and symptom scores were recorded 90 minutes after the fourth and tenth doses of each drug.

Hydroxyzine significantly prolonged simple and choice reaction times, whereas terfenadine did not. Neither drug prolonged decision time, the time to process 1 bit of spatial information. This indicates that hydroxyzine prolonged the interpretation and response to stimuli of the CNS without prolonging single-bit processing time. Hydroxyzine produced significant drowsiness, dry mouth, and irritability, whereas terfenadine was no different from placebo for any of these symptoms. Neither objective nor subjective symptom tolerance developed in the 5 days of hydroxyzine treatment. No association was noted between the subjective symptoms and prolongation of reaction times by hydroxyzine, which suggests that side effects reported with traditional antihistamines are unreliable predictors of objective performance. Terfenadine, a new, nonsedating antihistamine, is a promising therapeutic alternative to traditional antihistamines, particularly for patients performing critical tasks.

▶ A new generation of $H_1$-receptor antagonists for histamine has been developed, including terfenadine (Merrill Dow), cetirizine (Pfizer), astemizole (Janssen), azelastine (Wallace), loratidine (Schering-Plough), and acrivastine (Burroughs Wellcome) (1, 2). Most of these agents either have been released recently for clinical use or will be shortly. These compounds may differ from one another in a number of respects (whether or not they also inhibit mediator release from mast cells, for example), but all of them except azelastine have been described as low-sedating or nonsedating. The article abstracted above demonstrates that hydroxyzine, but not terfenadine, prolongs simple and choice reaction times. Of interest was the finding that subjective symptoms were not associated with the prolongation of reaction times produced by hydroxyzine. A study by Meador and associates (3) in the same journal reported that chlorpheniramine, but not terfenadine, increased the latency of the P300 or $P_3$ wave of the endogenous auditory-evoked potential, a measure of cognitive skill that recently has gained favor by cognitive scientists.

As pointed out in a thoughtful editorial by Shucard (4), these 2 studies demonstrate that terfenadine, in comparison with traditional antihistamines, produces little effect on simple cognitive processes but they provide no information concerning the effects of these drugs on higher cognitive processes such as memory. However, this new generation of antihistamines should prove to be useful, particularly for those patients in whom side effects from traditional antihistamines have proved troublesome. Whether astemizole in particular will prove to be of unusual clinical benefit (with its 120-hour serum elimination half-life) remains to be determined.—S.P. Peters, M.D., Ph.D.

*References*

1. Dockhorn RJ, Shellenberger MK: Antihistamines: The new generation. *Immunol Allergy Pract* 9:124, 1987.
2. Simons FER, Simons KJ: New $H_1$-receptor antagonists: A review. *Am J Rhinol* 2:21–25, 1988.
3. Meador KJ, Loring DW, Thompson EE, et al: Differential cognitive effects of terfenadine and chlorpheniramine. *J Allergy Clin Immunol* 84:322–325, 1989.
4. Shucard DW: The effect of antihistamines on electrophysiologic and behavioral measures of cognition. *J Allergy Clin Immunol* 84:284–285, 1989.

---

**A Self Management Plan in the Treatment of Adult Asthma**

Beasley R, Cushley M, Holgate ST (Southampton Gen Hosp, Southampton, England)

*Thorax* 44:200–204, March 1989 2–27

---

How effective is the self-management of adult asthma? Thirty-six consecutively seen asthmatic adults attending an outpatient chest clinic were included in an open prospective trial based on steroid inhalation and measurements of peak expiratory flow (PEF). Inhaled salbutamol and be-

Management Plan Based on Measurement of PEF

***PEF measured every morning, or more frequently if unstable***

**PEF ≥ 70% potential normal value, continue "maintenance regimen" of**
- **(*a*) inhaled beta sympathomimetic, twice daily and as required**
- **(*b*) inhaled beclomethasone dipropionate twice daily**

**PEF < 70% potential normal value:**
- **(*a*) double dose of beclomethasone dipropionate for number of days required to achieve previous baseline**
- **(*b*) continue this increased dose for same number of days**
- **(*c*) return to previous dose of maintenance regimen**

**PEF < 50% potential normal value**
- **(*a*) start oral prednisolone 40 mg daily and contact general practitioner**
- **(*b*) continue this dose for the number of days required to achieve previous baseline**
- **(*c*) reduce oral prednisolone to 20 mg daily for same number of days**
- **(*d*) stop prednisolone**

**PEF < 150–200 l/min**
- **(*a*) contact general practitioner urgently or, if he is unavailable,**
- **(*b*) contact ambulance service or, if it is unavailable,**
- **(*c*) go directly to hospital**

(Courtesy of Beasley R, Cushley M, Holgate ST: *Thorax* 44:200–204, March 1989.)

clomethasone dipropionate were used with the goal of achieving normal lung function. Patients measured their PEF each morning, aiming at the predicted normal PEF or the maximum achieved PEF, whichever was higher. The dose of beclomethasone was doubled if the measured PEF fell by more than 30% below the "potential norm," and prednisolone therapy was begun if it dropped by more than half (table).

Thirty patients remained in the trial for a mean of 7 months. All measures of asthma severity indicated significant improvement at the final clinic visit regardless of previous inhaled steroid therapy. Drug requirements declined significantly after home management was instituted. Most patients preferred to contact their physician when the PEF fell below 50%.

Adults with severe chronic asthma can manage their disease effectively using inhaled steroid and regular assessments of airflow obstruction. Most such patients can achieve relatively normal lung function. Patients in the trial slept better than before and lost less time from work as a result of asthma.

▶ In the 1989 YEAR BOOK OF PULMONARY DISEASE (pp 94–96) we discussed an article by Woolcock and co-workers (1) in which the goal of therapy was to maintain lung function as close to normal as possible. The article abstracted above had a similar goal and involved patients in the active management of the treatment of their disease. Using the strategy outlined in the table, these patients demonstrated, after a mean of 7 months, an improvement in lung function (mean $FEV_1$ improved from 75.6% to 91.9% predicted), a decrease in the mean time lost from school or work during the prior 6 months (from 12.9 to 1.7 days), and a decrease in mean number of courses of oral corticosteroids required (from 0.97 to 0.37). The use of high dose (250 μg/actuation) inhaled steroids increased an average of approximately 350 μg/day per patient. The patients in the article by Woolcock and colleagues demonstrated a decrease in symptoms, a decrease in nonspecific bronchial responsiveness, and a decrease in the variability of peak flow measurements, all of which suggested clinical improvement. These studies were not rigorously controlled (and the study abstracted above contained *no* control group), but they do suggest that therapy for asthmatic patients aimed at normalizing pulmonary function has important clinical benefits. This hypothesis needs to be rigorously tested, particularly from the point of view of long-term morbidity that might (unexpectedly) be associated with such intensive treatment.—S.P. Peters, M.D., Ph.D.

*Reference*

1. Woolcock AJ, Yan K, Salome CM: Effect of therapy on bronchial hyperresponsiveness in the long-term management of asthma. *Clin Allergy* 18:165–176, 1988.

Β-AGONISTS

**β-Adrenoceptor Responses to High Doses of Inhaled Salbutamol in Patients With Bronchial Asthma**

Lipworth BJ, Clark RA, Dhillon DP, Brown RA, McDevitt DG (Ninewells Hosp; Kings Cross Hosp; Univ of Dundee, Scotland)

*Br J Clin Pharmacol* 26:527–533, 1988 2–28

Doses of salbutamol ranging from 100 to 4,000 μg were administered by metered-dose inhaler to 14 stable asthmatic patients (mean age, 38 years). Airway parameters, tremor, and hemodynamic responses as well

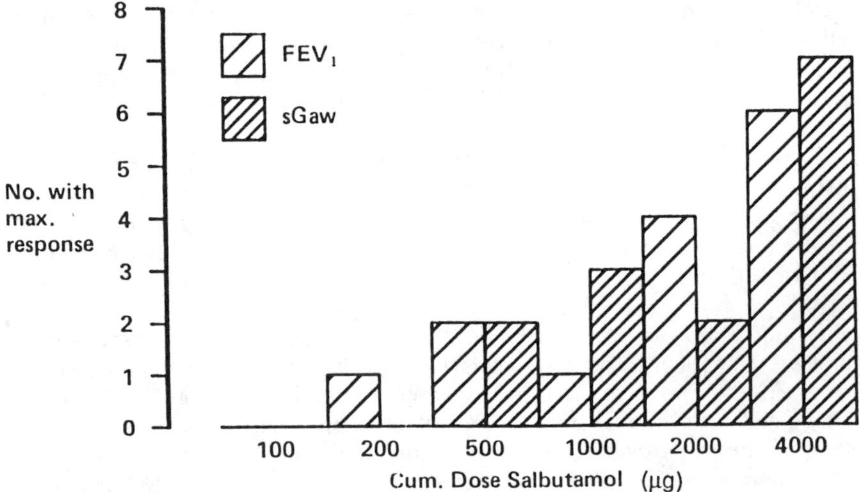


Fig 2–10.—Number of patients who had maximum airway response at each dose of salbutamol. (Courtesy of Lipworth BJ, Clark RA, Dhillon DP, et al: *Br J Clin Pharmacol* 26:527–533, 1988.)

as cyclic adenosine monophosphate (cAMP) were measured at each dose increment.

Peak responses for all airway parameters occurred at the highest dose of salbutamol. Most patients required this dose to achieve maximal bronchodilation (Fig 2–10). The heart response was linear after administration of salbutamol, 500 μg. No patient reported palpitations. No significant effect on tremor was seen at doses of less than 1,000 μg. Values for cAMP increased significantly after the first dose and were linear up to the highest dose.

Higher than usual doses of salbutamol may lead to substantially better airway responses in asthmatic patients. Tremor and heart rate responses have not been dose limiting up to 4,000 μg. The severity of asthma does not always indicate the dose needed to achieve maximal bronchodilation, but most patients require higher doses for a maximal effect.

---

**Tachyphylaxis to Systemic But Not to Airway Responses During Prolonged Therapy With High Dose Inhaled Salbutamol in Asthmatics**
Lipworth BJ, Struthers AD, McDevitt DG (Ninewells Hosp, Dundee, Scotland)
*Am Rev Respir Dis* 140:586–592, September 1989 2–29

---

High doses of inhaled salbutamol can produce marked improvements in airway response in asthma patients. Such treatment is associated with dose dependent systemic β-adrenoceptor reactions. To determine

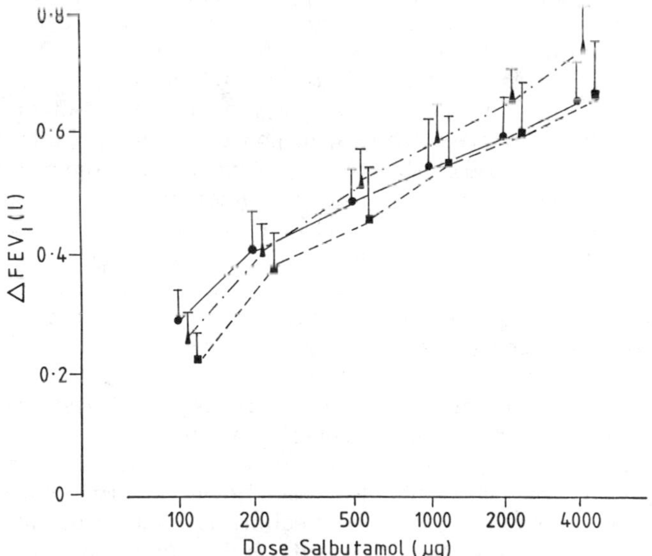


**Fig 2–11.**—Change in $FEV_1$ in response to cumulative doubling doses of inhaled salbutamol (100–4,000 μg on a log scale) in 12 asthmatic patients after pretreatment with placebo *(circles)*, low-dose inhaled salbutamol *(triangles)*, and high-dose salbutamol *(squares)*. Values are shown as mean and SEM. (Courtesy of Lipworth BJ, Struthers AD, McDevitt DG: *Am Rev Respir Dis* 140:586–592, September 1989.)

whether tachyphylaxis occurs during long-term treatment with high doses of inhaled salbutamol, 12 patients with asthma were examined.

The patients required only occasional inhaled β-agonists for treatment. For 14 days the patients received salbutamol, 4,000 μg daily; salbutamol, 800 μg daily; or placebo by metered-dose inhaler. A 14-day run-in and a washout period was provided in which inhaled β-agonists were withheld and ipratropium bromide was substituted for rescue purposes. At the end of each 14-day treatment, airway, chronotropic, tremor, and metabolic responses were determined.

The treatment did not significantly effect baseline values. Dose-dependent rises were noted in forced expiratory volume in 1 second ($FEV_1$) and forced expiratory flow at 25% to 75%. Pretreatment with high-dose inhaled salbutamol did not displace the dose-response curve to the right. The dose-response curves for the chronotropic and metabolic responses were attenuated after administration of high-dose salbutamol as compared with placebo. There also were differences between high- and low-dose salbutamol in these values. The frequency and severity of subjective adverse effects were diminished after treatment with high-dose salbutamol (Fig 2–11).

Improvements in asthmatic airway responses are maintained in the first 14 days of therapy with high-dose inhaled salbutamol. Tachyphylaxis develops to systemic adverse effects. Further trials are needed to determine whether the same is true of much longer courses of treatment.

▶ A single actuation of an albuterol (salbutamol) inhaler as packaged for sale in the United States delivers 90 μg of drug. Therefore, the highest dose of drug administered in these 2 studies would represent more than 40 puffs of albuterol. These 2 articles (Abstracts 2–28 and 2–29) by the same investigators contained information that was surprising to me. First, only 4 of 14 asthmatic patients achieved their maximal airway response (as determined by measurement of $FEV_1$) with a dose of albuterol comparable to the maximal *daily* recommended dose, approximately 1,000 μg; the other subjects required an even higher dose, and 6 of the 14 may not have reached a maximal bronchodilation at all because their greatest response occurred at the highest dose of albuterol tested, 4,000 μg. Second, even at a dose of 4,000 μg per day for 14 days, no airway tachyphylaxis to albuterol was noted, in spite of a tachyphylaxis to some of the adverse systemic effects (heart rate, metabolic effects, tremor, and palpitations). Whether such a high daily dose of albuterol administered for a longer time would also produce no airway tachyphylaxis is under investigation.

These data have rather limited practical applicability at present because it would be unwise to suggest that patients take severalfold more than the maximal daily dose of this or any other β-agonist. However, in light of this information, it would *not* be unreasonable to treat status asthmaticus with frequent doses of albuterol while waiting for the effects of other therapy, such as parenteral corticosteroids, to have an effect.—S.P. Peters, M.D., Ph.D.

**Nocturnal Asthma Therapy: Inhaled Bitolterol Versus Sustained-Release Theophylline**

Zwillich CW, Neagley SR, Cicutto L, White DP, Martin RJ (Pennsylvania State Univ; Hershey Med Ctr, Hershey, Pa: Natl Jewish Ctr for Immunology and Lung Disease, Denver)

*Am Rev Respir Dis* 139:470–474, February 1989 2–30

Many asthmatic persons report increased respiratory symptoms and need for additional medications during sleeping hours. Sustained-release theophylline (THEO) may prevent nocturnal asthma symptoms and early morning decrement in lung function, but may also delay sleep onset and alter normal sleep stage distribution. The electroencephalographic, cardiac, and gas exchange indices during sleep were evaluated during treatment with THEO and long-acting inhaled $\beta_2$-agonist. In this double-blind, crossover, placebo-controlled trial, 26 patients with mild to moderate asthma and a history of frequent nocturnal symptoms who had had decrements in morning lung function received either THEO or 3 puffs of bitolterol (BITOL) for 2 weeks ending with 2 consecutive nights of sleep evaluation followed by crossover to the alternate drug regimen.

Plasma concentrations on awakening were 11.4 μg/mL during THEO and 0.00 μg/mL during BITOL therapy. The electroencephalographic characteristics of sleep did not differ significantly between patients during THEO and inhaled BITOL therapy. Mean number of apneas and hypopneas were also similar between regimens. However, on awakening, mean forced expiratory volume in 1 second was significantly higher after THEO than BITOL (Fig 2–12). Furthermore, time spent with an oxyhemoglobin saturation of 4% or more below the control level was significantly less during THEO than BITOL (Fig 2–13). Asthmatic patients reported significantly fewer daytime complaints of wheezing, cough, and dyspnea, claimed better sleep quality, and showed an overall preference for THEO over BITOL.

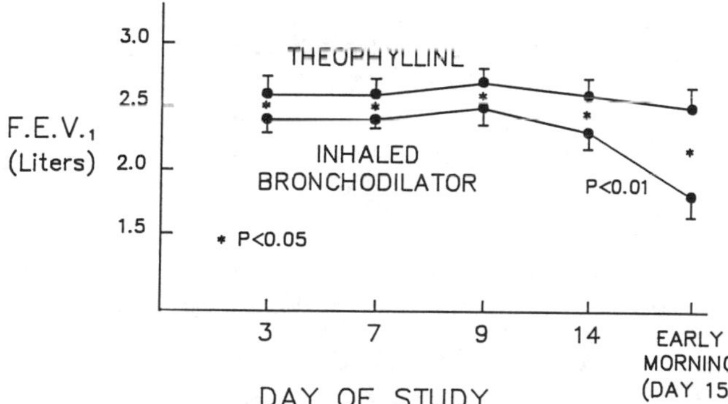


**Fig 2–12.**—Mean forced expiratory volume ($FEV_1$) during each phase of the study is shown. Theophylline therapy was associated with a consistently higher $FEV_1$. A significant decrease ($P < .01$) in lung function occurred in the early morning during inhaled bronchodilator therapy, but it was not present during theophylline administration. (Courtesy of Zwillich CW, Neagley SR, Cicutto L, et al: *Am Rev Respir Dis* 139:470–474, February 1989.)

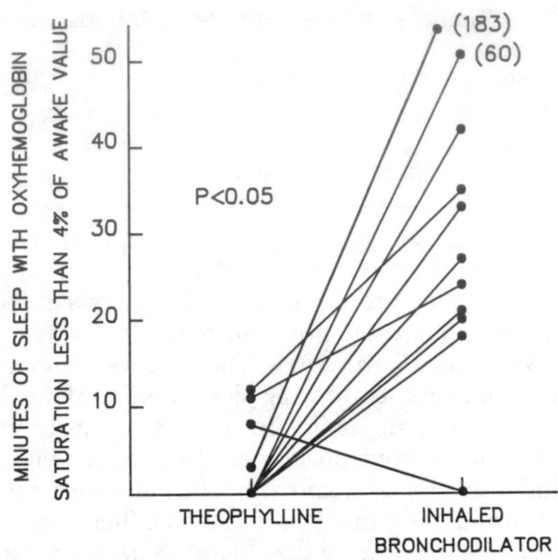


Fig 2–13.—Oxyhemoglobin desaturation episodes occurred in only 4 of the 26 patients during theophylline therapy. However, during inhaled bronchodilator, 10 patients had more frequent and more prolonged desaturation events. Most patients (not shown) did not have desaturation during sleep in either phase of the study. (Courtesy of Zwillich CW, Neagley SR, Cicutto L, et al: *Am Rev Respir Dis* 139:470–474, February 1989.)

Sustained-release theophylline results in better objective and subjective measures of asthma control than the long-acting inhaled $\beta_2$-agonist BITOL.

▶ That a sustained-release theophylline preparation was more effective than bitolterol in asthmatic patients with nocturnal symptoms may have been caused by the pharmacokinetics of the 2 drugs involved. As the authors noted, plasma theophylline concentrations were therapeutic upon awakening (11.4 ± 0.69 μg/mL) when patients were on the sustained-release preparation of theophylline. However, although bitolterol has been touted as a "long-acting" β-agonist, it has been reported to have a duration of action of 8 or more hours in only 25% to 35% of patients (1). A number of β-agonists that will meet anyone's definition of "long-acting" are now in clinical trials. It would be of interest to compare those agents with a sustained-release theophylline preparation in this protocol.—S.P. Peters, M.D., Ph.D.

*Reference*

1. *Physicians' Desk Reference*, ed 44. Oradell, NJ, Medical Economics Inc, 1990, p 2339.

---

**Long-Term Treatment of Severe Asthma With Subcutaneous Terbutaline**

O'Driscoll BRC, Ruffles SP, Ayres JG, Cochrane GM (East Birmingham Hosp, Birmingham, England)

*Br J Dis Chest* 82:360–367, October 1988 2–31

Despite large doses of bronchodilator drugs and corticosteroids given orally and by inhalation, patients with severe brittle asthma have frequent episodes of wheezing and breathlessness. Previously, greatly improved control of asthma was achieved in some of these patients when treated with terbutaline in 6-hourly subcutaneous injections (QDST) or as a continuous subcutaneous infusion (CSIT). It was possible to reduce or discontinue oral steroid and nebulized bronchodilator therapy, and early morning peak flow rates were increased. Terbutaline was administered subcutaneously to 17 patients with brittle asthma and 5 patients with chronic severe asthma.

Of the 17 patients with brittle asthma, 13 derived subjective and objective benefit from subcutaneous terbutaline treatment. The mean lowest daily peak expiratory flow (PEF) for all patients increased from 142 to 297 L per minute. This improvement was reflected in a reduction in steroid dose, nebulized β-agonist dose, and hospital admissions. Only 1 of 5 patients with chronic asthma had any lasting response; 18 patients continued to use terbutaline subcutaneously over long periods. Side effects have been minimal.

Terbutaline administered by infusion or by intermittent injections is a useful addition to the therapy of some patients with brittle asthma, especially when troublesome "morning dips" cannot be controlled by other means.

▶ This article suggests that subcutaneous terbutaline can be added to intramuscular triamcinolone (1987 YEAR BOOK OF PULMONARY DISEASE, pp 89–91) as a possible treatment of recalcitrant asthma. Side effects of terbutaline therapy included painful lumps at sites of infusion in 4 of 11 patients. It is not clear to me whether the distinctions in the patient population in which these 2 modalities have been suggested to be useful (terbutaline in "brittle asthma" [variation in diurnal peak flow rates of >50% on at least 3 days per week despite maximal therapy]; intramuscular triamcinolone in "chronic severe asthma") are important in the success of these agents; however, these patient characteristics should be kept in mind should a clinician be forced to consider such therapies. Perhaps longer-acting β-agonists, now under development as noted above, will prove to be as effective as subcutaneous terbutaline in "brittle asthma."—S.P. Peters, M.D., Ph.D.

CORTICOSTEROIDS

---

**Comparison of Inhaled Budesonide With Oral Prednisolone At Two Dose-Levels Commonly Used for the Treatment of Moderate Asthma**

Namsirikul P, Chaisupamongkollarp S, Chantadisai N, Bamberg P (Pramongkutklao Hosp, Pramongkutklao Med College, Bangkok, Thailand; Astra Pharmaceuticals Intnatl, Herts, England)

*Eur Respir J* 2:317–324, April 1989 2–32

---

The antiasthmatic efficacy of 2 doses of budesonide and 2 doses of oral prednisolone commonly used in clinical practice were compared in 2 randomized, double-blind, crossover trials. Twenty-eight asthmatic patients

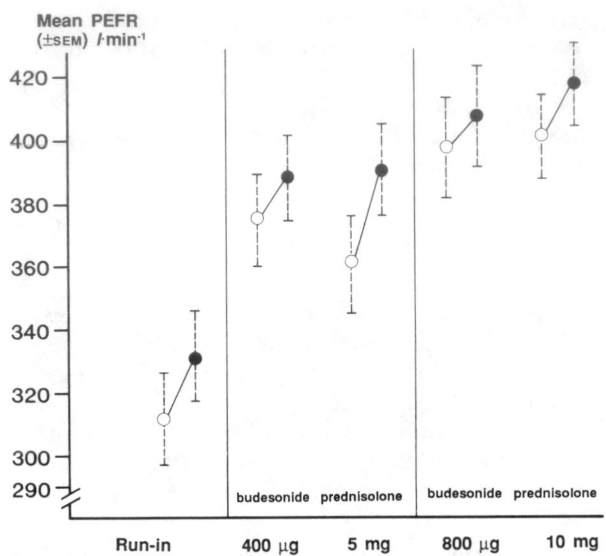


**Fig 2–14.**—Mean diary card peak expiratory flow rate (PEFR) values (±SEM). *Open circles,* A.M. (morning) PEFR; *filled circles,* P.M. (evening) PEFR at run-in and during each treatment period. Difference between open and filled circles represents mean diurnal variation. (Courtesy of Namsirikul P, Chaisupamongkollarp S, Chantadisai N, et al: *Eur Respir J* 2:317–324, April 1989.)

who had not received any regular inhaled glucocorticosteroids previously were treated with either 200 μg of budesonide or 5 mg of prednisolone daily for 3 weeks. This was followed by a washout period during which all patients received 400 μg of budesonide daily, followed by another 3-week treatment period with 800 μg of budesonide or 10 mg of prednisolone.

Lung function and symptoms improved significantly on all treatments, but the improvement was dose-dependent. When low-dose treatments were compared, mean morning peak expiratory flow rate was significantly higher during budesonide than prednisolone treatment (Fig 2–14). As a result, diurnal variation was significantly less during budesonide treatment. This trend was also visible with the high doses, but the difference was not significant. It is possible that the differences between the higher doses of the 2 drugs were masked because a "ceiling effect" had been reached. No serious side effects were noted.

Use of budesonide is recommended as the first additional treatment for asthmatic patients who are not adequately controlled by bronchodilators alone. Adequate control can be achieved with 400 μg/day of budesonide in most patients. The dose of budesonide can be increased to 800 μg/day with almost negligible side effects.

▶ Budesonide is an anti-inflammatory steroid with a potency approximately equal to that of beclomethasone. This article demonstrates that 5 mg of oral prednisolone is therapeutically equivalent to 400 μg of inhaled budesonide (approximately equal to 9 puffs of beclomethasone a day), whereas 10 mg of prednisolone is equal to 800 μg of budesonide (equivalent to the maximum recommended daily dose of beclomethasone). These equivalencies are helpful for a physician who contemplates adding an inhaled steroid to the treatment plan of a patient not well controlled with other agents, such as β-agonists or theophylline, or both, or who is planning to switch a patient from parenteral to inhaled steroid. In the latter case, we would suggest adding inhaled steroid at a time when the patient has been stabilized on a fixed dose of oral medication, then slowly tapering the oral agent. This should maximize chances of a successful conversion to an inhaled agent. In addition, it has been reported that inhaled steroids can further improve lung function in patients already on oral steroids (1). The goal in using inhaled steroids is, of course, to avoid steroid-related side effects.

It has been reported recently that posterior subcapsular cataracts developed in 3 patients on steroid aerosols (2). Whether steroids played an etiologic role in these patients is not known for certain, but this was their only known risk factor. Because it has been suggested that any dose of oral prednisolone over 10 mg per day may predispose a patient to cataract formation, steroid aerosols are still preferred over systemic steroids, even if they could be shown to produce this complication in a small number of patients.—S.P. Peters, M.D., Ph.D.

*References*

1. Tukiainen P, Lahdensuo A: Effect of inhaled budesonide on severe steroid-dependent asthma. *Eur J Respir Dis* 70:239–244, 1987.
2. Allen MB, Ray SG, Leitch AG, et al: Steroid aerosols and cataract formation. *Br Med J* 299:432–433, 1989.

---

**High Doses of Inhaled Corticosteroids in Unstable Chronic Asthma: A Multicenter, Double-Blind, Placebo-Controlled Study**

Salmeron S, Guerin J-C, Godard P, Renon D, Henry-Amar M, Duroux P, Taytard A (Hôpital Antoine Béclère, Clamart; Hôpital de la Croix Rousse, Lyon; Hôpital l'Aiguelongue, Montpellier; Hôpital du Haut Lévêque, Pessac, France)

*Am Rev Respir Dis* 140:167–171, July 1989 2–33

---

Corticosteroids are important in the treatment of chronic asthma. Corticosteroid aerosols minimize the systemic effects of the drug while maintaining topical activity. However, the usual doses of inhaled corticosteroids are not always effective in patients whose asthma is poorly controlled by standard bronchodilator treatment. High doses of beclomethasone dipropionate (BDP) were compared with placebo in noncorticosteroid-dependent patients whose moderately severe asthma was uncontrolled by $\beta_2$-agonist aerosols and oral theophylline.

Inhaled BDP, 1,500 μg/day, or placebo was administered to 43 chronic asthmatic patients. Before the trial, a test of maximal steroid reversibility (improvement ≥ 20%) with oral prednisolone, 0.5 mg/kg/day for 14 days, was done. Therapeutic responses were measured for 8 weeks as the ability to maintain the clinical improvement and the optimal pulmonary function induced by prednisolone. One of 21 patients receiving BDP had

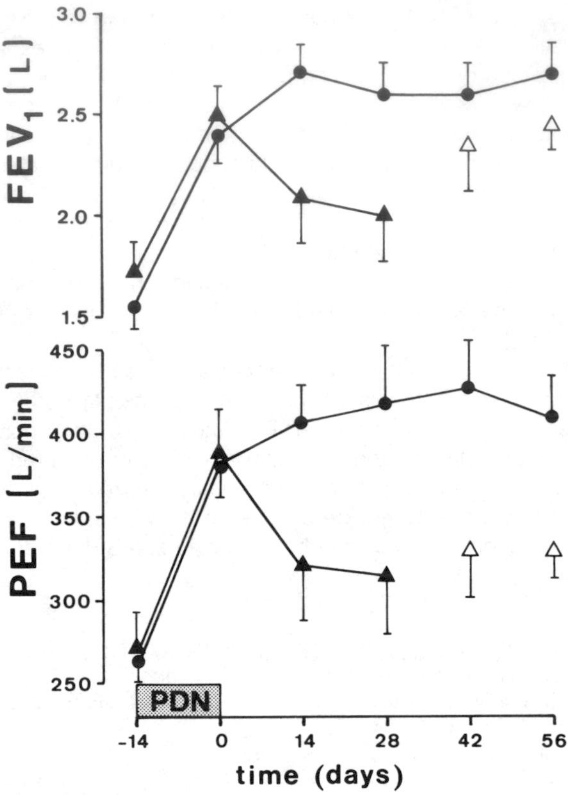


**Fig 2–15.**—Time course of $FEV_1$ (**top**) and peak expiratory flow (*PEF*, **bottom**) during the prestudy and study periods. The prednisolone *(PDN)* prestudy test is indicated between days −14 and zero. Data are shown as mean ± SEM. *Solid circles* represent the BDP group, and *solid triangles,* the placebo group, when comparisons between the 2 groups are possible, and *open triangles,* the placebo group when the low number of patients does not allow comparisons. (Courtesy of Salmeron S, Guerin J-C, Godard P, et al: *Am Rev Respir Dis* 140:167–171, July 1989.)

a severe asthma exacerbation, compared with 15 of 22 patients receiving placebo. Among those receiving BDP, forced expiratory volume in 1 second ($FEV_1$) and peak expiratory flow remained above the optimal post-prednisolone value. There was a trend toward improvement during the 8 weeks. In the placebo group, $FEV_1$ and peak expiratory flow decreased and remained below the optimal level (Fig 2–15).

Inhaled BDP, 1,500 μg daily, maintains the optimal pulmonary function in addition to the clinical benefit of a short course of oral corticosteroids. It may be valuable in the treatment of patients with unstable noncorticosteroid-dependent asthma.

▶ An important aspect of this article was the selection criteria used for patient inclusion: 1 or more asthma attacks per week during the 2-week observation period (off steroids but still taking a β-agonist and theophylline preparation), and basal peak flow rates and $FEV_1$ less than 80% predicted with an improvement of at least 20% after 2 weeks of oral prednisolone (0.5 mg/kg/day). Patients were excluded if they required continuous oral prednisolone therapy during the previous year. In these steroid responsive patients, high-dose inhaled beclomethasone (twice the recommended maximum daily dose in the United States) maintained lung function to the same degree, in general, as the oral prednisolone. Only 1 of the 21 beclomethasone-treated patients experienced a severe exacerbation of asthma, whereas 15 of 22 of placebo treated patients experienced a severe exacerbation.

These results should encourage us in our attempts to provide steroid-dependent asthmatic patients with optimal care. However, we cannot provide this treatment alternative to patients in the United States because high-dose preparations of inhaled steroids are not available for use. (The standard beclomethasone inhaler provides 42 μg of drug per actuation; 1,500 μg of drug would provide 36 puffs of medication per day.) In the 1988 YEAR BOOK OF PULMONARY DISEASE (pp 143–145), we discussed high-dose inhaled beclomethasone therapy and expressed our hope that such agents would soon be available for use in the United States. We reiterate this wish now, 2 years later.—S.P. Peters, M.D., Ph.D.

---

**Morphological Studies of Bronchial Mucosal Biopsies From Asthmatics Before and After Ten Years of Treatment With Inhaled Steroids**

Lundgren R, Söderberg M, Hörstedt P, Stenling R (Univ Hosp, Umeå, Sweden)
*Eur Respir J* 1:883–889, December 1988 2–34

---

Bronchial mucosal inflammation and epithelial damage have been implicated in the development of bronchial asthma, and inhaled steroids are thought to have an anti-inflammatory effect. To examine the effects of inhaled steroids on the bronchial mucosa, biopsy specimens from 6 nonsmokers aged 42–63 years with severe bronchial asthma were studied before and after 10 years of daily treatment with inhaled steroid. The results were compared with biopsy specimens from 6 healthy control persons.

In specimens obtained from the asthmatic patients before treatment, there was a significant increase in inflammatory cells compared with controls. Electron microscopy demonstrated reduced coverage by cilia in all patients. Squamous cell metaplasia was seen in 2 patients. After 10 years of treatment, the number of inflammatory cells was significantly reduced to that before treatment and was similar to that from the control biopsy specimens. In the 2 patients with squamous cell metaplasia before treatment, small areas of metaplasia could still be seen. Nonciliated areas decreased, and 3 patients had small areas with both nonciliated and ciliated cells (Fig 2–16). Bronchial hyperreactivity to methacholine remained.

The alleviation of epithelial damage and bronchial inflammation by long-term steroid inhalation does not seem to affect the bronchial hyperreactivity associated with bronchial asthma. The relation between mucosal inflammation, inhaled steroids, and bronchial hyperresponsiveness awaits clarification.

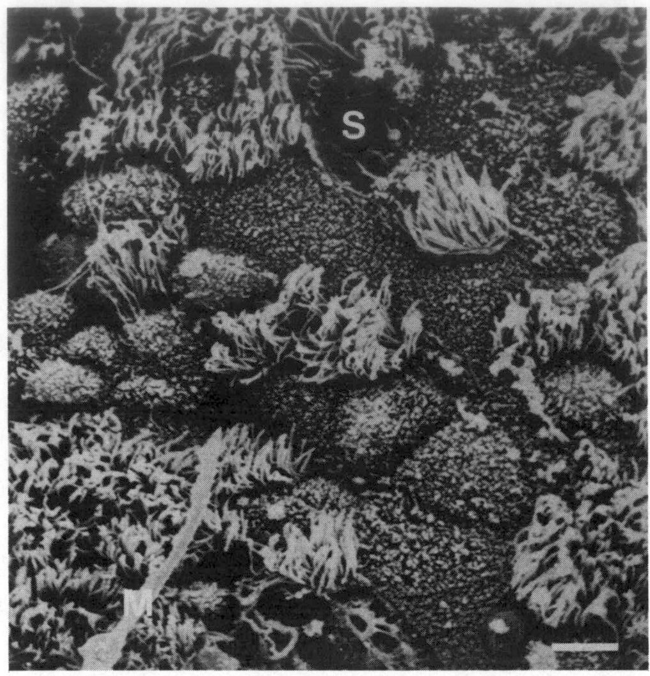


**Fig 2–16.**—Biopsy specimen from an asthmatic patient treated for 10 years with inhaled steroids showing bronchial epithelium with a mixture of ciliated and nonciliated cells. *S,* secretory cell; *M,* mucus; SEM ×2,400; *bar,* 5μm. (Courtesy of Lundgren R, Söderberg M, Hörstedt P, et al: *Eur Respir J* 1:883–889, December 1988.)

▶ We discussed in the section above on pathogenesis that damage to the bronchial epithelium appears common in asthmatic patients. This article confirms those results and also documents that treatment with inhaled steroids (up to 400 μg of beclomethasone per day) was associated with a reduction in the number of inflammatory cells present in the bronchial mucosa. The 10-year patient follow-up in this study is impressive. It is likely that this resulted from the anti-inflammatory effects of treatment, but it cannot be ruled out that this effect might have been part of the natural history of disease in these asthmatic patients. It is also reassuring to note that steroid use was not associated with histologic or ultrastructural abnormalities in bronchial mucosa.—S.P. Peters, M.D., Ph.D.

## Chronic Fatigue Syndrome

### Liver Extract–Folic Acid–Cyanocobalamin vs. Placebo for Chronic Fatigue Syndrome

Kaslow JE, Rucker L, Onishi R (Univ of California Irvine Med Ctr, Orange; Long Beach VA Hosp, Long Beach, Calif)
*Arch Intern Med* 149:2501–2503, November 1989 2–35

A variety of unproved treatments have been advocated for patients complaining of chronic fatigue syndrome (CFS). One widely used treatment is intramuscular injection of liver extract–folic acid–cyanocobalamin (LEFAC). A double-blind, randomized, crossover trial was done to determine the efficacy of LEFAC in 15 patients with CFS, 14 of whom completed the trial and 3 questionnaires. An elective open-label phase and a fourth questionnaire were completed by 11 patients. At entry 9 patients had documented fevers, with temperatures of less than 38.3 C. The patients had tried a variety of unsuccessful treatments.

The patients reported significant improvement in energy after both LEFAC and placebo administration. No significant differences between LEFAC and placebo were noted on any measure. Significant improvement occurred on all measures after unblinded LEFAC administration when compared with baseline values. No adverse reactions to the injections occurred. One patient ended open-label use of LEFAC after 2 days because of a temperature of 38.9 C, which appeared to be related to a viral illness.

Although liver extracts appear to have an in vitro effect on mononuclear cell function, LEFAC was no more effective than placebo in improving patients' functional status or relieving CFS symptoms. Physicians treating patients with CFS should carefully scrutinize the claims of untested therapies.

► In 1988 a group of investigators, including representatives from the Centers for Disease Control in Atlanta, proposed a working definition for the chronic Epstein-Barr virus syndrome, and proposed changing its name to the "chronic fatigue syndrome" because the etiologic role of Epstein-Barr virus infection in producing this disorder remains in doubt (1). Basically, the working definition requires that a patient's fatigue or symptom complex reduce his daily activity by at least 50% for at least 6 months without an etiologic medical or psychiatric condition being identified. In addition, at least 8 of the following signs or symptoms need to be present: patient-documented mild fever (37.5 to 38.6 C) or chills; sore throat; painful cervical or axillary lymph nodes; generalized muscle weakness; myalgia; prolonged (at least 24 hours) general fatigue after exercise that would not have produced it previously; generalized headaches; migratory arthralgia without arthritis; neuropsychiatric complaints; sleep disturbance; description of the major symptom complex as having developed over a few hours to a few days; physician-documented low-grade fever; nonexudative pharyngitis; palpable cervical or axillary lymphadenopathy.

The article abstracted above reports that the vitamin complex was no more effective than placebo in this syndrome. However, both treatments, and particularly open-label administration of the vitamin complex at the end of the study, improved level of daily activity, mental health, energy level, and symptoms. However, the authors do not state whether the subjects became reasonably functional at this point (after open-label administration of the complex). The authors stress that controlled studies will be hard to perform because of the large placebo effect in this syndrome. We agree, but would also suggest that this or similar therapy, if it appears to be without significant side effects, should be considered if it can make nonfunctional persons functional again.—S.P. Peters, M.D., Ph.D.

*Reference*

1. Holmes GP, Kaplan JE, Gantz NM, et al: Chronic fatigue syndrome: A working case definition. *Ann Intern Med* 108:387–389, 1988.

# 3 Chronic Obstructive Pulmonary Diseases

## Introduction

Chronic obstructive and restrictive diseases continue to receive more attention in pulmonary medicine as infectious diseases become less of a problem in the antibiotic era (AIDS-related pulmonary disease excluded). As the pathophysiology becomes better understood, researchers are turning their attention more to prevention, risk factors, and new therapeutic alternatives. This year's papers are not an exception, for they reflect these continued interests.

The big news in chronic obstructive pulmonary diseases this year is the increasing incidence of death from these diseases. I suggest that those interested in a complete review of this subject read the series of papers in the supplement to *The American Review of Respiratory Diseases* entitled "The Rise in Chronic Obstructive Pulmonary Disease Mortality" (vol 140, no. 3, part II, September 1989).

The series of papers on chronic obstructive pulmonary diseases chosen for this year's YEAR BOOK range from those focusing on risk factors to the effect of weight gain and loss and to the effect of inhaled morphine sulfate on breathlessness. The papers on interstitial lung disease focus primarily on treatment; the series on lung transplantation reviews new information about the value of transplantation in emphysema patients. Four papers on cigarette smoking review changes in smoking patterns, the addictive quality of smoking, and the risks of passive smoking on airline flights. Three papers in the field of bronchoscopy address the use of this procedure in tuberculosis patients, in evaluating hemoptysis, and in evaluating pleural effusions. Finally, a group of miscellaneous papers cover a broad spectrum including preoperative evaluations, bronchiectasis, ventilator-related work, and the use of noninvasive techniques in assessing pulmonary hypertension. All in all, these papers represent interesting additions to their particular spheres of knowledge.

**Peter B. Terry, M.D.**

# Chronic Obstructive Pulmonary Diseases

## Risk Factors and Pathogenesis

### A Reexamination of Risk Factors for Ventilatory Impairment

Burrows B, Knudson RJ, Cline MG, Lebowitz MD (Univ of Arizona)

*Am Rev Respir Dis* 138:829–836, October 1988 3–1

Cross-sectional analyses of data from the Tucson Epidemiological Study of Airways Obstructive Diseases have shown that ventilatory impairment is significantly related to various risk factors such as smoking, chronic productive cough, a history of childhood respiratory illnesses, atopy, blood eosionophilia, and high serum levels of immunoglobulin E (IgE). Later observations have suggested that 2 quite different types of airway obstructive disease can be distinguished partly by the presence or absence of asthma. The relationship of potential risk factors to ventilatory impairment was reexamined in research subjects aged 40 to 74 years to determine the effect of excluding known asthmatics.

After such exclusion, previously noted relationships of atopy, high serum levels of IgE, and eosinophilia to reduced ventilatory function were no longer evident, and nonasthmatic nonsmokers showed almost no remaining ventilatory impairment. Pack-years of smoking and chronic productive cough remained significant predictors of forced expiratory volume in 1 second ($FEV_1$) in current smokers, even after excluding asthmatic persons. However, for nonasthmatic ex-smokers, age at quitting smoking was a significant predictor of $FEV_1$ after accounting for pack-years. Young ex-smokers closely resembled nonsmokers, but they became increasingly similar to current smokers as their age at quitting increased. Even after exclusion of asthmatic persons, a history of childhood respiratory illnesses appeared to increase susceptibility to the effects of smoking, but the possible bias of preferential recall of childhood diseases limits interpretation of this observation.

Risk factors such as atopy, eosinophilia, and elevated serum level of IgE serve only to identify known asthmatic persons, but they have no relationship to nonasthmatic forms of chronic obstructive pulmonary disease (COPD). Hence the "Dutch hypothesis" appears relevant primarily to a syndrome called "chronic asthmatic bronchitis," but not to the more typical emphysematous forms of COPD that are characteristic of smokers without asthmatic background.

### The Relation of Airways Responsiveness and Atopy to the Development of Chronic Obstructive Lung Disease

Sparrow D, O'Connor G, Weiss ST (VA Outpatient Clinic, Boston; Harvard Med School)

*Epidemiol Rev* 10:29–47, 1988 3–2

Early studies produced 2 views of the origin of chronic obstructive lung disease. The "British hypothesis" is based on the effects of cigarette smoking, whereas the Dutch hypothesis posits that intrinsic host features (e.g., atopy and airway responsiveness) are important determinants of the response to later exposure. Current data suggest that both nonspecific airway responsiveness and atopy may well be risk factors for chronic obstructive lung disease. It is possible that the associations are noncausal and are all factors resulting from inflammation; that atopy and hyperresponsiveness are effect modifiers; or that smoking, atopy, and hyperresponsiveness independently influence the development of disease.

Population-based longitudinal studies that prospectively relate airway responsiveness and atopy to the course of lung function and the occurrence of respiratory symptoms would be helpful. The effects of smoking on nonspecific airway responsiveness and atopic status require further study. Available information on atopy and lung function comes mostly from cross-sectional studies.

▶ These first 2 papers represent our state-of-the-art understanding of airways reactivity, or the lack thereof, in the development of chronic airways obstruction. The prospective study by Burrow and colleagues (Abstract 3–1) is one in a series from a group that addresses the relationship between airways obstruction and atopy, eosinophilia, and elevated serum IgE levels (1, 2).

The paper by Sparrow and associates (Abstract 3–2) gives a nice overview of the contending risk factors for the development of airways obstruction. This complicated relationship probably will not be worked out in the near future, but has extraordinary important implications for both prevention and treatment of disabling airways obstruction.—P.B. Terry, M.D.

*References*

1. Burrows B: Possible pathogenetic mechanisms in chronic airflow obstruction. *Chest 85(suppl):13–15, 1984.*
2. Burrows B, Bloom JW, Traver GA, et al: The course and prognosis of different forms of chronic airways obstruction in a sample from the general population. *N Engl J Med* 317:1309–1314, 1987.

---

### Effects of Elastase-Induced Emphysema on Airway Responsiveness to Methacholine in Rats

Bellofiore S, Eidelman DH, Macklem PT, Martin JG (McGill Univ)
*J Appl Physiol* 66:606–612, February 1989 3–3

---

The limit to shortening of the airway smooth muscle may result from the elastic load imposed by the lung parenchyma on the muscle when it contracts. Because the effects of lung elastic recoil likely are mediated by parenchymal attachments on the airways, disruption of the parenchyma and the airway attachments in emphysema should lead to increased airway responses to methacholine. Emphysema also should attenuate the bronchodilating effects of increased lung volume. The effects of elastase-induced emphysema were examined in rats. Porcine pancreatic elastase was given intratracheally.

The peak airway response to methacholine was enhanced 3 weeks after instillation of elastase, and no plateau was noted as in baseline recordings. An increase in end-expiratory lung volume lowered peak pulmonary resistance before receiving elastase, but not afterward.

The enhanced airway response to methacholine in emphysematous rats may result from loss of elastic recoil of the lungs and lessened impedance to shortening of airway smooth muscle. A similar effect may explain some of the change in airway responsiveness associated with chronic obstructive lung disease.

▶ This study may have implications that extend beyond the obvious application to emphysema patients. It suggests that persons who have bronchospasm and small lung volumes for whatever reason may have more dyspnea for a given level of bronchial smooth muscle constriction. For example, the obese asthmatic patient may enter a vicious cycle by being given steroids to temporarily reduce bronchospasm with a resultant weight gain that reduces functional residual capacity and further accentuates the effect of bronchospasm. For the emphysema patient, this may imply reconsideration of an old British idea of giving whole lung radiation to emphysema patients to increase their elastic recoil.—P.B. Terry, M.D.

*References*

1. Ding DJ, Martin JG, Macklem PT: Effects of lung volume on maximal methacholine-induced bronchoconstriction in normal humans. *J Appl Physiol* 62:1324–1330, 1987.
2. Linhartova A, Anderson AE, Foraker AG: Radial traction and bronchial obstruction in pulmonary emphysema. *Arch Pathol* 92:384–391, 1971.

---

## Observations on Sputum Production in Patients With Variable Airflow Obstruction: Implications for the Diagnosis of Asthma and Chronic Bronchitis

Openshaw PJM, Turner-Warwick M (Brompton Hosp, London)
*Respir Med* 83:25–31, January 1989 3–4

A wide clinical spectrum characterizes patients with episodic wheezy breathlessness and physiologic evidence of airflow limitation. The present study focused on production of sputum by 145 patients aged 10 to 60 years who had clear histories of episodic wheezy breathlessness. The mean age at time of study was 35 years, and the mean age at onset of the attacks was 17 years. Ninety-eight of 130 patients (75%) had positive skin reactions. About the same proportion reported production of sputum.

Eighty-eight (68%) of 130 patients reported no marked change in production of sputum after the onset of asthmatic symptoms. Many patients produced most of their sputum during recovery rather than at the peak of an episode. Copious production of sputum was associated with more time away from school or work. Persistent airflow limitation did not correlate significantly with production of sputum. Although patients with chronic bronchitis were more likely to have smoked, the volume of sputum was unrelated to smoking.

That hypersecretion is a common feature of asthma supports the view that asthma and chronic bronchitis are not mutually exclusive diagnoses. Both hypersecretion of mucus and lowered mucus clearance may lead to accumulation within the bronchi in chronic asthma and contribute to persistent airflow limitation.

▶ Classifying patients with obstructive lung disease into the categories of asthma, bronchitis, and emphysema is comforting. There is growing recognition, however, that these are not mutually exclusive categories. As the present study shows, many patients who fulfill criteria for asthma also fulfill criteria for bronchitis. To confuse things more, original diagnoses of asthma increasingly are being changed to persistent airflow limitation (1). The heterogeneity may reflect the multiplicity of mechanisms in the development of asthma.—P.B. Terry M.D.

*References*

1. Brown PJ, Grenville HW, Finucaine KE: Asthma and the irreversible airflow obstruction. *Thorax* 39:131–136, 1984.
2. Tschopp JM, Turner-Warwick M: Persistent airflow obstruction in asthmatics receiving routine self-adjusted medication. *Eur J Respir Dis* 65:346–353, 1984.

**Morphometric Analysis of Intraluminal Mucus in Airways in Chronic Obstructive Pulmonary Disease**

Aikawa T, Shimura S, Sasaki H, Takishima T, Yaegashi H, Takahashi T (Tohoku Univ, Sendai, Japan)

*Am Rev Respir Dis* 140:477–482, August 1989 3–5

Hypersecretion of mucus is characteristic of chronic obstructive lung disease. Because fixation via the bronchus washes out mucus and alters its distribution in the airways, immersion was used for measuring intraluminal airway mucus. Autopsied lungs from 13 patients with chronic obstructive pulmonary disease and 4 normal lungs were examined morphometrically. Six study patients had chronic bronchitis, and 7 had chronic pulmonary emphysema.

Obstructive impairment in the 2 patient groups was comparable, but hypersecretion of mucus during periods of remission was much more marked in the lungs of patients with chronic bronchitis. The volume ratio of mucus to airway lumen in both the central and peripheral airways was significantly higher in the group with chronic bronchitis than in normal lungs. No comparable increase was found in lungs of patients with emphysema.

Hypersecretion of mucus leads to accumulation of mucus in the airways, which this could be a prominent contributor to airway obstruction in patients with chronic bronchitis. In contrast, mucus accumulation in the airways is not a prominent factor in chronic emphysema.

▶ This study suggests that a technical mistake in the way autopsy specimens were processed in the past led us to erroneous conclusions about the amount and distribution of mucus in the airways of patients with bronchitis and emphysema. This conclusion is supported by the fact that, when the authors fixed 1 of each pair of the lungs by the 2 methods, there was a significant difference in the amount of mucus noted in the airways of the separate lungs. The most important implication is that obstructive bronchitis may be completely reversible if mucus production can be controlled.—P.B. Terry, M.D.

*References*

1. Reid L: Measurement of the bronchial mucous gland layer: A diagnostic yardstick in chronic bronchitis. *Thorax* 15:132–141, 1960.
2. Annesi I, Kauffman F: Is respiratory mucus hypersecretion really an innocent disorder? A 22-year mortality survey of 1,061 working men. *Am Rev Respir Dis* 134:688–693, 1986.

---

**Oxygen Consumption of the Respiratory Muscles in Normal and in Malnourished Patients With Chronic Pulmonary Disease**

Donahoe M, Rogers RM, Wilson DO, Pennock BE (Univ of Pittsburgh; Presbyterian-Univ Hosp; Oakland VA Hosp, Pittsburgh)

*Am Rev Respir Dis* 140:385–391, August 1989 3–6

---

Patients with severe chronic obstructive pulmonary disease (COPD) often lose weight. An increased energy expenditure for respiration may account for the increased caloric requirements and weight loss. The oxygen cost of increasing ventilation in a group of 19 patients with COPD, 9 normally nourished and 10 malnourished, was measured to determine whether malnourished COPD patients have an increased $O_2$ cost for augmenting ventilation, whether the relative increase in resting energy expenditure in these patients is associated with an increased $O_2$ cost, and whether a relationship exists between standard pulmonary function tests and measured $O_2$ cost. Seven healthy controls were examined as well. The $O_2$ cost was measured using an open circuit method with dead-space stimulation of ventilation.

The $O_2$ cost was increased significantly in the malnourished patients compared with that in normally nourished patients and controls. Measured resting energy expenditure also was higher than predicted in the malnourished patients. Malnourished patients had a higher degree of hyperinflation and inspiratory muscle weakness.

Malnourished patients with COPD have a relative increase in resting energy requirements and elevated energy requirements for augmenting ventilation. This increase may be caused by the increased mechanical workload associated with severe COPD or a decreased ventilatory muscle efficiency, or both.

▶ This study, if confirmed by others, would explain the relationship between weight loss and mortality among patients with COPD. Its suggests that COPD patients consume their bodies to continue living with advanced lung disease.

One factor not understood is why these patients do not replenish their caloric needs. It may be that discomfort associated with eating is the limiting factor. Alternatively, hypercarbia or hypoxia, or both may be anorexigenic.—P.B. Terry, M.D.

*References*

1. Goldstein S, Askanazi J, Weissman C, et al: Energy expenditure in patient with chronic obstructive pulmonary disease. *Chest* 91:222–224, 1987.
2. Cherniack RM: The oxygen consumption and efficiency of the respiratory muscles in health and emphysema. *J Clin Invest* 38:494–499, 1959.

## Effect of Weight Gain

### Adverse Effect of Additional Weight on Exercise Against Gravity in Patients with Chronic Obstructive Airways Disease

Swinburn CR, Cooper BG, Mould H, Corris PA, Gibson GJ (Freeman Hosp, Newcastle upon Tyne, England)

*Thorax* 44:716–720, September 1989 3–7

The primary symptoms of chronic obstructive airways disease are breathlessness and effort intolerance. Excess weight in patients with this disease may have an adverse effect on exercise capacity. The effects of a small, acute, artificially induced increase in body weight on the ventilatory response to exercise and exercise capacity were determined for 14 patients with chronic obstructive airways disease and 6 healthy controls. Patients performed a 6-minute walking test and a symptom-limited step-climbing test with and without 2 leaded aprons attached, comprising 10 kg of extra weight. The controls performed a step test with and without the leaded aprons.

The additional weight did not change resting spirometric values. The median number of steps climbed by patients decreased from 67.5 to 44.5 with the additional weight. Mean ventilation and oxygen consumption rose during weighted step climbing by 14% and 13%, respectively. However, the maximal levels of ventilation and oxygen consumption attained during weighted and unweighted exercise were similar. The controls were easily able to complete 150 steps with and without the extra weight. The 6-minute walking distance in patients dropped only slightly with the added weight.

A small, acute increase in weight may substantially worsen an already decreased exercise tolerance in patients with chronic obstructive airways disease. Most physicians advise weight loss in visibly obese patients with respiratory disease; in addition, modest weight loss may benefit slightly overweight patients with symptomatic chronic obstructive airways disease.

▶ This study suggests that reduction in weight may be good for patients with chronic obstructive pulmonary disease and may increase exercise tolerance against gravity. At first glance the study appears to contradict the previous one (Abstract 3–6), which suggested that low weight was associated with increased mortality among patients with chronic obstructive pulmonary disease. The contradiction may be more apparent than real, for the weight loss in this case would not put persons at less than 90% of their ideal weights and they would be losing the weight purposefully. In the prior study, weight loss was an apparent effect of the underlying pathophysiology. To truly test the hypothesis, the author would have to make a group of slightly overweight patients lose 20 lb and then demonstrate improved exercise tolerance against gravity.

*References*

1. Hanson JS: Exercise responses following production of experimental obesity. *J Appl Physiol* 35:587–591, 1973.
2. Fairbrother MJB: Respiratory function and cardiorespiratory response to exercise in obesity. *Br J Dis Chest* 73:211–229, 1979.

---

**Body Weight in Chronic Obstructive Pulmonary Disease: The National Institutes of Health Intermittent Positive-Pressure Breathing Trial**

Wilson DO, Rogers RM, Wright EC, Antonisen NR (Univ of Pittsburgh; Univ of Manitoba; George Washington Univ, Rockville, Md)

*Am Rev Respir Dis* 139:1435–1438, June 1989 3–8

---

Physicians long have recognized the association between malnutrition and chronic obstructive pulmonary disease (COPD). However, it is unclear whether low weight is a marker of more severely impaired lung function. The effect of nutritional state on the course and prognosis of COPD was investigated retrospectively in 985 patients enrolled in the Clinical Trial of Intermittent Positive-Pressure Breathing sponsored by the National Institutes of Health. Body weight, expressed as a percentage of ideal weight, was related to numerous other features of the disease recorded.

Body weight was related directly to forced expiratory volume in 1 second ($FEV_1$); therefore, all subsequent analyses of body weight had to consider $FEV_1$. Body weight independent of $FEV_1$ appeared to influence mortality. Among patients with $FEV_1$ of less than 35%, death rates increased as body weights decreased. This relationship was stronger among patients with $FEV_1$ of 35% to 47% and strongest among patients with $FEV_1$ of more than 47%. Body weight was correlated positively with exercise capacity and was related inversely to the percent total lung capacity after adjusting for $FEV_1$. Among patients with the same $FEV_1$, body weight was strongly predictive of diffusing capacity.

Body weight influenced mortality and was inversely related to total lung capacity and diffusing capacity after adjusting for $FEV_1$. These findings support the suggestion that factors related to a patient's nutritional status independently affect the course of COPD.

▶ This retrospective study suggests that low ideal body weight is a predictor of mortality among patients with COPD. The key question is whether weight reduction is a cause of the mortality or an epiphenomenon correlated with some other factor closely associated with mortality. The direct way to determine the importance of weight is to do a randomized study in which half of the underweight, obstructed patients were fed a diet that increased their weights to within the range of ideal body weight. These persons then would be observed for evidence of clinical improvement in contrast with a control group.—P.B. Terry, M.D.

*References*

1. Wilson DO, Rogers RM, Hoffman RM: Nutrition and chronic lung disease. *Am Rev Respir Dis* 132:1347–1365, 1985.
2. Arora N, Rochester D: Effect of body weight and muscularity on human diaphragm muscle mass thickness and area. *J Appl Physiol* 52:64–70, 1982.
3. Edelman NM, Rucker RB, Deavy MM: NIH workshop summary: Nutrition and the respiratory system. *Am Rev Respir Dis* 134:347–352, 1986.

**Nutritional Repletion in Malnourished Patients With Emphysema**

Otte KE, Ahlburg P, D'Amore F, Stellfeld M (Vejle County Hosp, Denmark)

*J Parenter Enteral Nutr* 13:152–156, March–April 1989 3–9

A relationship between malnutrition and lung dysfunction has been shown in patients with emphysema pulmonum (EP). It is assumed that nutritional repletion may prove beneficial to these patients.

The effect of nutritional supplementation on the indices of anthropometrics, pulmonary function, immunologic status, and subjective well-being was assessed in 28 ambulatory malnourished patients with EP allocated into 2 groups. The 13 patients in the fed group were supplied with a nutritional formula providing 20% protein, 30% fat, and 50% carbohydrate, 1 Kcal/mL, whereas the 15 controls were given a reference product of the same consistency and taste containing 0.1 Kcal/mL. All patients drank 400 ml/day of the supplement for 13 weeks, in addition to consuming the foods in their usual diet.

The mean weight gain was significantly higher for the fed group than for the control group (mean, 1.5 vs. 0.16 kg). The mean sum of 4 skinfolds (triceps, biceps, subscapular, and suprailiac) increased significantly to 2.7 mm in the fed group but decreased by 0.9 mm in the control group. A significantly higher serum albumin difference for the fed group also was observed. Pulmonary function, immunologic status, and subjective well-being, however, did not differ between groups. A habitual high intake of energy (204% Basal Energy Expenditure) was observed in the fed group.

Although nutritional supplementation produces weight gain in malnourished patients with EP, it does not alter other indices of well-being.

▶ When emphysema patients begin losing weight steadily, they have an average of 3 years to live (1, 2). Thus, interest in the effects of the malnourished state on lung function recently has been considerable. (YEAR BOOK OF PULMONARY DISEASE, p 54, 1988.) This study, well done in that it is double-blinded, randomized, and controlled, failed to show any respiratory improvements, in contrast with previous studies. The amount of weight gain in the experimental group was small. This may account for the lack of physiologic improvement. Further well-designed studies with larger weight gains perhaps would settle this issue.—P.B. Terry, M.D.

*References*

1. VandenBerg E, VandeWoestinje KP, Gysclen A: Weight changes in the terminal stages of chronic obstructive pulmonary disease. *Am Rev Respir Dis* 95:556, 1967.
2. Renzetti AD, McClement JH, Litt BD: Veterans Administration cooperative study of pulmonary function: Mortality in relation to respiratory function in chronic obstructive pulmonary disease. *Am J Med* 41:115, 1966.
3. Wilson DO, Rogers RM, Hoffman RM: State of the art: Nutrition in chronic lung disease. *Am Rev Respir Dis* 132:1347, 1985.

## TREATMENT

### *Medical*

---

**Naloxone Does Not Alter Response to Hypercapnia or Resistive Loading in Chronic Obstructive Pulmonary Disease**

Simon PM, Pope A, Lahive K, Steinbrook RA, Schwartzstein RM, Weiss JW, Fencl V, Weinberger SE (Beth Israel Hosp; Brigham and Women's Hosp; Harvard Med School, Boston)

*Am Rev Respir Dis* 139:134–138, January 1989 3–10

---

The physiologic role of endogenous opioid peptides in ventilatory control seems to be limited, despite the well-documented ability of opiates to suppress ventilation. In recent studies it was postulated that the stress of chronic airflow obstruction in patients with chronic obstructive pulmonary disease (COPD) results in release of endogenous opioid peptides, which suppress the response to the resistive load. In a randomized, double-blind controlled trial, the role of endogenous opioid peptides and ventilatory control was assessed in 11 male patients with COPD by measuring the ventilatory and mouth occlusion pressure responses to hypercapnia and the compensatory response to an inspiratory resistive load before and after intravenous administration of naloxone or placebo on 2 separate days.

While breathing air, all 11 patients had $P_{CO_2} < 45$ mm Hg and $P_{O_2} > 70$ mm Hg. No statistically significant differences between naloxone and placebo administration were found in any index of ventilatory response to $CO_2$ or resistive loading. Minute ventilation at end-tidal $PCO_2$ ($PETco_2$ equaled 50 mm Hg in all 11 patients decreased significantly with placebo and naloxone when an inspiratory resistive load was added during $CO_2$ breathing. In 8 of the 11 patients, mouth occlusion pressure did not increase in response to the inspiratory resistive load. Those 8 patients were classified as noncompensators. Neither in the group as a whole nor in the subgroup of 8 patients classified as noncompensators, did naloxone affect the mouth occlusion pressure response to inspiratory resistive loading.

Increased activity of endogenous opioid peptides suppressing the ventilatory response to resistive loading in patients with COPD was not demonstrated. The potential role that endogenous opioid peptides play in modulating ventilation in adults with or without COPD appears to be small as shown in previous studies.

▶ There has been much interest in the role of endogenous opiates in regulating respiration. Speculation has centered on the possibility of an increased release of endogenous opiates in response to loading of the respiratory system. At present, study results present a mixed picture. Some human and animal studies have shown evidence of opioid secretion, and some have not. This study, well done in that it was double-blind and placebo-controlled, failed to show any role of endogenous opioids in the regulation of respiration. This result may, however, be the result of selection of subjects. Little work has been done in the study of endogenous opioids in persons with restrictive lung disease. At present, no role in clinical medicine is apparent for opioid antagonists in the management of obstructive lung disease.—P.B. Terry, M.D

*References*

1. Fleetham JA, Clark H, Dhingra S, et al: Endogenous opiates and chemical control of breathing in humans. *Am Rev Respir Dis* 121:1045–1049, 1980.
2. Scardella AT, Parisi RA, Dilshad PK, et al: The role of endogenous opioids in the ventilatory response to acute flow resistive loads. *Am Rev Respir Dis* 133:26–31, 1986.
3. Santiago TV, Remolina C, Scoles V, et al: Endorphins in the control of breathing. *N Engl J Med* 304:1190–1195, 1981.

**Effects of Oral Morphine on Breathlessness and Exercise Tolerance in Patients With Chronic Obstructive Pulmonary Disease**

Light RW, Muro JR, Sato RI, Stansbury DW, Fischer CE, Brown SE (VA Med Ctr, Long Beach, Calif; Univ of California, Irvine)

*Am Rev Respir Dis* 139:126–133, January 1989 3–11

Administration of opiates increases the exercise tolerance of patients with chronic obstructive pulmonary disease (COPD), but the mechanism responsible for the improved exercise tolerance has not been identified. The effects of oral opiate administration on exercise tolerance, dyspnea, and arterial blood gas levels were evaluated in patients with COPD.

Thirteen eucapnic men aged 58–70 years with stable COPD performed duplicate incremental cycle ergometer tests to exhaustion after ingesting a placebo or morphine solution. Arterial lines were inserted for testing blood on the day of active medication.

After ingestion of the morphine solution, the mean maximal work load increased by 18.6% from 78.5 to 93.1 W, and thc mean duration of exercise increased from 6.5 to 7.5 minutes (table). The mean oxygen uptake increased by 19.3%, and the mean carbon dioxide output increased by 13%. Despite the higher ventilation at maximal work load after morphine ingestion, the mean Borg score was not significantly higher. The improved exercise tolerance appears to be related to a higher arterial carbon dioxide pressure and a reduced perception of breathlessness for a given level of ventilation.

▶ Narcotics have fallen in and out of favor as dyspnea modifiers for patients with COPD. Initially, in the 1950s, narcotics were avoided when their suppression of respiration in obstructed patients was recognized. In 1981, Woodcock

Comparison of Data at Highest Equivalent Work Load After the Patients Received Placebo and Morphine

| Measurement | Placebo | Morphine |
|---|---|---|
| $\dot{V}O_2$, L/min | 0.88 ± 0.23 | 0.94 ± 0.26* |
| $\dot{V}CO_2$, L/min | 0.99 ± 0.35 | 0.95 ± 0.37 |
| Ventilation, L/min | 41.7 ± 12.7 | 38.4 ± 11.5* |
| Respiratory rate | 32.0 ± 4.55 | 28.0 ± 4.83† |
| Tidal volume, L | 1.22 ± 0.42 | 1.29 ± 0.45 |
| Borg score | 8.59 ± 2.31 | 7.08 ± 2.35‡ |
| $P_{0.1}$, cm $H_2O$ | 7.88 ± 3.45 | 6.14 ± 2.08† |
| $Pa_{CO_2}$, mm Hg | 38.3 ± 8.52 | 41.9 ± 7.83† |
| $Pa_{O_2}$, mm Hg | 71.9 ± 15.5 | 66.7 ± 11.6* |
| pH | 7.33 ± 0.05 | 7.33 ± 0.05 |
| $HCO_3^-$, mEq/L | 20.1 ± 3.38 | 21.6 ± 2.44* |
| Base excess | −4.65 ± 3.19 | −3.56 ± 2.39* |
| $Sa_{O_2}$, % | 91.4 ± 6.25 | 89.9 ± 6.40† |
| Hemoglobin | 13.5 ± 1.76 | 14.7 ± 1.65† |
| $Ca_{CO_2}$ | 17.1 ± 2.10 | 18.3 ± 2.32* |
| $\dot{V}E/\dot{V}O_2$ | 48.1 ± 8.64 | 41.5 ± 7.40‡ |
| $\dot{V}E/\dot{V}CO_2$ | 43.3 ± 5.58 | 41.9 ± 6.86 |
| VD/VT | 0.39 ± 0.12 | 0.44 ± 0.09* |
| R | 1.11 ± 0.18 | 0.99 ± 0.17‡ |
| Heart rate | 129.4 ± 21.2 | 132.3 ± 19.7 |
| Blood pressure | 146.7 ± 23.9 | 140.0 ± 15.3 |
| $O_2$ pulse | 6.81 ± 1.71 | 7.13 ± 2.03 |
| $PA_{O_2}$ | 111.9 ± 10.8 | 104.5 ± 9.89‡ |
| A-a $O_2$ | 40.0 ± 9.07 | 38.6 ± 8.74 |

*$P < .05$.
†$P < .01$.
‡$P < .001$.
(Courtesy of Light RW, Muro JR, Sato RI, et al: *Am Rev Respir Dis* 139:126–133, January 1989.)

(1) rekindled interest by reporting increased exercise tolerance in obstructed patients treated with small doses of dihydrocodeine. Subsequent studies have confirmed these initial findings. The present study suggests that the increased exercise tolerance is partially explained by a reduced amount of ventilation for a given work load and a reduced sensation of dyspnea for a given degree of ventilation.

This reviewer takes issue with a conclusion of this article, which states that narcotics should be used only in a research setting to treat obstructive pulmonary disease. Enough evidence shows that narcotics work. The issues of dosage, tolerance, and sleep-related desaturation and others can be addressed in individual patients by careful and prudent physicians. To deny patients relief when they have end-stage lung disease is not to act in the best interests of these patients.—P.B. Terry, M.D.

*References*

1. Woodcock AA, Gross ER, Gellert A, et al: Effects of dihydrocodeine, alcohol, and caffeine on breathlessness and exercise tolerance in patients with chronic obstructive lung disease and normal blood gases. *N Engl J Med* 305:1611–1616, 1981.
2. Robin ED, Burke CM: Single-patient randomized clinical trial: Opiate for intractable dyspnea. *Chest* 90:888–892, 1986.

---

**Effect of Low Dose Nebulised Morphine on Exercise Endurance in Patients With Chronic Lung Disease**

Young IH, Daviskas E, Keena VA (Royal Prince Alfred Hosp, Camperdown, Australia)

*Thorax* 44:;387–390, May 1989 3–12

---

Small doses of nebulized morphine can improve dyspnea at rest in patients with primary pulmonary hypertension. Low-dose nebulized morphine may relieve dyspnea through a direct effect on lung afferent nerves. The effects of low-dose nebulized morphine on exercise endurance were assessed in 11 adults with advanced chronic lung disease. One hour after a control endurance exercise test at 80% of maximum work load, the patients inhaled from a jet nebulizer either 5 mL of morphine, 1 mg/mL, or isotonic saline for 12 minutes. Fifteen minutes later the patients repeated the exercise test, and endurance time was recorded. The same procedure was repeated on a separate day with inhalation of the alternative solution. All patients breathed 100% oxygen from a demand valve during all exercise tests.

The mean increase in endurance time was significantly greater after morphine than after placebo inhalation (mean, 64.6 seconds vs. 8.9 seconds). The mean dose of morphine nebulized was 1.7 mg, giving a mean inhaled dose of about 0.6 mg, assuming a 30% retention of the nebulized dose by each patient. No side effects were reported.

Nebulized morphine may act directly on lung afferent nerves to reduce dyspnea. Low-dose nebulized morphine may have a role in the management of distressing dyspnea.

▶ This randomized, double-blind, placebo-controlled study suggests that very small doses of inhaled morphine can affect the sensation of dyspnea with exercise. This further suggests that opiate receptors would have to be available in the lining cells of alveoli or airways. In fact, opioid receptor immunoreactivity has been documented in bronchial mucosa. This study sets the stage for a larger trial, perhaps using larger doses of opiates or opiate-antagonists to see whether dyspnea can be increased or decreased via this mechanism.—P.B. Terry, M.D.

*Reference*

1. Bostwick DG, Null WE, Homes D, et al: Expression of opioid peptides in tumors. *N Engl J Med* 317:1439–1443, 1987.

---

**A Randomized Controlled Trial of Methylprednisolone in the Emergency Treatment of Acute Exacerbations of COPD**

Emerman CL, Connors AF, Lukens TW, May ME, Effron D (Cleveland Metropolitan Gen Hosp; Case Western Reserve Univ)

*Chest* 95:563–567, March 1989 3–13

---

Corticosteroids have an established role in the emergency treatment of acute asthma, but their role in acute exacerbations of chronic obstructive pulmonary disease (COPD) remains to be defined. In a randomized, controlled double-blind study to determine whether intravenous administration of methyprednisolone early in the treatment of acute exacerbations of COPD would improve pulmonary function in the emergency department and reduce the need for hospitalization, 96 patients aged 50 years and older age and with no history of asthma received either methyprednisolone, 100 mg, or placebo within 30 minutes after arrival in the emergency department.

Patients also received aminophylline and hourly administration of aerosolized isoetharine. Spirometry was performed initially and after the third and fifth aerosol treatments.

There was no greater improvement in pulmonary function in the steroid group than in the placebo group and there was no difference between the groups in the rate of hospitalization. In patients with eosinophilia or more severe COPD, methyprednisolone therapy did not result in a lower rate of hospitalization or greater improvement in pulmonary function.

Early administration of methylprednisolone does not affect the outcome of the emergency phase of treatment for acute exacerbations of COPD.

▶ Several studies have suggested that giving steroids to patients with COPD results in more rapid improvement in pulmonary function and shorter stays in intensive care units. These studies have suggested that certain characteristics of patients are predictive of success. Predictors that have been sited are blood eosinophilia, response to bronchodilators, and baseline variability in spirometry. The study by Albert and co-workers (3) is quoted most frequently. It suggested that the length of stay in an intensive care unit could be shortened by the use of steroids.

The present study fails to show any benefit from steroids. It must be remembered, however, that patients were observed only in an emergency room for a short period before a decision was made to admit them. The apparent failure of steroids may reflect only an inadequate period of observation.—P.B. Terry, M.D.

*References*

1. Blair GP, Light RW: Treatment of chronic obstructive pulmonary disease with corticosteroids. *Chest* 86:524–528, 1984.
2. Mandella LA, Manfreda J, Warren CP, et al: Steroid response in stable chronic obstructive pulmonary disease. *Ann Intern Med* 96:17–21, 1982.
3. Albert RK, Martin TR, Lewis SW: Controlled clinical trial of methylprednisolone in patients with chronic bronchitis and acute respiratory insufficiency. *Ann Intern Med* 92:753–758, 1980.

**Nifedipine Reduces Pulmonary Pressure and Vascular Tone During Short- but Not Long-Term Treatment of Pulmonary Hypertension in Patients With Chronic Obstructive Pulmonary Disease**

Agostoni P, Doria E, Galli C, Tamborini G, Guazzi MD (Univ of Milan)

*Am Rev Respir Dis* 139:120–125, January 1989 3–14

Nifedipine induces pulmonary vasodilation in pulmonary hypertension caused by chronic obstructive pulmonary disease (COPD). Whether the drug lowers pulmonary vascular pressure and resistance during short-term and long-term therapy, and whether pulmonary transmural pressure may be further reduced by the combined use of nifedipine and oxygen, were studied in 15 patients with COPD-related pulmonary hypertension. Changes in the pulmonary vascular tone were determined on the pulmonary driving pressure–flow curve during upright maximal exercise test.

In the short-term study the 15 patients received nifedipine, 180 mg daily, for 1 week. Short-term nifedipine therapy significantly reduced pulmonary arterial pressure (Ppa) through active pulmonary vasodilation because the pulmonary driving pressure–flow curve was shifted right and downward. That is, the right ventricle was shifted into a more advantageous preload/flow (Starling) curve. In the long-term study, 10 patients were able to continue the same nifedipine daily dosage for 2 months. They were reevaluated after 8 weeks of treatment and after nifedipine withdrawl in the following week. Both the reduction of Ppa and the active pulmonary vasodilation observed in the short-term study regressed during long-term nifedipine therapy. Oxygen inhalation was ineffective in further lowering Ppa in both short-term and long-term nifedipine therapy. On the contrary, after nifedipine withdrawl, oxygen induced Ppa reduction.

Nifedipine should not be used as long-term treatment for COPD-related pulmonary hypertension. Furthermore, because nifedipine inhibits the oxygen capability to reduce pulmonary pressure, it should be avoided for patients who need oxygen therapy.

▶ This study was not the first to suggest that pulmonary vasodilation occurs in patients with COPD who are taking nifedipine (1,2). It does suggest that long-term treatment with nifedipine is of no benefit, a statement some would dispute.

Physicians should remember that nifedipine tends to promote ventilation-profusions imbalance and hypoxemia in patients with COPD (1986 YEAR BOOK OF PULMONARY DISEASE, p 178); thus, such patients may require more supplemental oxygen.— P.B. Terry, M.D.

*References*

1. Muramoto A, Caldwell J, Albert RK, et al: Nifedipine dilates the pulmonary vasculature without producing symptomatic systemic hypotension in upright resting and exercising patients with pulmonary hypertension secondary to chronic obstructive pulmonary disesae. *Am Rev Respir Dis* 132:963–966, 1985.
2. Kennedy G, Michael J, Huang C, et al: Nifedipine inhibits hypoxic pulmonary vasoconstriction during rest and exercise in patients with chronic obstructive pulmonary disease. *Am Rev Respir Dis* 129:544–551, 1984.

---

**Prescription of Oxygen Concentrators for Long Term Oxygen Treatment: Reassessment in One District**

Walshaw MJ, Lim R, Evans CC, Hind CRK (Royal Liverpool Hosp; Univ of Liverpool, England)

*Br Med J* 297:1030–1032, Oct 22, 1988 3–15

---

When oxygen concentrators became available on Form FP10 in 1985, the Department of Health and Social Security (DHSS) issued clear guidelines for prescribing long-term oxygen treatment ($PaO_2 < 7.3$ kilopascals, $FEV_1 < 1.5$ L, forced vital capacity $< 2.0$ L). The minimal criteria included patient evaluation within a hospital setting to select those suitable for treatment, use of the oxygen concentrator for at least 15 hours a day, and cessation of smoking. Patients for whom an oxygen concentrator was prescribed in the first 22 months of their availability were reassessed to determine whether DHSS requirements were met and whether concentrators were used properly.

Only 32 of 61 patients restudied fulfilled the DHSS criteria for long-term oxygen treatment. In 17 patients the concentrator was prescribed by the general practitioner without advice from a hospital physician. For these patients the prescribed number of hours of use of the concentrator was lower than for patients who had prescriptions from a respiratory physician on the advice of a general physician.

Only 28 patients ran their concentrators for at least 15 hours a day, but this was the result of inadequate prescribing instructions rather than poor patient compliance. Twelve of 54 smokers continued to smoke. Overall only 18 of 61 patients fulfilled the minimal DHSS criteria for long-term oxygen treatment.

There is a need for better cooperation between the general practitioner and the hospital in the initial assessment of patients for long-term oxygen treatment. Both physicians and patients need better education in the use of oxygen concentrators, particularly the clinical need for a minimum of 15 hours of oxygen daily.

▶ This interesting study suggests that physicians and patients can't or won't follow simple guidelines in adopting an expensive form of long-term treatment. Some of the patients who failed to meet the criteria developed by the Department of Health and Social Security in fact may have met the criteria initially but improved sufficiently to be no longer eligible. This has been noted before, when initial hypoxia improved with additional bronchodilator therapy or other modes of therapy. The study suggests that periodic reevaluation of patients on supplemental oxygen is appropriate, both in terms of meeting physiologic criteria and in terms of comprehension of physician directions.—P.B. Terry, M.D.

*Reference*

1. Nocturnal Oxygen Therapy Trial Group: Continuous or nocturnal oxygen therapy in hypoxaemic chronic obstructive lung disease. A clinical trial. *Ann Intern Med* 93:391–398, 1980

---

**External Work Output and Force Generation During Synchronized Intermittent Mechanical Ventilation: Effect of Machine Assistance on Breathing Effort**

Marini JJ, Smith TC, Lamb VJ (Vanderbilt Univ)
*Am Rev Respir Dis* 138:1169–1179, November 1988 3–16

---

In intermittent mandatory ventilation (IMV) mechanically assisted breathing is intermixed with spontaneous breaths. The additon of timing circuitry to IMV synchronizes the onset of each machine cycle to patient effort (SIMV).

The total mechanical work performed by the patient across the spectrum of patient-initiated machine support was determined and the patient's work output and force development during consecutive spontaneous and machine-assisted breaths were compared in 12 critically ill patients who were receiving volume-cycled machine support. Over a 60- to 90-minute interval, patients were tested under 6 conditions applied in random order: fully assisted mechanical ventilation (AMV) and SIMV calculated to provide 80%, 60%, 40%, 20%, and 0% of the ventilation during AMV.

The frequency and tidal volume of spontaneous breaths increased at lower levels of mechanical ventilation; however, the inspiratory time fraction was similar across the spectrum of machine support. Inspiratory work and pressure-time product increased progressively for both spontaneous and assisted breathing cycles as machine support was withdrawn. On a per cycle basis work output was greater for assisted than for spontaneous breaths at all levels of comparison. Patients taxed their maximal ventilatory capability at all but the highest levels of support.

Patients perform substantial work at all levels of machine-assisted breathing. On a breath-by-breath basis, there appears to be little effort adaptation to machine support during SIMV.

▶ This elegant study reminds us that ventilated patients aren't being rested completely when a machine intermittently or continuously breathes for them. This is of consequence only when a patient is on a ventilator for a long period and weaning is necessary, or cardiac output is so tenuous that any redistribution of blood flow away from the diaphragm is critical to raising the mixed venous $PO_2$

The critical unanswered questions in this equation are how much and how long a rest the diaphragm must have to recover from a fatigued state. Certainly, many patients are weaned from ventilators using an intermittent mandatory ventilation mode, suggesting that the degree of rest needed for the diaphragm is less than expected if the present study is accurate. An alternative explanation is that many of these patients in fact do not have fatigued diaphragms.

*References*

1. Marini JJ, Rodriguez RM, Lamb V: The inspiratory workload of patient-initiated mechanical ventilation. *Am Rev Respir Dis* 134:902–909, 1986.
2. Roussos C, Macklem PT: Diaphragmatic fatigue in man. *J Appl Physiol* 43:189–197, 1977.

---

**Combined Use of Non-Invasive Techniques to Predict Pulmonary Arterial Pressure in Chronic Respiratory Disease**

Bishop JM, Csukas M (European Office of World Health Organization, Copenhagen)

*Thorax* 44:85–96, February 1989 3–17

---

Pulmonary arterial hypertension is known to occur in various forms of chronic respiratory disease, but complete information is lacking. The value of noninvasive procedures in predicting pulmonary arterial pressure was investigated in 370 patients with chronic obstructive lung disease and in 73 others with fibrosing alveolitis in a study conducted at 9 centers in 6 European countries.

Patients were tested for forced expiratory volume in 1 second and for arterial blood gas tensions. They also had clinical examination, electrocardiography, radiography of the pulmonary artery, echocardiography of the right ventricle, and myocardial scintigraphy.

No single variable accurately predicted pulmonary arterial pressure. Multiple stepwise regression explained nearly half the variance in pulmonary arterial pressure in patients with chronic obstructive lung disease, but it was not a useful technique for prediction. It was possible to allocate patients to bands of pulmonary arterial pressure by discriminant analysis.

Decision trees established by using either the Kolmogoroff-Smirnoff statistic or Fisher's exact test were also useful. Fisher's exact test had a sensitivity of 83% and a specificity of 91% in patients with a pulmonary artery pressure of 30 mm Hg or greater. The nonparametric tests gave better results than studies of discriminant function. In patients with fibrosing alveolitis results were similar.

The mathematical functions described in this study allow the use of combinations of noninvasive procedures to identify patients at risk for pulmonary arterial hypertension who should be studied by direct measurement. As other noninvasive methods are developed, the results can be incorporated into new functions whose value can be tested.

▶ Attempts to accurately predict pulmonary hypertension with noninvasive techniques have been made and will continue to be made. This study, flawed by lack of contemporary technology and failure of standardization between centers in a multicenter study, nevertheless raises interesting questions. One is whether incorporating contemporary technology such as the single-breath diffusing capacity and measurements of right ventricular wall thickness might help predict more accurately the presence of pulmonary hypertension.—P.B. Torry, M.D.

*References*

1. Keller CA, Shepard JW, Chun DS, et al: Pulmonary hypertension in chronic obstructive pulmonary disease: Multivariate analysis. *Chest* 90:185–192, 1986.
2. Oswald-Mammosser M, Oswald T, Nyankiye E, et al: Non-invasive diagnosis of pulmonary hypertension in chronic obstructive pulmonary disease: Comparison of ECG, radiological measurements, echocardiography, and myocardial scintography. *Eur J Respir Dis* 71:419–429, 1987.

## *Surgical*

▶ The next 2 articles (Abstracts 3–18 and 3–19) describe treatment of patients with large lung bullae. This is a particularly vexing problem for both the patient and physician. A number of articles have addressed the surgical indications for the removal of bullae and their likelihood of success.

As a general rule, dyspneic patients with bullae occupying more than a third of the hemithorax and associated with otherwise normal lung parenchyma in the nonbullous parts of the lung, are thought to benefit most from removal of large bullae. These 2 articles suggest methods less invasive than resectional surgery. Furthermore, their success rates appear to be comparable.

Bullae have been known to shrink spontaneously after being filled with inflammatory material associated with infection. Thus, one might even consider introduction of a sclerosing agent into a bullous lesion via a bronchoscope and a transbronchial needle aspiration technique.—P.B. Terry, M.D.

*References*

1. MaCarthur AM, Fountain SW: Intracavitary suction and drainage in the treatment of emphysematous bullae. *Thorax* 32:668–672, 1977.
2. Head JR: Intracavitary (Monaldi) suction. *J Thorac Surg* 15:153–161, 1946.

---

**Drainage of Giant Bulla With Balloon Catheter Using Chemical Irritant and Fibrin Glue**

Uyama T, Monden Y, Harada K, Kimura S, Taniki T (Univ of Tokushima, Japan)
*Chest* 94:1289–1290, December 1988 3–18

---

Surgery usually is contraindicated for giant bullous emphysema in compromised patients. A simple technique has been developed for draining a giant bulla with a balloon catheter, chemical irritants, and fibrin glue.

This procedure is similar to that reported by Macarthur and Fountain. The balloon catheter is connected to a water-sealed tube, and continuous negative pressure (−10 cm of $H_2O$) is applied until the bulla is diminished in size. Then OK-432, produced by incubating cultures of the low virulent Su strain of group A *Streptococcus pyogenes* treated penicillin G, is injected as an irritant into the bulla with concurrent administration of antibiotic. OK-432 facilitates aseptic inflammation to harden the wall of the bulla and the lung tissue near the bulla. After cessation of air leakage through the catheter, fibrin glue is administered into the bulla.

This method provided physical and functional improvement without major surgery for a man aged 60 years with a giant bulla and a history of pneumoconiosis and severe emphysema. Chest roentgenograms showed no progression of the bulla 2 years after this simple and safe procedure for treating a compromised patients with a giant bulla.

---

**Intracavitary Drainage for Bullous, Emphysematous Lung Disease: Experience With the Brompton Technique**

Venn GE, Williams PR, Goldstraw P (Brompton Hosp, London)
*Thorax* 43:998–1002, December 1988 3–19

---

Dominant bullae are associated with advanced and generalized emphysematous lung disease. Various surgical methods have been designed to excise the dominant bullae. Although many patients benefit from surgery, it has sometimes proved difficult to equate symptomatic improvement with improvement in respiratory function. Techniques involving intracavitary intubation have potential advantages for the treatment of bullous disease. No lung tissue is removed, and the limited incision and brief anesthesia required for the procedure are tolerated better by patients with poor lung function. To explore the limits of this technique, 22 procedures were performed on 20 patients to relieve symptoms caused by bullous lung disease.

Open intubation drainage of the bullae was used in all patients. A technique initially developed by Monaldi for treating intrapulmonay tuberculosis abscesses was modified and involves a single stage: instilling sclerosant directly into the bulla to produce rapid contraction and fibrosis within the bulla and inducing pleurodesis to minimize the immediate effect of any air leak in the pleural space.

Of the 20 patients, 3 died after surgery. Death was associated with low preoperative forced expiratory volume in 1 second and higher preoperative arterial carbon dioxide tension. Symptomatic improvement was achieved in 16 of the 17 surviving patients and was maintained for a median of 1.6 years. This improvement was accompanied by an objective improvement in lung function, with a 22% median improvement in forced expiratory volume in 1 second, an 11% decrease in total lung capacity, and a 26% median decrease in residual volume. One patient's symptoms were unchanged after surgery.

The procedure described is a simple method of decompressing bullae by means of minimally invasive surgery. It also permits treatment of further bullae later by closed intubation under local anesthetic. It is suitable for all patients but those with the poorest lung function.

## Interstitial Lung Disease

### Diagnosis

**Does Open Lung Biopsy Affect Treatment In Patients With Diffuse Pulmonary Infiltrates?**

Walker WA, Cole FH Jr, Khandekar A, Mahfood SS, Watson DC (Univ of Tennessee, Memphis)

*J Thorac Cardiovasc Surg* 97:534–540, April 1989 3–20

Open lung biopsy usually establishes a definite diagnosis in a patient with a diffuse pulmonary infiltrate; however, many clinicians eschew this procedure unless they are certain that results will lead to a change in treatment. Data on 61 patients who underwent open lung biopsy were retrospectively reviewed to determine the impact of the procedure on diagnosis and treatment of diffuse pulmonary infiltrates.

Data obtained included prior diagnostic studies, immunologic status, preoperative treatment, biopsy site, histologic and culture results, the effect of biopsy on patient management, complications, and in-hospital mortality. Of 61 patients, 22 were considered immunocompromised. Interstitial pneumonitis was diagnosed in 20 patients and interstitial fibrosis was diagnoed in 17 patients; both were nonspecific diagnoses. A total of 8 neoplastic, 7 autoimmune, and 6 infectious diseases were specifically diagnosed in 21 patients. Treatment was changed as a result of the biopsy findings for 54% of patients. In the immunocompromised group, a specific diagnosis was obtained for 59% of patients and 77% had their treatments changed. In the noncompromised group, a specific diagnosis was obtained for 21% of patients; treatment was changed for 41%. There was no difference in hospital mortality whether the diagnosis was specific or nonspecific or whether treatment was altered or not.

If diagnosis by less invasive means fails, open lung biopsy provides accurate and reliable diagnoses for both immunocompromised and noncompromised patients with diffuse pulmonary infiltrates. The morbidity and mortality associated with biopsy are acceptable. The pathologic findings will lead to a change in treatment for a large percentage of patients.

▶ This abstracted article is one of many about open lung biopsy that have been reviewed over the years in the YEAR BOOK OF PULMONARY DISEASES (1986, pp 202–204; 1989, p 198). The conclusion of this paper is similar to that of the prior papers (i.e., open lung biopsy usually offers a definitive diagnosis, but it does not appreciably affect patient outcome). This conclusion has exceptions (1), but a meta-analysis of all the papers likely would conclude no affect on patient outcome. This conclusion may be strengthened in subsequent years as the role of bronchoalveolar lavage becomes more defined.—P.B. Terry, M.D.

*References*

1. Greenman RL, Goodoll PT, King D: Lung biopsy in immunocompromised hosts. *Am J Med* 59:488–496, 1975.
2. Gaensler EA, Carrington CB: Open biopsy for chronic infiltrative lung disease: Clinical, roentgenographic, and physiologic correlation in 502 patients. *Ann Thorac Surg* 30:411–426, 1980.
3. Wall CP, Gaensler EA, Carrington CB, et al: Comparison of transbronchial and open biopsies in chronic infiltrative lung diseases. *Am Rev Respir Dis* 123:280–285, 1981.

---

**Methotrexate Pneumonitis: Bronchoalveolar Lavage Findings Suggest an Immunologic Disorder**

White DA, Rankin JA, Stover DE, Gellene RA, Gupta S (Mem Sloan-Kettering Cancer Ctr, New York; Yale Univ)

*Am Rev Respir Dis* 139:18–21, January 1989 3–21

---

Bronchoalveolar lavage specimens were taken from 6 patients with metotrexate pneumonitis to clarify the pathogenesis of this disorder. Two of the 6 were smokers. The mean dose of methotrexate was 35 mg. In addition, 3 patients with breast cancer who had bilateral infiltrates during methotrexate therapy were studied, along with 7 patients with underlying malignancy and 7 healthy persons.

The total number of cells per 100 mL of bronchoalveolar lavage fluid was significantly increased in the group with methotrexate pneumonitis; a significant increase in the absolute number of lymphocytes was responsible. There was a significant decrease in the percentage of macrophages in patients with methotrexate pneumonitis because of the increase in proportion of lymphocytes. The number of suppressor T cells was reduced and the number of helper T cells was increased in the study group, but not significantly.

Methotrexate pneumonitis is characterized by lymphocytic alveolitis with a proponderance of helper T cells. An immunologically mediated injury more likely may be a pathophysiologic mechanism than a direct toxic effect of methotrexate.

▶ This study suggests that an immunosuppressive agent can cause immunologic hypersensitivity in the lungs of some patients. The immunologic response is not unlike that of sarcoidosis. The response of "methotrexate lung" to steroids is in keeping with this analogy. That this does not occur in all patients taking methotrexates suggests a genetic co-factor as has been suggested in sarcoidosis. Against an immunologic hypersensitivity response is that rechallenge has not consistently shown recurrence of the pneumonitis. More patients must be studied to confirm this observation.—P.B. Terry, M.D.

*References*

1. Jolivet J, Cowan KH, Curt GA, et al: The pharmacology and clinical use of methotrexate. *N Engl J Med* 309:1094–1104, 1983.
2. Sostman HD, Matthay RA, Putman CE, et al: Methotrexate-induced pneumonitis. *Medicine* (Baltimore) 55:371–388, 1976.

**Long-Term Follow-Up of Drug Abusers With Intravenous Talcosis**

Paré JP, Cote G, Fraser RS (Montreal Chest Hosp Ctr; Royal Victoria Hosp, Montreal; Montreal Gen Hosp)

*Am Rev Respir Dis* 139:233–241, January 1989 3–22

In the mid-1970s data on 17 drug addicts who had injected varying quantities of methadone intravenously were reported. The degree of dyspnea, presence of talc particles in the fundi, and severity of radiographic and pulmonary function abnormalities were related to the quantity of drug abused. Six of these 17 patients were followed for 10 or more years.

Although all the addicts stopped abusing drugs, all had severe respiratory disability. Three died of respiratory disease. The evolving spectrum of radiographic and functional patterns noted was considered to be virtually diagnostic. Radiographically, an initial diffuse, pinpoint micronodularity eventually becomes associated with conglomerates, usually in the upper lobes, closely resembling the progressive massive fibrosis of the pneumoconioses. The lower lobes become relatively translucent, in some cases with bulla formation and the development of pneumothorax. Pulmonary function, which initially has both restrictive and obstructive features, is eventually markedly obstructive with hyperinflation and air trapping. In this late stage pathologic assessment shows emphysema in addition to the granulomatous inflammation and fibrosis surrounding the talc particles in the pulmonary interstitium.

This complication associated with the intravenous injection of talc may be a clue to the pathogenesis of the more common type of emphysema related to cigarette smoke.

▶ This study suggests that talc injected intravenously can, in some instances, give a radiographic picture similar to that of inhaled silica exposure and a physiologic response similar to that of smoking-induced emphysema. Curiously, the authors don't contrast the typical radiographic, physiologic, and pathologic changes of talc inhalation with those of intravenous talc use. Talc inhalation usually is associated with a radiographic pattern of interstitial lung disease and a physiologic pattern of restriction.

The conclusion of the study is flawed, however, because all the patients for whom smoking status was reported were smokers (smoking status of the last patient in this series is unknown) and it may be that smoking is a necessary co-factor in the development of this pattern of disease. This might be analogous to the evidence that smoking asbestos workers have a higher incidence of radiographic abnormalities than nonsmoking asbestos workers.—P.B. Terry, M.D.

*References*

1. Stern WZ, Subbarao K: Pulmonary complications of drug addiction. *Sem Roentgenol* 18:183–197, 1983.
2. Hunt AC: Massive pulmonary fibrosis from the inhalation of talc. *Thorax* 11:287–294, 1956.

## Treatment

### Randomised Controlled Trial Comparing Prednisolone Alone With Cyclophosphamide and Low Dose Prednisolone in Combination in Cryptogenic Fibrosing Alveolitis

Johnson MA, Kwan S, Snell NJC, Nunn AJ, Darbyshire JH, Turner-Warwick M (Brompton Hosp, London)

*Thorax* 44:280–288, April 1989 3–23

Several uncontrolled studies show that immunosuppressant drugs may be as effective as corticosteroids in treatment of cryptogenic fibrosing alveolitis, as well as have less serious side effects. In a randomized, controlled study, 43 patients with previously untreated fibrosing alveolitis were treated with either cyclophosphamide plus alternate-day low-dose prednisolone (Cyclophosphamide-Prednisolone series) (no. = 21), or alternate-day prednisolone with an initial high-dose phase (prednisolone alone series) (no. = 22). All patients had been followed for at least 3 years.

Seven patients in the prednisolone-alone series and 5 patients in the cyclophosphamide-prednisolone series improved. At 3 years, only 5 in the prednisolone series were either improved or stable and still in their allocated regimen, as were 5 of the patients in the cyclophosphamide-prednisolone series. Three patients from the latter group stopped taking cyclophosphamide because of toxicity.

Life-table analysis suggested better survival in patients in the cyclophosphamide-prednisolone series, but this was not significant. At 3 years, 10 of the 22 patients in the prednisolone series died compared with 3 of the 21 patients in the cyclophosphamide-prednisolone series. Time until failure of the first treatment regimen or death was significantly longer for patients in the cyclophosphamide-prednisolone series, partly because of the better lung volumes in this group on admission. Patients with initial total lung capacity (TLC) less than 60% predicted did badly, whereas those with a TLC of 80% or more predicted did well with both regimens. Patients with a TLC of 60% to 79% predicted did significantly better with the cyclophosphamide regimen. Although the dose of cyclophosphamide used was moderately low, 6 patients had a fall in the neutrophil or platelet count and microscopic hematuria developed in 1; these effects were rapidly reversed when the drug was discontinued. It is interesting that 5 of these patients remained stable for up to 6 years after stopping or reducing cyclophosphamide and continued with low-dose prednisolone.

Cyclophosphamide in combination with low-dose prednisolone is at least as effective as prednisolone alone with an initial high-dose phase in the treatment of cryptogenic fibrosing alveolitis. Toxicity is limited and rapidly reversible with reduction or termination of drug usage. Unfortunately, many patients failed to respond to both these drug regimens.

▶ The dismal prognosis of cryptogenic fibrosing alveolitis (idiopathic pulmonary fibrosis) has led to a variety of immunosuppressive agents being given in an attempt to suppress the inflammatory process. This well-done study explores the value of cyclophosphamide as an adjunct to low-dose prednisolone therapy. The conclusion is mixed. No major difference was seen between the prednisolone-only group and the cyclophosphamide-treated patients, but there was a hint that stability may persist longer in some of the cyclophosphamide-treated group.—P.B. Terry, M.D.

*References*

1. Crystal RG, Fulmer JD, Roberts WC, et al: Idiopathic pulmonary fibrosis: Clinical, histologic, radiographic, physiologic, scintographic, cytologic, and biochemical aspects. *Ann Intern Med* 85:769–788, 1976.
2. Brown CH, Turner-Warwick M: Treatment of cryptogenic fibrosis alveolitis with immunosuppressant drugs. *Q J Med* 40:289–302, 1971.
3. Turner-Warwick M: Future possibilities of therapeutic intervention, in Bouhys A (ed): *Lung Cells in Disease*. Amsterdam, North-Holland, 1976, pp 329–340.

---

**Advanced Cryptogenic Fibrosing Alveolitis: Preliminary Report on Treatment With Cyclosporin A**

Alton EWFW, Johnson M, Turner-Warwick M (Brompton Hosp, London)

*Respir Med* 83:277–279, July 1989 3–24

---

The etiology of cryptogenic fibrosing alveolitis (CFA) is unknown, but the immune system has been implicated. Seven patients with CFA who failed to respond to corticosteroids or immunosuppressives were treated with cyclosporin A. The patients were not responding to prednisolone and cyclophosphamide and were deteriorating. At the beginning of cyclosporin A therapy, 6 had progressive breathlessness for at least the preceding 3 months.

After 1 month of cyclosporin A therapy 6 patients reported improvement or no further worsening of dyspnea. No substantial changes were seen on chest radiographs. Results from 3 patients fit enough to undergo tests confirmed reports of improvement, with a more than 15% increase in lung function. However, the initial favorable response was not maintained. When compared with a control group matched for severity of disease, survival among the cyclosporin A group was doubled, from 2.5 to 5 months. Side effects, although generally not substantial, occurred in almost all patients. In 1 patient dose adjustment controlled the adverse effects.

Cyclosporin A therapy was attempted at a late stage in these patients when any substantial improvement was unlikely. Initially many patients had a favorable response to treatment, but this response was not maintained. Cyclosporin A treatment of patients with less severe disease seems justified.

▶ This interesting study may be a ray of hope in the otherwise gloomy world of idiopathic pulmonary fibrosis. Because one hypothesis is that idiopathic pulmonary fibrosis is a T cell-mediated disease, it is reasonable to try a drug such as cyclosporin A, which interferes with T cell function. These preliminary results are encouraging. The mean survival of idiopathic pulmonary fibrosis is approximately 4.5 years after diagnosis. This reviewer treated a single patient with cyclosporin A for 8 years before he died. More studies are needed to clarify this drug's value.— P.B. Terry, M.D.

*Reference*

1. Borel JF, Fever C, Gubler HU, et al: Biological effects of cyclosporin A: New anti-lymphocytic agent. *Agents Actions* 6:432–440, 1976.

---

**Inhaled Corticosteroids Can Modulate the Immunopathogenesis of Pulmonary Sarcoidosis**

Spiteri MA, Newman SP, Clarke SW, Poulter LW (Royal Free Hosp and School of Medicine, London)

*Eur Respir J* 2:218–224, March 1989 3–25

---

Pulmonary sarcoidosis, a chronic inflammatory disease characterized by a T cell alveolitis and the formation of granulomas within the lung interstitium, has a variable clinical course. Aberrant immunologic reactions apparently cause the inflammatory response seen in patients. In most patients sarcoidosis is self-limiting and resolves with or without treatment. However, the granulomas persist in 20% of patients, leading to an insidious development of fibrosis, which produces significant morbidity and mortality. On the hypothesis that persistence of granulomas and fibrosis observed in pulmonary sarcoidosis are features determined as much by alveolar macrophages as by T-lymphocytes, the effect of inhaled corticosteroids on the phenotypes and functional capacity of macrophages obtained by bronchoalveolar lavage from 10 patients with pulmonary sarcoidosis was studied.

Ten patients with previously untreated symptomatic sarcoidosis having radiologic parenchymal shadowing and abnormal pulmonary function received 800 μg of budesonide twice daily through a pressurized metered dose inhaler for 16 weeks. Five other patients with sarcoidosis and similar features received placebo as did 10 healthy volunteers. Results were correlated with clinical status and therapeutic effectiveness.

In the 10 patients receiving budesonide therapy 10% of the inhaled drug appeared in the alveoli. Symptomatic relief was noted in all 10 treated patients with sarcoidosis; there were no adverse effects. Significant resolution of radiologic shadowing was seen in 3 of the 10. No significant change in pulmonary function occurred in any group. A marked decrease in bronchoalveolar lavage lymphocytosis was observed in those patients receiving budesonide, but no such change was seen in the other 2 groups. Inhaled budesonide produced a reduction in the proportion of RFD1+ cells after 16 weeks with a dramatic decrease in the proportion of macrophages expressing RFD1+D7+, which was not seen in either placebo group.

In pulmonary sarcoidosis, inhaled budesonide can modulate the aberrant immunologic reactions present, and it may provide concomitant symptomatic relief without side effects. A significant decrease in lavage lymphocytes was produced concurrently with a change in the phenotype and functional characteristics of the alveolar macrophage population.

▶ This interesting study raises the question of the value of inhaled steroids in treating inflammatory diseases in the lung. Inhalational therapy has received mixed reviews. Although beneficial for asthma and the treatment of *Pneumocystis carinii* pneumonia, it has not been as successful in the treatment of bacterial infections. Part of the problem may be the method of delivery or the dose available at the alveolar level. Aerosol therapy may be much more effective than we think, but may simply lack technicologic development.—P.B. Terry, M.D.

*Reference*

1. Selroos OB: Use of budesonide in the treatment of pulmonary sarcoidosis. *Ann NY Acad Sci* 465:713–721, 1986.

## Lung Transplantation

▶ ↓ The next 3 articles (Abstracts 3–26 through 3–28) address the value of single- and double-lung transplantation in emphysema patients. This patient population has not been considered recently for lung transplantation because of poor results in the early 1970s and because of presumed accentuation of the ventilation-perfusion mismatch that, theoretically, occurs with unilateral transplantation. An additional factor is the usual age of most emphysema patients, which is beyond that considered acceptable in transplant programs. The 3 abstracts that follow suggest that the questions of both unilateral and bilateral transplantation in emphysema patients should be reexplored from the physiologic point of view. Still, the advanced stage of most emphysema patients may preclude the use of these techniques.

The expenditure of enormous sums of money for patients near the end of their lives already is being questioned in intensive care medicine and in transplant programs in general. This issue undoubtedly will arise concerning lung transplantation in older persons.—P.B. Terry, M.D.

*References*


1. Vanderhoeft PJ, Rocmans P, Nemry C, et al: Left lung transplantation in a patient with emphysema. *Surgery* 103:505–509, 1971.
2. Wildevuur CRH, Benfield JR: A review of 23 human lung transplantations by 20 surgeons. *Ann Thorac Surg* 9:489–515, 1970.
3. Veith FJ, Koerner SK: Problems in the management of human lung transplant patients. *Vasc Surg* 8:273–282, 1974.
4. Cooper JD, Ginsberg RJ, Goldberg M: The Toronto Lung Transplant Group: Unilateral transplantation for pulmonary fibrosis. *N Engl J Med* 314:1140–1145, 1986.


---

**Unilateral Lung Transplantation in Panlobular Emphysema**

Pariente R, Mal H, Andreassian B (Hôp Beaujon, Clichy, France)

*Presse Med* 18:347–349, Feb 18, 1989 3–26

---

The first successful unilateral lung transplantation was performed in 1971 in a patient who survived for 10 months. However, few subsequent lung transplantations have been successful. Since 1983 unilateral lung transplantation has been restricted to patients with diffuse pulmonary fibrosis, whereas panlobular emphysema (PLE) has been rejected by other investigators as an indication for unilateral lung transplantation. This policy is based on the belief that the contralateral emphysematous lung will expand, compress the pulmonary graft, and interfere with the functioning of the lung transplant.

Because of the limited number of heart-lung transplantations being done, and because the authors take issue with the belief that unilateral lung transplantation is contraindicated for patients with PLE, 5 unilateral lung transplantations in patients with PLE were performed. All 5 patients were given cyclosporine and azathioprine postoperatively for immunosuppression.

The patients, 4 men and 1 woman, aged 51–65 years, had uneventful postoperative courses and are still alive. One patient has survived for 9 months, despite 2 episodes of rejection, and 1 patient has survived for 8 months. Follow-up for the other 3 patients has been short, ranging from 21 to 40 days. One patient is in guarded condition, but the others are in good condition. The lung grafts are functioning well by both subjective and objective criteria. The long-term outcome cannot be predicted on the basis of these few patients. However, the results to date suggest that PLE does not need to be considered a contraindication to unilateral lung transplantation.

**Single Lung Transplantation for Severe Chronic Obstructive Pulmonary Disease**

Trulock EP, Egan TM, Kouchoukos NT, Kaiser LR, Pasque MK, Ettinger N, Cooper JD, Washington Univ Lung Transplant Group (Washington Univ)

*Chest* 96:738–742, October 1989 3–27

Single lung transplantation has been considered inappropriate for patients with chronic obstructive lung disease (COPD). The high compliance and increased vascular resistance of the native lung presumably could cause unacceptable ventilation-perfusion mismatching or overinflation of the native lung, with consequent encroachment on expansion of the transplanted lung. One man with severe COPD who underwent a single-lung transplant in March 1989 has returned to an active life.

A man, 60, with COPD was referred for double-lung transplantation. He had severe airflow obstruction with minimal hypercapnia; oxygenation was adequate on 1.5 L/min of oxygen. Results of a radionuclide ventriculogram were normal. Single lung transplantation was offered because of a shortage of donor material. After a structured pulmonary rehabilitation program a left lung transplant was carried out without complications. Despite ventilation-perfusion mismatching in the first postoperative weeks, resting gas exchange was normal on breathing room after the second week. At 14 weeks the peak oxygen uptake was 37% of predicted maximum, and there was no evidence of ventilatory limitation. There were 2 episodes of presumed acute allograft rejection. The patient was doing well in the fifth posttransplant month and has returned to work and to an active lifestyle.

Single lung transplantation may be a reasonable approach to selected patients with COPD who are not candidates for double-lung transplantation. The procedure is not, however, suitable for patients with generalized bronchiectasis.

**Double-Lung Transplant for Advanced Chronic Obstructive Lung Disease**

Cooper JD, Patterson GA, Grossman R, Maurer J, Toronto Lung Transplant Group (Univ of Toronto)

*Am Rev Respir Dis* 139:303–307, February 1989 3–28

Four women and 2 men aged 33 to 47 years with chronic obstructive lung disease underwent double-lung transplantation between November 1986 and October 1987. Only patients who had progressive, disabling illness and a life expectancy of 12 to 18 months were considered for the operation. All were oxygen dependent or had had life-threatening respiratory failure in the past year.

Marked thoracic hyperinflation rapidly resolved after lung transplantation. In 3 cases the lungs were retrieved some distance from the surgical center. Oral cyclosporine and intravenous injections of azathioprine were used for immunosuppression, along with antilymphoblast globulin. Suspected rejection episodes were managed with intravenous injections of methylprednisolone.

Ischemic airway complications occurred in 3 patients; 1 had a short circumferential stricture at the origin of the left main bronchus, in another the membranous part of the tracheal anastomosis failed to heal satisfactorily and a retrotracheal air space formed, and 1 had ischemic necrosis of the membranous wall of the donor trachea with dehiscence of part of the anastomosis. All 6 recipients were well 5 to 15 months after operation. A seventh transplant failed in a patient with primary pulmonary hypertension.

The en bloc double-lung transplant procedure is suitable for patients with adequate right ventricular function. For these patients the cardiac component of the heart-lung transplant adds significant liability and limits the number of suitable donors. Heart-lung transplantation remains ideal for patients with pulmonary hypertension and irreversible right ventricular failure.

## Cigarette Smoking

**Trends in Cigarette Smoking in the United States: The Changing Influence of Gender and Race**

Fiore MC, Novotny TE, Pierce JP, Hatziandreu EJ, Patel KM, Davis RM (Ctrs for Disease Control, Atlanta)

*JAMA* 261:49–55, Jan 6, 1989 3–29

To determine the trends in prevalence, initiation, and cessation of cigarette smoking in the United States, weighted and age-standardized data from 7 National Health Interview Surveys taken from 1974 to 1985 were reviewed. Smokers were identified as "ever" smokers, current smokers, or former smokers. All results were stratified by race and sex to evaluate differences between black and white persons and men and women. Other racial groups were excluded because of insufficient sample size.

There was a linear decline in smoking prevalence, with the prevalence for men decreasing at .91 percentage point per year to a smoking rate of 33.5% in 1985. The prevalence for women decreased by .33 percentage point per year to 27.6% in 1985. The smoking rate for white persons declined .57 percentage point per year to 29.4% in 1985, and the smoking rate for black persons declined by .67 percentage point per year to 35.6% in 1985 (Fig 3–1).

From 1974 tp 1985 cessation of smoking increased among all sex–race groups. The rates for white and black persons were similar, but the smoking cessation rate was higher for women than for men. The rate of smoking initiation declined among young men; for young women, it re-

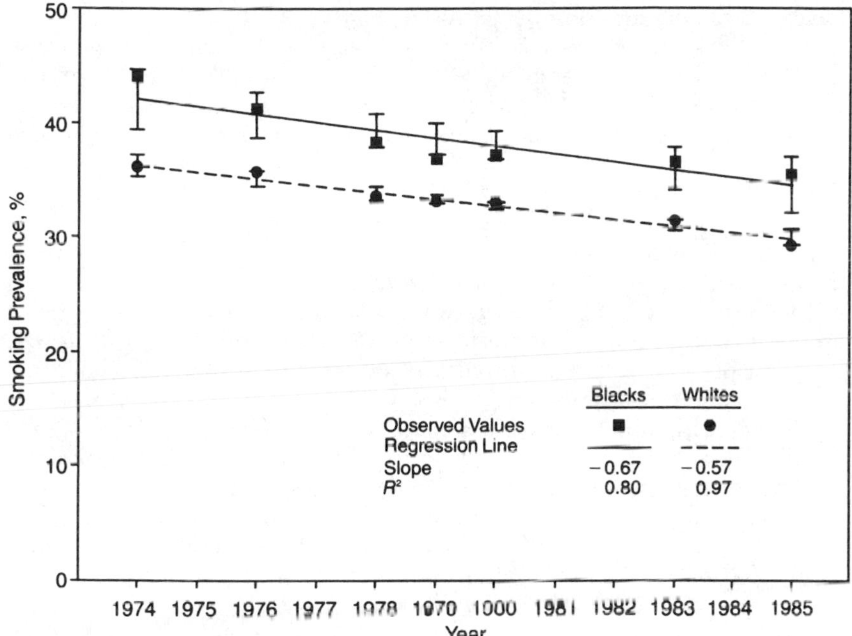


Fig 3–1.—Weighted and age-standardized smoking prevalence among blacks and whites aged 20 years and more from 1974 to 1985 in National Health Interview Surveys in United States. (Courtesy of Fiore MC, Novotny TE, Pierce JP, et al: *JAMA* 261:49–55, Jan 6, 1989.)

mained about the same. Initiation of smoking decreased more rapidly among black persons than among white persons.

Smoking is decreasing among all sex–race groups, but smoking prevalence is declining at a slower rate for women than for men. Converging prevalence rates among men and women are occasioned more by differences in initiation than by differences in cessation.

▶ It is hard to imagine, but if the trends projected in this study continue into the 1990s, women eventually will smoke more than men in the United States. This may result in a significant change in the sexual distribution of smoking-related diseases. Already, male lung cancer rates appear to be declining while female rates continue to rise. Postmenopausal coronary artery disease may increase significantly as may other smoking-related diseases in women.—P.B. Terry, M.D.

*References*

1. Devesa SS, Diamond EL: Socioeconomic and racial differences in lung cancer incidence. *Am J Epidemiol* 118:818–831, 1983.
2. Davis RM: Current trends in cigarette advertising and marketing. *N Engl J Med* 316:725–732, 1987.

### Passive Smoking on Commercial Airline Flights

Mattson ME, Boyd G, Byar D, Brown C, Callahan JF, Corle D, Cullen JW, Greenblatt J, Haley NJ, Hammond SK, Lewtas J, Reeves W (Natl Cancer Inst, Bethesda, Md; Prospect Associates, Rockville, Md; American Health Found, Valhalla, NY; Univ of Massachusetts, Worcester; Environmental Protection Agency, Research Triangle Park, NC, et al)

*JAMA* 261:867–872, Feb 10, 1989 3–30

Data on in-flight exposure to nicotine and urinary levels of cotinine, a major metabolite of nicotine, and symptom self-reports were obtained from 4 attendants and 5 passengers on 4 routine commercial flights of approximately 4 hours' duration. Exposures to nicotine were measured by using personal exposure monitors, and urine samples were collected for 72 hours after each flight.

All persons had measurable exposure to environmental tobacco smoke on all flights, but exposure was highly variable, with some nonsmoking areas having levels comparable to or higher than those in smoking sections. The type of aircraft ventilation was an important factor in the levels of in-flight nicotine exposure. Those with 100% fresh air had significantly less ambient nicotine than those with 50% fresh air and 50% recirculating air. The levels of environmental tobacco smoke led to increased urinary levels of cotinine in both passengers and attendants, with the highest levels of cotinine occurring in passengers with the greatest smoke exposure. Changes in eye and nose symptoms between the beginning and end of the flights and perception of annoyance and smokiness in the airplane cabin were related to both in-flight nicotine exposure and urinary excretion of cotinine.

Total separation of smoking and nonsmoking sections was not achieved on the flights that were studied. This presents another contributor to the cumulative health risk, acute irritation, and annoyance that nonsmoking persons receive from passive smoking.

### Controlled Trial of Transdermal Nicotine Patch in Tobacco Withdrawal

Abelin T, Buehler A, Müller P. Vesanen K, Imhof PR (Univ of Berne; Ciba-Geigy, Basel, Switzerland)

*Lancet* 1:7–10, Jan 7, 1989 3–31

Substitution of nicotine for cigarettes can lessen abstinence symptoms and the craving for tobacco. A transdermal nicotine patch system (TNS) was evaluated in a double-blind study of patients from 21 general medical practices. The patch delivers 0.7 mg/cm$^2$ of nicotine per 24 hours and is available in 10-, 20-, and 30-cm$^2$ sizes. The large patch was used in persons smoking more than a pack a day and the 20-cm$^2$ patch in the others.

The effect of the TNS was most marked in persons with high Fagerström tolerance scores. Of 100 actively treated persons, 36% were abstinent at 3 months, compared with 23% of the 99 placebo recipients. Body weight increased only in placebo recipients. Craving and withdrawal symptoms decreased more in the TNS group. The patches were generally well tolerated. The important question remains of whether the TNS promotes continuing abstinence from smoking.

▶ This study, which superficially shows promising results, should be viewed with skepticism. First, the study is reported after only 3 months of follow-up. Those steeped in the smoking literature will acknowledge that 9- to 12-month follow-up generally is considered the gold standard. It is interesting that the authors say this is a 9-month study, raising the question why they presented the material at this time. Second, the difference between the placebo and nicotine patch groups, although statistically significant, is not dramatic. Third, the recidivism rate for the placebo group is not typical of the usual placebo group, which generally shows a decline in the number of successful quitters with time. Fourth, a drug company apparently was involved actively with the study to the extent that the company is acknowledged in the authorship section of the paper.—P.B. Terry, M.D.

*References*

1. Hughes JR, Hatsukami DK, Pickens RW, et al: Effect of nicotine on the tobacco withdrawal syndrome. *Phys Pharmacol* 83:82–87, 1984.
2. Lam W, Sze PC, Sacks HS, et al: Meta-analysis of randomized controlled trials of nicotine chewing-gum. *Lancet* 2:27–30, 1987.

---

**Persistent Increase in Caffeine Concentrations in People Who Stop Smoking**

Benowitz NL, Hall SM, Modin G (San Francisco Gen Hosp Med Ctr; Univ of California, San Francisco; San Francisco VA Med Ctr)
*Br Med J* 298:1075–1076, Apr 22, 1989 3–32

---

Recent reports have shown that cigarette smokers drink more coffee on average than nonsmokers and metabolize caffeine much more rapidly. The rate at which caffeine is metabolized declines when smokers stop smoking, and concentrations of caffeine in the body should rise if consumption of caffeine remains the same. In view of recent data showing increased risks of coronary heart disease in and low birth weights of children of heavy coffee drinkers, persistent increases in caffeine concentrations may cause concern. Plasma caffeine concentrations and caffeine consumption before and 6 months after persons gave up smoking were studied. Sixty-four persons were evaluated at 12 weeks, and 61 persons, at 26 weeks.

Persons who continued smoking were significantly older, with a mean of 42.8 years, vs. 36.2 years for nonsmokers. Cigarette consumption, number of years of smoking, and plasma cotinine and caffeine concentrations were not significantly different between those who gave up and those who continued smoking. Plasma caffeine concentrations in persons who stopped smoking were more than double the baseline value at 12 and 26 weeks. Throughout the study caffeine concentrations in smokers changed little. At 26 weeks persons who stopped smoking had significantly decreased their caffeine consumption.

The hypotheses that plasma caffeine concentrations increase after people give up smoking and remain increased for at least 6 months were confirmed. The increase was substantial and averaged more than 250%. Caffeine concentrations were unchanged, as expected for persons who continued to smoke. In caffeine concentrations, an increase of 250% is equivalent to drinking 2.5 times as many cups of coffee or tea each day. Therefore, smokers who abstain would be at continuing high risk because of their caffeine consumption if there is a dose response relation between coffee consumption and coronary heart disease or infants with low birth weights that is mediated by caffeine. Patients should be advised that continuing to consume coffee at the same level may exacerbate the tobacco withdrawal syndrome and contribute to increased health risks. They should be encouraged to reduce their consumption.

▶ This paper presents a hypothesis to explain why smokers drink more coffee (to maintain a certain caffeine level) but fails to point out that, if that were the prime regulator, they should be expected to dramatically increase coffee consumption after smoking cessation. Because the authors show that caffeine levels are increased after smoking cessation, it is unlikely that one can accept the initial hypothesis that they drink more coffee to maintain a certain caffeine level. Social factors may be much more important in explaining coffee drinking habits in smokers.—P.B. Terry, M.D.

*References*


1. Parsons WD, Neims AH: Effect of smoking on caffeine clearance. *Clin Pharmacol Ther* 24:40–45, 1978.
2. LaCroix AZ, Mead LA, Liang K-Y, et al: Coffee consumption in the incidence of coronary heart disease. *N Engl J Med* 315:977–982, 1986.


## Bronchoscopy

**Bronchoscopy to Evaluate Hemoptysis in Older Men With Nonsuspicious Chest Roentgenograms**

Lederle FA, Nichol KL, Parenti CM (Minneapolis VA Med Ctr; Univ of Minnesota)

*Chest* 95:1043–1047, May 1989 3–33

Whether the risk of cancer is high enough to warrant bronchoscopy in patients with hemoptysis and a nonsuspicious chest roentgenogram is debatable. The rate of cancer detection and the yield of treatable disease identified with bronchoscopy was determined in 106 men aged more than 40 years (mean age, 61 years) who underwent fiberoptic bronchoscopy for hemoptysis and had a nonsuspicious chest roentgenogram.

Six patients (5.7%) had cancer diagnosed at bronchoscopy, representing 1 cancer for every 18 bronchoscopic examinations performed. Of the

5 bronchogenic carcinomas, 4 appeared to be surgically resectable. Cancer patients were significantly older (mean age, 70 years), had smoked within the last 5 years, and had a significantly higher frequency of central abnormalities on chest roentgenogram that might prevent clear visualization of the central lung fields. Six additional bronchogenic carcinomas were diagnosed during the 32-month follow-up period; 2 of these were probably present but not detected at the time of bronchoscopy. Apart fom the diagnosis of cancer, fiberoptic bronchoscopy contributed little to the evaluation of hemoptysis.

Because of the appreciable risk of cancer, hemoptysis with a nonsuspicious roentgenogram remains an indication for bronchoscopy in older men with substantial history of smoking. Most of these cancers are in early development and surgically resectable. A chest roentgenogram in which the central lung fields are obscured in any way should not be considered negative in patients with hemoptysis. In addition, a negative bronchoscopic examination does not exclude the possibility of cancer in these patients.

▶ This study presents an interesting question. When does the yield of a procedure become so low that it is no longer worth doing? In this study, 5.7% of the patients had diagnoses of cancer; 4.6% of these cancers were surgically resectable. Would 2% or 1% have been an unacceptably low yield? When the yield of a procedure is low but the outcome of the study is extremely important, rather than screen large numbers of patients to find the small percentage who are positive, it is extremely important to develop studies that examine all the historical, physical, and laboratory information so risk factors that increase the probability of a positive test will be found. Thus, a history of symptoms compatible with acute bronchitis accompanying the hemoptysis may decrease the probability that the hemoptysis is tumor-associated. The authors have looked at and found some discriminating factors. It is important to look for more to reduce the number of unnecessary bronchoscopies.—P.B. Terry, M.D.

*References*

1. Peters J, McClung HC, Teague RB: Evaluation of hemoptysis in patients with normal chest roentgenograms. *West J Med* 141:624–626, 1984.
2. Snider GL: When not to use the bronchoscope for hemoptysis. *Chest* 76:1–2, 1979.
3. Adelman M, Haponik EF, Bleecker ER, et al: Cryptogenic hemoptysis: Clinical features, bronchoscopic findings, and natural history in 67 patients. *Ann Intern Med* 102:829–834, 1985.

---

**Fibreoptic Bronchoscopy in Smear-Negative Pulmonary Tuberculosis**

Chawla R, Pant K, Jaggi OP, Chandrashekhar S, Thukral SS (Univ of Delhi, India)

*Eur Respir J* 1:804–806, October 1988 3–34

---

The role of fiberoptic bronchoscopy in reaching an early bacteriologic diagnosis of pulmonary tuberculosis was studied in 50 sputum smear-negative patients. Positive smears for the acid-fast bacilli (AFB) were obtained in 28 brushings, 12 bronchial aspirates, and 14 postbronchoscopic sputum samples. Bronchial biopsy specimens provided the diagnosis in 9 of 30 patients. After combining all these results, diagnoses were established rapidly for 36 of 50 patients. When culture results were available, definite diagnoses of pulmonary tuberculosis were made for 45 patients. The yield of AFB was significantly better from brush smears than from bronchial aspirate smears and postbronchoscopic smears.

Fiberoptic bronchoscopy is a useful ancillary procedure in making the diagnosis of pulmonary tuberculosis in smear-negative patients. Brush smears provide a high yield of AFB, particularly when they are made exclusively from the caseous material in the bronchi.

▶ This study and others clearly have shown that fiberoptic bronchoscopy is an appropriate secondary diagnostic technique when the clinical suspicion of tuberculosis is high but sputum smears are negative. This approach poses a health hazard to bronchoscopists, however. When the index of suspicion is high, it is not unreasonable to begin antituberculous therapy for 5–10 days before bronchoscopy is performed. This generally will not interfere with culture or stain results.

*References*

1. Danek SJ, Bower JS: Diagnosis of pulmonary tuberculosis by flexible fiberoptic bronchoscopy. *Am Rev Respir Dis* 119:677–679, 1979.
2. Wallace JM, Deutsch AL, Harell JH, et al: Bronchoscopy and transbronchial biopsy in evaluation of patients with suspected active tuberculosis. *Am J Med* 70:1189–1191, 1981.
3. Russell MD, Kenneth GT, Michael FT: A ten-year experience with fiberoptic bronchoscopy for mycobacterial isolation: Impact of Bactec system. *Am Rev Respir Dis* 131:1069–1071, 1986.

---

## The Role of Fiberoptic Bronchoscopy in Evaluating the Causes of Pleural Effusions

Chang S-C, Perng R-P (Natl Yang-Ming Med College, Taipei, Taiwan)
*Arch Intern Med* 149:855–857, April 1989 3–35

---

Fiberoptic bronchoscopy, in addition to thoracentesis and closed pleural biopsy, was performed in 140 consecutive adults with pleural effusion of unknown origin, seen in 1983–1985. Thirty-nine patients had various nonneoplastic disorders, and 95 had a diagnosis of malignancy. In 6 patients, no definite diagnosis was made, despite an aggressive work-up and follow-up for a year or longer.

A final diagnosis was provided by pleural examination in 68 patients and fiberoptic bronchoscopy in 58. Bronchoscopy was used to diagnose malignancies in 56 patients and tuberculosis in 2. Bronchoscopy or pleural examination established the final diagnosis in 100 of the 140 patients. All 52 patients with abnormal bronchoscopic findings proved to have malignant tumors.

Fiberoptic bronchoscopy was especially productive in patients first seen with hemoptysis or concurrent pulmonary lesions on chest radiography. Thoracentesis with closed pleural biopsy was more productive in the absence of hemoptysis or roentgenographic abnormalties other than effusions.

▶ This very practical study documents what one would suspect intuitively. However, 1 group of patients with tumors may have negative pleural and bronchoscopic evaluations. Those patients have neoplastic involvement of hilar lymphatics who are first seen with pleural effusions. It is not surprising that process-oriented studies that document the appropriate sequence of diagnostic studies were seldom done in the past. As cost constraints become more important, it is likely that we are going to see more such studies.—P.B. Terry, M.D.

*References*

1. Williams T, Thomas P: The diagnosis of pleural effusion by fiberoptic bronchoscopy and pleuroscopy. *Chest* 80:566–569, 1981.
2. Feinsilver SH, Barrows AA, Braman SS: Fiberoptic bronchoscopy and pleural effusion of unknown origin. *Chest* 90:516–519, 1986.
3. LeRoux BT: Bronchial carcinoma with pleural effusion. *S Afr Med J* 42:865–866, 1968.

## Miscellaneous

### Submaximal Invasive Exercise Testing and Quantitative Lung Scanning in the Evaluation for Tolerance of Lung Resection.

Olsen GN, Weiman DS, Bolton JWR, Gass GD, McLain WC, Schoonover GA, Hornung CA (Univ of South Carolina)

*Chest* 95:267–273, February 1989 3–36

Lung resection is a hazardous procedure in patients with cardiopulmonary dysfunction. The value of submaximal exercise testing and lung scanning is evaluating patients before lung resection was studied in 52 elderly men with lung masses and airflow obstruction. After resting ventilatory assessment and quantitative lung scanning, cycle exercise was done at work loads of 25 and 40 W.

Seven of 29 patients who had operation could not tolerate lung resection and died within 60 days or were ventilator dependent for a prolonged time. The cardiac index, oxygen delivery, and calculated peak oxygen uptake during exercise most clearly separated patients who tolerated surgery from those who did not. Peak oxygen consumption during exercise appeared to be an important predictor of tolerance for lung resection.

Submaximal exercise testing can help identify those patients who can survive the stress of lung resection. It does not, however, predict the likelihood or the type of complications. Peak oxygen uptake reflects both cardiac function and oxygen transport.

▶ This is one of a variety of studies over the years that have been done to determine risk factors for postoperative mortality after resectional surgery in patients with pulmonary dysfunction. Some of the factors that have been thought to be helpful are maximal voluntary ventilation less than 50% of predicted, forced vital capacity less than 70% of predicted, maximal oxygen consumption, pulmonary vascular resistance greater than 190 dynes/sec/cm$^5$, and postoperative $FEV_1$ less than 0.8 L. All have some utility, but none are perfect. The attractive feature of this study is its suggestion that a certain level of cardiovascular reserve may be necessary to help one through the complications that may occur after surgery. Further refinement obviously is necessary.—P.B. Terry, M.D.

*References*


1. Gass GD, Olsen GN: Preoperative pulmonary function testing to predict postoperative morbidity and mortality. *Chest* 89:127–135, 1986.
2. Smith TP, Kinasewitz GT, Tucker WY, et al: Exercise capacity as a predictor of post-thoracotomy morbidity. *Am Rev Respir Dis* 129:730–734, 1984.


---

**Low Glucose and pH Levels in Malignant Pleural Effusions: Diagnostic Significance and Prognostic Value in Respect to Pleurodesis**

Rodríguez-Panadero F, López Mejías J (Virgen del Rocío Univ Hosp, Seville, Spain)

*Am Rev Respir Dis* 139:663–667, March 1989 3–37

---

Results of a previous study suggested that a low pH level is indicative of the extension of a malignant pleural lesion. These findings, however, were based on only a small number of patients. A larger study was conducted to investigate the diagnostic and prognostic significance of low pleural glucose and pH levels in 77 patients with malignant pleural effusions.

Patients underwent chest roentgenography and thoracoscopic exploration. Pleural and arterial gases, blood cell count, glucose, lactate dehydrogenase, total protein count, and the cytologic yield of the pleural fluid were determined. Cultures were evaluted for tuberculous organisms. Some patients underwent pleurodesis, followed by clinical and radiographic evaluation after 1 month. Patients underwent periodic examinations until they died; when possible, the final cause of death was investigated. Seventy-seven pleural neoplasms were diagnosed from 116 thoracoscopic examinations. Cancer of the lung and breast were the most common findings. Sixteen patients had pleural glucose levels less than 60 mg/dL; pleural pH was less than 7.30 in 18 patients. There were highly significant differences in the extent of lesions when the group with low glucose values was compared with those with high glucose values; differences were even greater when pH was considered. There was a statistically significant relationship between positive cytologic results and extension of the lesions. Mean glucose values in patients with failed pleurodesis was 66 mg/dL compared with values of 108 mg/dL in those for whom pleurodesis was successful (Fig 3–2).

Both pH levels and pleural glucose are valuable predictors of the out-

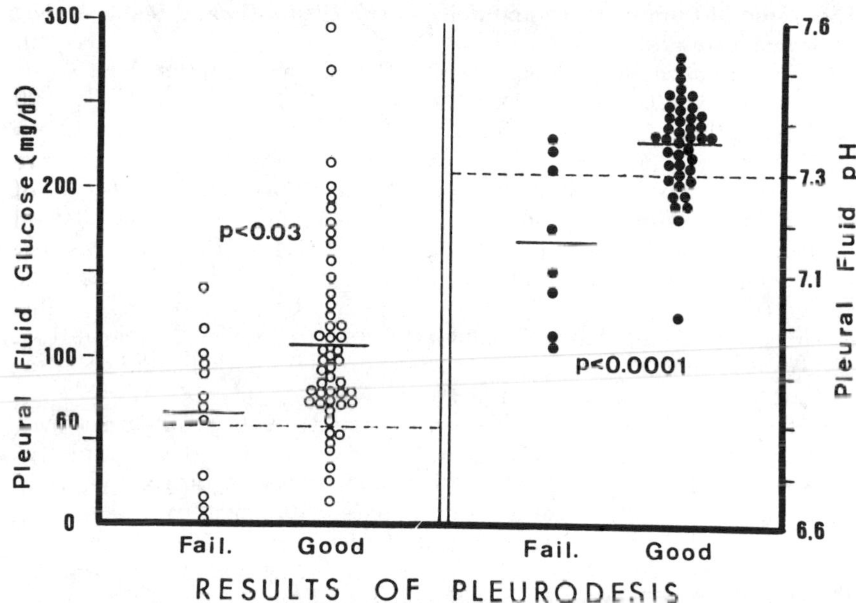


Fig 3–2.—Results of pleurodesis. *Horizontal short lines,* means of the groups. The low glucose group (less than 60 mg/dL) had 42% fail, and the low pH group (less than 7.30) had 36% fail, against 15% and 8% respectively, in the higher groups. (Courtesy of Rodríguez-Panadero F, López Mejías J: *Am Rev Respir Dis* 139:663–667, March 1989.)

come of pleurodesis; approximately half the attempts will fail if glucose or pH levels, or both, are low. When levels are high, the outcome will be good in about 90% of patients; when glucose levels are less than 60 mg/dL, the cytologic yields will be positive in approximately 87% of patients.

▶ The management of malignant pleural effusions continues to be problematic, for a significant number of patients do not achieve permanent obliteration of pleural space after the instillation of a substance introduced to create pleural inflammation. Failure of pleurodesis usually reflects an inability to keep the inflamed pleural surfaces together long enough to achieve adherence. This is more likely to occur with greater neoplastic involvement of the pleural surface. Thus, the findings of this study are consistent, for the low pH and glucose reflect a greater extent of pleural involvement with tumor.—P.B. Terry, M.D.

*Reference*

1. Sahn SA, Good JT: Pleural fluid pH in malignant effusions: Diagnostic, prognostic, and therapeutic implications. *Ann Intern Med* 108:345–349, 1988.

## The Value of Computed Tomography in the Diagnosis and Management of Bronchiectasis

Pang JA, Hamilton-Wood C, Metreweli C (The Chinese Univ of Hong Kong; Prince of Wales Hosp, Shatin, Hong Kong)
*Clin Radiol* 40:40–44, January 1989 3–38

Conflicting results in the diagnosis of bronchiectasis with CT have been reported. Thus, the role of CT in the diagnosis and management of bronchiectasis is unclear. The effectiveness of CT in the diagnosis and management, as distinct from only the diagnosis, of bronchiectasis was evaluated.

The clinical, lung function, and radiologic data of 38 patients suspected of having the disease were reviewed. All 38 patients had chest radiographs, CT scans, and bronchograms.

The patients' radiologic studies were examined sequentially in 3 stages: stage I, chest radiograph; stage II, CT; and stage III, bronchography. A decision was made at the end of each stage either to proceed with the next stage or to stop because further investigation was considered unlikely to change patient management. Criteria for proceeding included apparent normality, equivocal abnormality, or unilateral abnormality. Criteria for stopping after a firm diagnosis had been made at the preceding stage included being unfit for surgery, unequivocal bilateral disease, or mild disease.

Radiographic studies were halted at stage I in 4 (11%) patients because chest radiographs revealed bilateral bronchiectasis and 2 patients had poor lung function. Studies were stopped at stage II in 15 (39%) patients, with 12 having bilateral disease on CT and 3 having unilateral disease on CT but with clinical features so mild that bronchography was considered unjustified. Scrutiny of the CT and bronchography films of the patients who were judged not to require CT or bronchography confirmed that no change in their management was needed. In the 19 remaining patients who proceeded to stage III, bronchography was not useful in 4 (11%) because of underfilling; however, it was useful in 15 (39%) patients because it confirmed or refuted CT findings.

In the investigation of patients suspected of having bronchiectasis, CT should precede bronchography despite its relative insensitivity compared with that procedure. Careful scrutiny of plain chest radiographs and CT findings as well as clinical data will show bronchography to be unnecessary in the diagnosis and management of a substantial proportion of patients.

▶ The diagnosis of bronchiectasis traditionally has required a bronchogram. With the advent of CT, it has become possible to make the diagnosis noninvasively. However, the sensitivity and specificity of CT scanning have been disputed. This study, in which both CT and bronchograms were done in all patients, shows that bronchograms still have a place in the evaluation of patients, but a preceding CT may obviate the need for this more invasive and risky test.—P.B. Terry, M.D.

*References*

1. Naidich DP, McCauley DI, Khouri NF, et al: Computed tomography of bronchiectasis. *J Comput Assist Tomogr 6:437–444, 1982.*
2. Phillips MS, Williams, MP, Flower CDR: How useful is computed tomography in the diagnosis and the assessment of bronchiectasis? *Clin Radiol* 37:321–325, 1986.

**The Development of Subsensitivity to Atropine Methylnitrate: A Double-Blind, Placebo-Controlled Crossover Study**

Vaughan TR, Bowen RE, Goodman DL, Weber RW, Nelson HS (Fitzsimons Army Med Ctr, Aurora, Colo)

*Am Rev Respir Dis* 138:771–774, October 1988 3–39

When combined with β-agonists or theophylline, anticholinergic agents have been found to provide additional bronchodilation. Subsensitivity to a variety of β-agonists has been reported as a decrease in the response to a drug or hormone resulting from chronic stimulation of its receptor. With anticholinergic agents the development of subsensitivity has not been reported previously. A double-blind, placebo-controlled crossover study was designed to assess the effectiveness of nebulized atropine methylnitrate (AMN) with chronic use in 22 patients with asthma. Ten received theophylline and inhaled β-agonists, and 12 were receiving corticosteroids in addition. Either spontaneously or after use of the bronchodilator, all patients had demonstrated at least a 15% change in forced expiratory volume in 1 second. For 4 hours after inhalation of the initial dose, and again after 2 weeks of 4-times-daily use, the bronchodilator effect was measured serially.

When compared with the effect of placebo, a significant bronchodilator effect was seen initially with AMN (Fig 3–3). The bronchodilator ef-

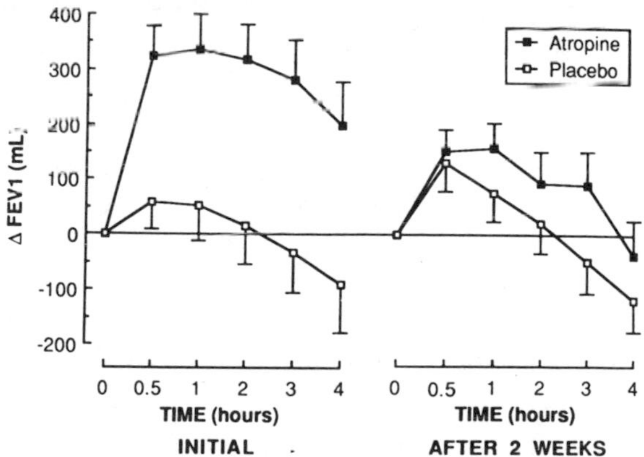


**Fig 3–3.**—The bronchodilator effect of 2 mg of atropine methylnitrate (AMN) compared with placebo when AMN was used for the first time (**left panel**) and after 2 weeks of 4-times-daily use (**right panel**). *Bar,* standard error of the mean. (Courtesy of Vaughan TR, Bowen RE, Goodman DL, et al: *Am Rev Respir Dis* 138:771–774, October 1988.)

fect of AMN was significantly diminished after 2 weeks of use compared with its initial effect, but was still better than placebo. Adverse side effects with AMN were minimal.

Prolonged administration of AMN resulted in a partial loss of the bronchodilator effect that was attainable when the drug was first used. The significance of the diminished effect clinically is not known. It remains to be determined whether continued loss of bronchodilator effect would occur with even longer use.

▶ Anticholinergics have become first-line therapy for many patients with chronic obstructive pulmonary disease. They are particularly attractive because of the relative absence of significant side effects in a population of patients who often have arrhythmias and occasional adverse responses to high-dose β-sympathomimetic therapy.

The study by Vaughn and colleagues is one of the first to suggest that anticholinergic responses may be similar to β-sympathomimetic responses in that there is a reduction in sensitivity with repetitive use. This observation needs to be verified but, if true, suggests that we may have to adjust our dosing schedules upward with time.—P.B. Terry, M.D.

*References*

1. Jenne JW, Chick TW, Stricklan RD, et al: Subsensitivity of beta-responses during therapy with a long acting beta-2 preparation. *J Allergy Clin Immunol* 59:383–390, 1977.
2. Storms WW, Bodman SF, Nathan RA, et al: Use of impratropium bromide in asthma. *Am J Med* 81:61–65, 1986.

# 4 Pulmonary Vascular Disease and Critical Care

## Introduction

Compared with the previous year, this year has not produced any easily recognizable landmark studies, such as the discovery of endothelin or the publication of large-scale clinical trials of steroid therapy in ARDS or septic shock. The articles this year offer refinements of familiar themes: the potential role of tumor necrosis factor, surfactant replacement therapy in acute lung injury, the use of inspiratory resistance in patients that are difficult to wean, a method to assess the optimal amount of pressure support, and the value of formalized weaning protocols. The selected articles are grouped into the following categories: pathophysiology and therapy of acute lung injury, weaning from the ventilator, pulmonary vascular disease, and general critical care.

**John R. Michael, M.D.**

## Acute Lung Injury

► ↓ The first 3 abstracts, as well as Abstract 4–11, discuss the potential role of tumor necrosis factor α in the pathophysiology of acute lung injury. The following three articles (Abstracts 4–4 through 4–6) emphasize rare but potentially treatable causes of acute lung injury; the next 4 articles (Abstracts 4–7 through 4–10) continue the theme that surfactant therapy may be helpful in patients with adult respiratory distress syndrome (ARDS); the subsequent 2 articles (Abstracts 4–11 and 4–12) illustrate the growing indications that the methylxanthine pentoxifylline may reduce acute lung injury; and the final 3 articles in this section (Abstracts 4–13 through 4–15) discuss fluid management, the development of pleural effusions, and residual impairment in ARDS.—J.R. Michael, M.D.

---

**Tumour Necrosis Factor in Bronchopulmonary Secretions of Patients With Adult Respiratory Distress Syndrome**

Millar AB, Foley NM, Singer M, Johnson NM, Meager A, Rook GAW (Univ College and Middlesex School of Medicine, London; Natl Inst for Biological Standards and Control, South Mimms, England)

*Lancet* 2:712–714, Sept 23, 1989 4–1

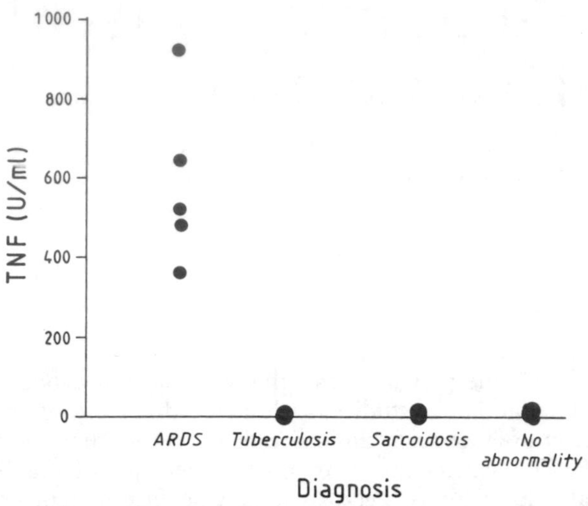


**Fig 4–1.**—Tumor necrosis factor *(TNF)* in bronchopulmonary secretions from patients with adult respiratory distress syndrome *(ARDS)* and controls. (Courtesy of Millar AB, Foley NM, Singer M, et al: *Lancet* 2:712–714, Sept 23, 1989.)

Concentrations of tumor necrosis factor (TNF) are elevated in patients with septicemia, and it has been suggested that TNF is a mediator of adult respiratory distress syndrome (ARDS). This possibility was examined in 5 adults who required mechanical ventilation for respiratory failure caused by ARDS. All were afebrile for at least 48 hours before the study. Bronchoscopic specimens were obtained from 24 control patients.

The mean level of TNF in bronchopulmonary secretions from patients with ARDS was 523 units/mL. In contrast, TNF was not detected in bronchopulmonary secretions or in bronchoalveolar lavage fluid from control patients (Fig 4–1). (The control patients had tuberculosis, sarcoidosis, or hemoptysis of unknown origin.)

Local production of TNF in the lungs appears to be important in the pathogenesis of ARDS. Treatment with anti-TNF antibody, intravenously or by nebulizer, may be beneficial to patients at risk or those with established ARDS.

---

**Tumor Necrosis Factor α-Induced Pulmonary Vascular Endothelial Injury**

Goldblum SE, Hennig B, Jay M, Yoneda K, McClain CJ (VA Med Ctr, Baltimore; Univ of Maryland; VA Med Ctr, Lexington, Ky; Univ of Kentucky)

*Infect Immun* 57:1218–1226, April 1989 4–2

---

Experimental models of acute lung injury have exhibited increased circulating tumor necrosis factor-alpha (TNF-α), and TNF-α has been shown to induce endothelium and monocytes to produce interleukin-1, a possible mediator of acute lung injury. The in vivo effects of infusion of human recombinant TNF-α were studied in rabbits preinfused with $^{125}$I-labeled albumin. A control group received saline infusions.

Infusions of TNF-α increased lung wet-dry weight ratios by about 150%, and the ratio of $^{125}$I activity in bronchoalveolar lavage fluid to plasma increased by 376%, compared with values for controls. Ultrastructural study of lung sections revealed endothelial injury, perivascular edema, and extravasation of a permeability tracer.

In vitro studies of porcine pulmonary artery endothelial cell monolayers showed increased transendothelial albumin flux in the absence of granulocyte effector cells.

Recombinant TNF-α can produce acute pulmonary vascular endothelial injury both in vitro and in vivo. It appears that TNF may have a role in the pathogenesis of acute lung injury and ARDS. It may act alone or in conjunction with other endogenous mediators to induce lung injury.

---

**Human Recombinant Tumor Necrosis Factor Alpha Infusion Mimics Endotoxemia in Awake Sheep**

Johnson J, Meyrick B, Jesmok G, Brigham KL (Vanderbilt Univ; Cetus Corp, Emeryville, Calif)

*J Appl Physiol* 66:1448–1454, March 1989 4–3

---

The most frequent and most lethal risk factor for adult respiratory distress syndrome is gram-negative bacterial sepsis. The endotoxin of bacterial cell walls is considered a major lung toxin, and it has been suggested that an endogenous monokine, tumor necrosis factor alpha (TNFα), mediates the injurious effects of endotoxin on the lungs. The effects of a single infusion of human recombinant TNFα were studied in 6 chronically instrumented awake sheep after a dose of 0.01 mg/kg was infused over 30 minutes.

Pulmonary artery pressure peaked within 15 minutes of the start of the infusion. The pulmonary hypertension was accompanied by hypoxemia and leukopenia in both the peripheral blood and lung lymph, which persisted during the 4-hour study. Flow of protein-rich lung lymph then increased, indicating increased pulmonary microvascular permeability. Cardiac output and left atrial pressure did not change significantly. Light-microscopic examination of lung tissue at autopsy showed congestion, sequestration of neutrophils, and patchy interstitial edema.

The pulmonary response to recombinant human TNFα in awake sheep is similar to the effects of endotoxemia. Because endotoxin is known to stimulate production of TNFα, it is reasonable to suppose that TNFα may mediate endotoxin-induced lung injury. In addition, endotoxin may well exert direct toxic effects on pulmonary endothelial cells.

▶ These 3 articles and Abstract 4–11 provide further evidence that TNFα may play an important pathophysiologic role in noncardiogenic pulmonary edema. See the 1989 YEAR BOOK OF PULMONARY DISEASE, pages 141–145, for related articles on TNFα. In Abstract 4–1, high levels of TNF were found in the bronchoalveolar lavage fluid from 5 intubated patients with ARDS, but not in control patients. Unfortunately, none of the control patients were intubated.

Abstracts 4–2, 4–3, and 4–11 demonstrate that TNFα can cause pulmonary edema and increase pulmonary vascular permeability in intact animals and increase albumin flux across pulmonary artery endothelial cells. Because endotoxin can stimulate the production of TNFα, it has been proposed to mediate some of endotoxin's physiologic effects. Abstract 4–3 demonstrates that infusion of TNFα into awake sheep reproduces many of the physiologic and biochemical effects caused by infusing *Escherichia coli* endotoxin. Pretreatment with a monoclonal antibody to TNFα, however, apparently prevents the effects of infusing TNFα, but does not prevent the effects of *E. coli* endotoxin. Thus, TNFα may cause lung injury, but its role in the pulmonary pathophysiology of *E. coli* endotoxin is unclear.—J.R. Michael, M.D.

**Acute Eosinophilic Pneumonia as a Reversible Cause of Noninfectious Respiratory Failure**

Allen JN, Pacht ER, Gadek JE, Davis WB (Ohio State Univ Hosps, Columbus)
*N Engl J Med* 321:569–574, Aug 31, 1989 4–4

Three men and 1 woman aged 20 to 64 years were seen in the past 2 years with a distinct form of idiopathic lung disease that appeared to be acute respiratory failure. The patients, all previously healthy, had marked eosinophilia in bronchoalveolar lavage fluid. Infectious causes of lung disease were excluded, and the 4 had prompt responses to steroid therapy.

These patients had had acute febrile illness for less than a week when first seen. All had severe hypoxemia and diffuse lung infiltrates. Eosinophils made up 28% to 50% of the effector cells recovered during lavage at admission. Erythromycin therapy was ineffective, but the dyspnea, in-

Results of Bronchoaveolar Lavage

| Patient No. | Time of Bronchoscopy | Macrophages | Lymphocytes | Neutrophils | Eosinophils* |
|---|---|---|---|---|---|
| | | | *percent* | | |
| 1 | Admission | 8 | 3 | 61 | 28 |
| | Day 3 | 15 | 17 | 21 | 47 (178) |
| | Day 5 | 62 | 1 | 0 | 37 |
| | Day 30 | 74 | 2 | 4 | 20 (243) |
| | Day 45 | 93 | 6 | 0 | 1 (7) |
| 2 | Admission | 15 | 30 | 5 | 50 |
| | Day 44 | 78 | 13 | 1 | 8 (5) |
| | Day 293 | 95 | 3 | 2 | 0 (0) |
| 3 | Admission | 3 | 36 | 17 | 44 |
| | Day 409 | 97 | 2 | 0 | 1 (3) |
| 4 | Admission | 54 | 0 | 0 | 46 (215) |
| | Day 96 | 97 | 2 | 1 | 0 (0) |

*Figures in parentheses are numbers of cells ($\times 10^{-3}$) per milliliter of lavage fluid.

(Courtesy of Allen JN, Pacht ER, Gadek JE, et al: *N Engl J Med* 321:569–574, Aug 31, 1989.)

filtrates, and hypoxemia resolved rapidly when steroid therapy was begun. Symptoms did not recur after prednisone was tapered or during follow-up ranging from 5 to 21 months. After steroids were discontinued, lavage fluid contained 1% or fewer eosinophils (table).

Differential cell counts should be routinely done on bronchoalveolar lavage specimens, because acute eosinophilic pneumonia may be clinically indistinguishable from acute infectious pneumonia and adult respiratory distress syndrome.

▶ In patients with acute respiratory failure, fever, and bilateral radiographic infiltrates, this treatable diagnosis should be considered. Many patients do not have peripheral eosinophilia (1). To avoid missing the diagnosis, the authors suggest that differential cell counts be done routinely on BAL secretions. Patients respond quickly to steroid therapy with 40 to 60 mg a day. When steroids were stopped after 10 days to 12 weeks of therapy, the illness did not reappear during follow-up for at least 5 months.—J.R. Michael, M.D.

*Reference*

1. Badesch DB, King TE Jr, Schwarz MI: Acute eosinophilic pneumonia: A hypersensitivity phenomenon? *Am Rev Respir Dis* 139:249–252, 1989.

**Wegener's Granulomatosis Presenting as Acute Respiratory Failure With Anti-Neutrophil-Cytoplasm Antibodies**

Lenclud C, De Vuyst P, Dupont F, Depierreux M, Ketelbant P, Goldman M (Free Univ of Brussels)

*Chest* 96:345–347, August 1989 4–5

Anti-neutrophil-cytoplasm antibodies (ANCA) recently have been found in sera of patients with Wegener's granulomatosis, and it has been proposed that the ANCA titer may reflect disease activity. Two patients with Wegener's granulomatosis had acute respiratory failure and circulating ANCA.

*Case 1.*—Woman, 69, had positive findings on immunofluorescence (IF) testing for serum ANCA at the time a lung biopsy specimen showed typical lesions of Wegener's disease, with granulomas and necrotizing vasculitis. Despite steroid and cyclophosphamide therapy the patient died of septic shock caused by *Staphylococcus aureus* infection from a central venous catheter.

*Case 2.*—Man, 70, with progressive dyspnea and hemoptysis had negative findings on immunologic tests except for ANCA in high titer by both indirect IF testing and enzyme-linked immunosorbent assay. The patient recovered satisfactory lung function on treatment but died 4 months later with pulmonary aspergillosis and gram-negative septicemia.

The presence of ANCA in a patient with acute respiratory failure suggests the possibility of necrotizing vasculitis, particularly Wegener's granulomatosis. Immunosuppressive therapy is appropriate when ANCA are demonstrated in sera.

▶ Anti-neutrophil-cytoplasm antibodies recently have been described as a marker of activity in Wegener's granulomatosis (1). Two types of antibodies have been identified. Antibodies that distribute in a perinuclear immunofluorescence pattern in alcohol-fixed neutrophils appear to bind myeloperoxidase. The antibodies that produce diffuse cytoplasmic immunostaining appear to bind to proteinase 3. Proteinase 3 is a recently described serine proteinase produced by human white cells that can cause emphysema (2). In addition to occurring in patients with Wegener's, ANCA have been reported in a few patients with polyarteritis nodosa, necrotizing and cresenteric glomerulonephritis, and systemic lupus erythematous (3–4).—J.R. Michael, M.D.

*References*

1. Van der Woude FJ, Rasmussen N, Lobatto S, et al: Autoantibodies against neutrophils and monocytes: Tool for diagnosis and marker of disease activity in Wegener's granulomatosis. *Lancet* 1:425–429, 1985.
2. Kao RC, Wehner NG, Gray BH, et al: Proteinase 3: A distinct human polymorphonuclear leukocyte proteinase which produces emphysema in hamsters. *J Clin Invest* 82:1963–1973, 1988.
3. Savage COS, Winearls CG, Jones S, et al: Prospective study of radioimmunoassay for antibodies against neutrophil cytoplasm in diagnosis of systemic vasculitis. *Lancet* 1:1389–1393, 1987.
4. Falk RJ, Jennette JC: Anti-neutrophil cytoplasmic autoantibodies with specificity for myeloperoxidase in patients with systemic vasculitis and idiopathic necrotizing and crescentic glomerulonephritis. *N Engl J Med* 318:1651–1657, 1988.

---

**Pulmonary Edema in Cocaine Smokers**

Hoffman CK, Goodman PC (San Francisco Gen Hosp)

*Radiology* 172:463–465, August 1989 4–6

---

The medical risks of cocaine smoking are well known. Pneumomediastinum and pneumothorax resulting from barotrauma are the most common reported radiographic abnormalities. Five patients aged 21–41 years were seen with pulmonary edema after smoking cocaine. All reported chest pain and shortness of breath on admission. Other symptoms included minimally productive cough, mild hemoptysis, pedal edema, and abdominal pain. All but 1 admitted cocaine smoking.

Arterial blood gas determinations showed decreased oxygenation and associated respiratory alkalosis. All 5 patients had chest radiographic findings compatible with pulmonary edema. These abnormalities resolved within 24–72 hours regardless of whether the patient received treatment. No other cause of pulmonary edema was found.

Pulmonary edema is another complication of cocaine smoking that first may be detected radiographically. Its presence in a young, otherwise healthy patient without predisposing factors should alert a radiologist to the possible diagnosis of cocaine abuse.

► Smoking cocaine can produce a variety of medical complications (1). The reported pulmonary complications include pneumothorax and pneumomediastinum (2), pulmonary hemorrhage (3), bronchiolitis obliterans organizing pneumonia (4), transient pulmonary infiltrates with eosinophilia (5), and noncardiogenic pulmonary edema (6). The finding of increased protein in the bronchoalveolar lavage fluid from 1 patient suggests that the pulmonary edema occurs because of an increase in vascular permeability (6). The development of pulmonary edema appears associated with cocaine smoking within the previous 24 hours. One patient had a history of multiple episodes of edema temporally related to cocaine smoking. The lung injury appears mild, with resolution within 24 to 48 hours. Fortunately, the incidence of pulmonary edema appears low (7). Because cocaine also may cause coronary vasoconstriction and myocardial infarction (8), this cause must be excluded for any cocaine smoker with pulmonary edema. (See the 1988 YEAR BOOK OF CRITICAL CARE MEDICINE, pp 301–302).—J.R. Michael, M.D.

*References*


1. Cregler L, Mark H: Medical complications of cocaine abuse. *N Engl J Med* 315:1495–1499, 1986.
2. Mundinger MO: Pneumopericardium from cocaine inhalation. *N Engl J Med* 313:46–47, 1985.
3. Murray RJ, Albin RJ, Mergner W, et al: Diffuse alveolar hemorrhage temporally related to cocaine smoking. *Chest* 93:427–429, 1988.
4. Patel RC, Dutta D, Schonfeld SA: Free base cocaine use associated with bronchiolitis obliterans pneumonia. *Ann Intern Med* 107:186–187, 1987.
5. Kissner DG, Lawrence DW, Selis JE, et al: Crack lung: Pulmonary disease caused by cocaine abuse. *Am Rev Respir Dis* 136:1250–1252, 1987.
6. Cucco RA, Ok HY, Cregler L, et al: Nonfatal pulmonary edema after "free base" cocaine smoking. *Am Rev Respir Dis* 136:179–181, 1987.
7. Eurman DW, Potash HI, Eyler WR, et al: Chest pain related to "crack" cocaine smoking: Value of chest radiography (abstract). *Radiology* 169(P):302, 1988.
8. Isner JM, Estes NAM, Thompson PD, et al: Acute cardiac events temporally related to cocaine abuse. *N Engl J Med* 315:1438–1443, 1986.


---

**Type II Pneumocyte Changes During Hyperoxic Lung Injury and Recovery**

Holm BA, Matalon S, Finkelstein JN, Notter RH (Univ of Rochester; Univ of Alabama, Birmingham)

*J Appl Physiol* 65:2672–2678, December 1988 4–7

---

Pulmonary oxygen toxicity involves surfactant-related pathology, but the degree of change in type II cell function is uncertain. Biochemical changes were examined in type II cells from the lungs of rabbits exposed for 64 hours to 100% oxygen and then allowed to recover for varying periods in room air. Laser flow cytometric analyses were performed on single cell suspensions of type II pneumocytes.

Lung injury was characterized by reduced levels of alveolar surfactant and a subsequent rebound. In vivo change in levels of alveolar phospholipid correlated well with the cellular lipid metabolic changes seen in isolated type II pneumocytes. The isolated cells had a 60% reduction in phosphatidylcholine synthesis, cell lipid content, and glycerol-3-phosphate (G-3-*P*) acyltransferase activity. This enzyme catalyzes 1 of the early reactions in phosphoglyceride synthesis. All variables then began to recover with rebound effects apparent about 3 days after exposure. The number of type II cells in S-phase was increased at this time.

The changes in lung phospholipids observed in vivo after toxic exposure to oxygen may be at least partly explained by changes in surfactant biosynthesis by type II pneumocytes.

**Effect of Exogenous Surfactant Instillation on Experimental Acute Lung Injury**

Harris JD, Jackson F Jr, Moxley MA, Longmore WJ (St Louis Univ)

*J Appl Physiol* 66:1846–1851, April 1989 4–8

Instillation of exogenous pulmonary surfactant is beneficial in the human neonatal respiratory distress syndrome. Its role in models of acute lung injury other than quantitative surfactant deficiency states is uncertain. The *N*-nitroso-*N*-methylurethane (NNNMU) model of acute lung injury in the rat was developed to simulate human adult respiratory distress syndrome. The effects of exogenous surfactant instillation on the biochemical and physiologic changes on these injured animals were investigated.

The NNNMU induced an acute lung injury in the rat characterized by gross lung injury, hypoxemia, increased mortality, a previously unreported alveolitis, and changes in the pulmonary surfactant system. These alterations in surfactant included a reduction in the ratio of phospholipid to protein, reduced surface activity, and alterations in the relative percentages of the individual phospholipids compared with controls. Treatment of the NNNMU lung injury with exogenous surfactant (100 mg/kg of Survanta) improved oxygenation, reduced mortality to control values, and returned to control values the surfactant phospholipid-to-protein ratio, surface activity, and with the exception of phosphatidylglycerol, the relative percentages of individual surfactant phospholipids.

Exogenous surfactant instillation may be valuable in the treatment of lung injury other than quantitative surfactant deficiency states. Exogenous surfactant instillation significantly improves both physiologic and biochemical derangements induced by injury with NNNMU in the rat lung.

**Alveolar Hyperoxic Injury in Rabbits Receiving Exogenous Surfactant**

Loewen GM, Holm BA, Milanowski L, Wild LM, Notter RH, Matalon S (State Univ of New York, Buffalo; Univ of Rochester, NY; Univ of Alabama, Birmingham)

*J Appl Physiol* 66:1087–1092, March 1989 4–9

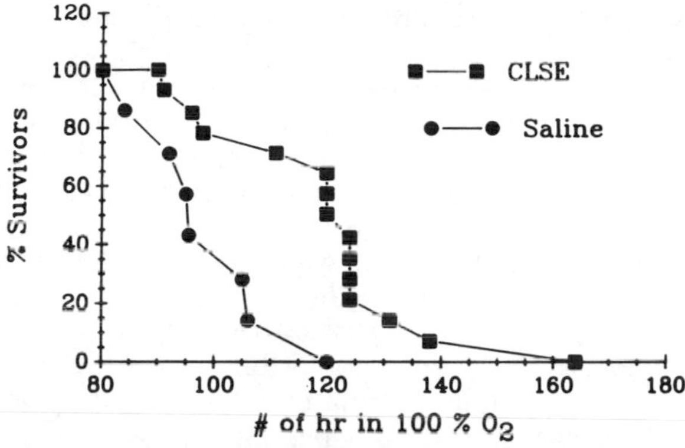


Fig 4–2.—Percentage of surviving rabbits vs. number of hours in 100% $O_2$. Calf-lung surfactant extract *(CLSE)* or saline was instilled as described in text of original article. Each *point* represents 1 animal. (Courtesy of Loewen GM, Holm BA, Milanowski L, et al: *J Appl Physiol* 66:1087–1092, March 1989.)

In a previous study, instillation of a calf-lung surfactant extract (CLSE) in rabbits exposed to 100% oxygen for 64 hours mitigated the progression of lung disease after return to room air. A new study was conducted to determine whether the onset and development of hyperoxic lung injury

Physiologic and Biochemical Variables After 72 Hours in 100% Oxygen or 66 Hours in Air

| | 72 h in 100% $O_2$ | | 66 h in Air |
|---|---|---|---|
| | Surfactant | Saline | Unexposed and uninstilled‡ |
| $Pa_{O_2}$, Torr | 333±28*† (19) | 281±29† (18) | 79±3 (5) |
| $P_L$, μm/kg | 12.5±1.5*† (7) | 5±1† (8) | 8.7±1.6 (5) |
| $P_r$, mg/kg | 24±3*† (7) | 52±8† (8) | 7.4±3 (5) |
| $T_{min}$, dyn/cm | 2±1* (7) | 26±1† (8) | 2±1 (5) |
| TLC, ml/kg | 41±2* (5) | 25±3.5† (4) | 42±1 (5) |
| CL, ml/cm$H_2O$ | 4.4±0.2 (5) | 4.3±0.2 (4) | 4.8±0.1 (5) |
| $W_L/W_D$ | 5.9±0.2*† (7) | 6.5±0.3† (6) | 4.1±0.3 (5) |

Values are means ± standard error with number of animals in parentheses.

*Abbreviations:* $O_2$, oxygen; $Pa_{O_2}$, partial pressure of $O_2$ in arterial blood; $P_L$ and $P_r$, total phospholipid and protein amounts in bronchoalveolar lavage, respectively; $T_{min}$, minimum surface tension of the bronchoalveolar lavage; TLC, total lung capacity; CL, lung compliance (measured as slope of linear portion of pressure-volume curve); $W_L/W_D$, lung wet-to-dry weights.

*$P < .05$ compared with corresponding saline value.

†$P < .05$ compared with corresponding uninstilled air value.

‡Data derived from Holm BA, et al: *J Appl Physiol* 59:1402–1409, 1985.

(Courtesy of Loewen GM, Holm BA, Milanowski L, et al: *J Appl Physiol* 66:1087–1092, March 1989.)

could be reduced or prevented by sequential instillations of CLSE during hyperoxic exposure.

After exposure to 100% oxygen, CLSE was instilled intratracheally into the rabbits' lungs at 24-hour intervals. Control animals were exposed to 100% oxygen and given equal volumes of saline or no instillations. Rabbits instilled with CLSE had higher arterial oxygen pressure values throughout the exposure period and survived longer than the control rabbits instilled with saline (Fig 4–2). After 72 hours in oxygen, CLSE-treated rabbits showed significantly greater lavageable alveolar phospholipid levels and total lung capacities and lower levels of alveolar protein, minimum surface tension, and lung wet-to-dry weights (table). After 72 hours in oxygen, lungs from both CLSE- and saline-instilled animals showed evidence of diffuse hyperoxic injury. However, atelectasis was less prominent in CLSE-treated animals. Instillation of CLSE limits the onset and development of hyperoxic lung injury to the alveolar epithelium of rabbits.

---

**Surfactant Replacement Attenuates the Increase in Alveolar Permeability in Hyperoxia**

Engstrom PC, Holm BA, Matalon S (Univ of Alabama, Birmingham; State Univ of New York, Buffalo)

*J Appl Physiol* 67:688–693, August 1989 4–10

---

The pulmonary microvasculature appears to be the primary site of lung injury in animals exposed to hyperoxia. Surfactant deficiency may promote the formation of pulmonary edema and increase alveolar permeability to solute. To determine whether intratracheal instillation of surfactant can mitigate the increase in solute flux of cyanocobalamin, which is lipid insoluble, across the alveolar epithelium, the distribution of instilled surfactant in rabbits exposed to 100% oxygen for 72 hours was determined.

A dose of 125 mg of calf lung surfactant extract (CLSE), equivalent to about 170 μmol of dipalmitoyl phosphatidylcholine, was instilled at 24 and 48 hours. Dipalmitoyl phosphatidylcholine liposes labeled with $^{14}C$ were used to quantify the distribution of CLSE.

The right lower lobe received the most CLSE in the hyperoxia group. Instillation of surfactant extract was associated with significantly increased 72-hour survival from hyperoxia, compared with survival of saline-treated control animals. The rate constant for movement of labeled cyanocobalamin out of the alveolar space was significantly reduced by treatment with surfactant.

Instillation of surfactant reduces the hyperoxia-related rise in lung protein permeability in this model, but it does not totally restore the integrity of the alveolar epithelium.

▶ These 4 articles (Abstracts 4–7 through 4–10) provide additional support for the concept that surfactant therapy may be useful in patients with adult respiratory distress syndrome. In response to acute lung injury, alveolar type II cells have at least 2 important functions: producing surfactant and serving as the source of alveolar type I and II cells to repopulate the alveoli. In intact rabbits, exposure to 100% oxygen for 64 hours causes mild lung injury and decreases alveolar surfactant. If the animals are removed from 100% oxygen for 3 days, recovery from lung injury occurs and the concentration of surfactant returns to control levels. Abstract 4–7 extends these observations to the cell level and indicates that exposure to 100% oxygen for 64 hours causes a reversible decrease in surfactant production and cell turnover in alveolar type II cells.

Abstracts 4–8 through 4–10 provide further evidence that acute lung injury can impair surfactant activity and that replacement therapy can effectively restore surfactant activity, reduce atelectasis, improve arterial oxygen pressure, and increase survival. The most likely etiology for the decrease in surfactant activity is inactivation by oxidants or by plasma proteins that have leaked into the alveolar space (1–3). To date surfactant therapy has been shown to reduce the lung injury caused by bilateral vagotomy (4), lung lavage (5), the intratracheal instillation of xanthine oxidase (6), the infusion of NNNMU (Abstract 4–8), and oxygen toxicity (7, 8). In addition to its ability to prevent alveolar collapse, the lipid in surfactant may scavenge oxygen radicals (9). Abstract 4–10 also indicates that surfactant therapy partially reduces the increase in alveolar epithelial injury caused by 100% oxygen. Previous studies also have found that surfactant therapy reduces the increase in alveolar-capillary permeability caused by acute lung injury (7, 10, and Abstract 4–9). For related articles see the 1988 YEAR BOOK OF CRITICAL CARE MEDICINE, pages 81 and 391–392, the 1988 YEAR BOOK OF PULMONARY DISEASE, pages 268–271, and the 1989 YEAR BOOK OF PULMONARY DISEASE, pages 130–132. J.R. Michael, M.D.

*References*


1. Ikegami M, Jobe A, Berry D: A protein that inhibits surfactant in respiratory distress syndrome. *Biol Neonate* 50:121–129, 1986.
2. Holm BA, Notter RH: Effects of hemoglobin and cell membrane lipids on pulmonary surfactant activity. *J Appl Physiol* 63:1434–1442, 1987.
3. Ikegami M, Jobe A, Jacobs H, et al: A protein from airways of premature lambs that inhibits surfactant function. *J Appl Physiol* 57:1134–1142, 1984.
4. Berry D, Ikegami M, Jobe A: Respiratory distress and surfactant inhibition following vagotomy in rabbits. *J Appl Physiol* 61:1741–1748, 1986.
5. Berggren P, Lachmann B, Curstedt T, et al: Gas exchange and lung morphology after surfactant replacement in experimental adult respiratory distress syndrome induced by repeated lung lavage. *Acta Anaesthesiol Scand* 30:321–328, 1986.
6. Lachmann B, Saugstad OD, Klein J, et al: Acute respiratory failure induced by tracheal instillation of xanthine oxidase, its prevention and therapy by exogenous surfactant instillation. *Adv Exp Med Biol* 215:351–354, 1987.
7. Matalon S, Holm BA, Notter RH: Mitigation of pulmonary hyperoxic injury by administration of exogenous surfactant. *J Appl Physiol* 62:756–761, 1987.
8. Holm, BA, Notter RH, Siegle J, et al: Pulmonary physiological and surfactant changes during injury and recovery from hyperoxia. *J Appl Physiol* 59:1402–1409, 1985.
9. Tanswell AK, Freeman BA: Liposome-entrapped antioxidant enzymes prevent lethal $O_2$ toxicity in the newborn rat. *J Appl Physiol* 63:347–352, 1987.
10. Jobe A, Ikegami M, Jacobs H, et al: Permeability of premature lamb lungs to protein and the effects of surfactant on that permeability. *J Appl Physiol* 55:169–176, 1983.

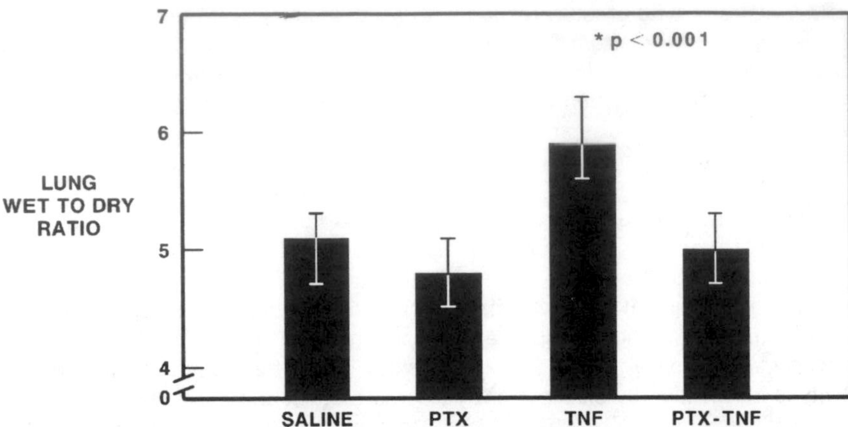


**Fig 4–3.**—The lung wet-to-dry weight was significantly increased in the TNF group ($P < .001$) compared with the PTX-TNF group, which was not significantly different from the control groups. Data are expressed as group means with 95% confidence intervals. (Courtesy of Lilly CM, Sandhu JS, Ishizaka A, et al: *Am Rev Respir Dis* 139:1361–1368, June 1989.)

---

**Pentoxifylline Prevents Tumor Necrosis Factor-Induced Lung Injury**

Lilly CM, Sandhu JS, Ishizaka A, Harada H, Yonemaru M, Larrick JW, Shi T-X, O'Hanley PT, Raffin TA (Stanford Univ; Cetus Immune Corp, Emeryville, Calif)

*Am Rev Respir Dis* 139:1361–1368, June 1989 4–11

---

Tumor necrosis factor (TNF) appears to be an important inflammatory mediator in acute lung injury. Because pentoxifylline (PTX) counters phagocyte activity and suproxide anion formation by human monocytes and neutrophils in vitro, a study was conducted to determine whether it protects against lung damage from TNF administration in a guinea pig

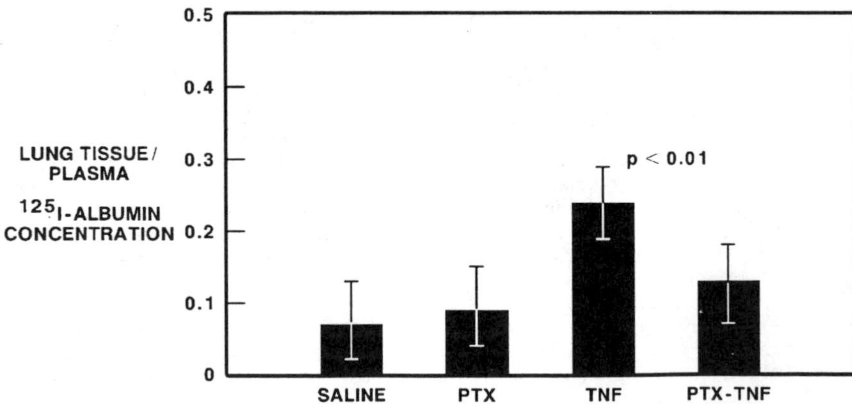


**Fig 4–4.**—The ratio of $^{111}$I-labeled albumin concentration in lung tissue to that in plasma (albumin index) was significantly increased in the TNF group ($P < .01$) compared with the PTX-TNF group, which was not significantly different from the control groups. Data are expressed as group means with 95% confidence intervals. (Courtesy of Lilly CM, Sandhu JS, Ishizaka A, et al: *Am Rev Respir Dis* 139:1361–1368, June 1989.)

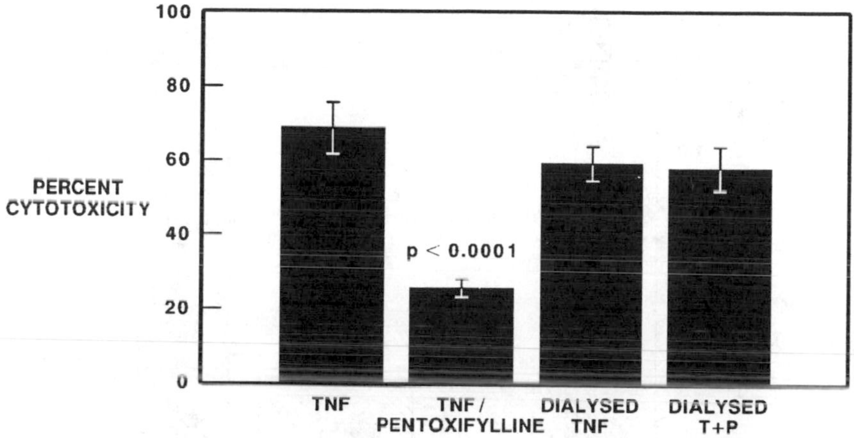


Fig 4–5.—The TNF-associated L929 cell cytotoxicity was significantly reduced by PTX ($P < .0001$). This protective effect of PTX was abolished by dialysis. Data are expressed as group means with 95% confidence intervals. (Courtesy of Lilly CM, Sandhu JS, Ishizaka A, et al: *Am Rev Respir Dis* 139:1361–1368, June 1989.)

model. Treated animals received a 20-mg/kg bolus of PTX, followed by infusion of 6 mg/kg/hour, after TNF in a dose of $3.75 \times 10^6$ units/kg.

The lung wet-to-dry ratio was elevated significantly only in TNF recipients (Fig 4–3); the same was true for the lung albumin index (Fig 4–4). Similarly, bronchoalveolar lavage leukocyte and polymorph counts were increased only in animals given TNF alone. Administration of PTX prevented a marked decrease in mean arterial pressure. An in vitro cytotoxicity assay indicated that PTX did not inhibit TNF in a general manner (Fig 4–5).

In this study, PTX protected against the adverse effects of TNF in guinea pigs. It is not unreasonable to assume that PTX might also ameliorate the effects of TNF in human beings. A generalized cytoprotective effect is not likely; Possibly, altered polymorph and mononuclear-cell function is an important means by which PTX prevents TNF-related tissue injury.

---

**Pentoxifylline Decreases Endotoxin-Induced Pulmonary Neutrophil Sequestration and Extravascular Protein Accumulation in the Dog**

Welsh CH, Lien D, Worthen GS, Weil JV (Univ of Colorado; Denver VA Med Ctr; Natl Jewish Ctr for Respiratory Medicine, Denver)

*Am Rev Respir Dis* 138:1106–1114, November 1988 4–12

---

The in vitro effects of pentoxifylline suggest that it may counter neutrophil sequestration and lung injury in vivo. Its use in treating rats with peritonitis has promoted survival and shortened the duration of bacteremia.

The effects of pentoxifyllin on pulmonary neutrophil retention and on

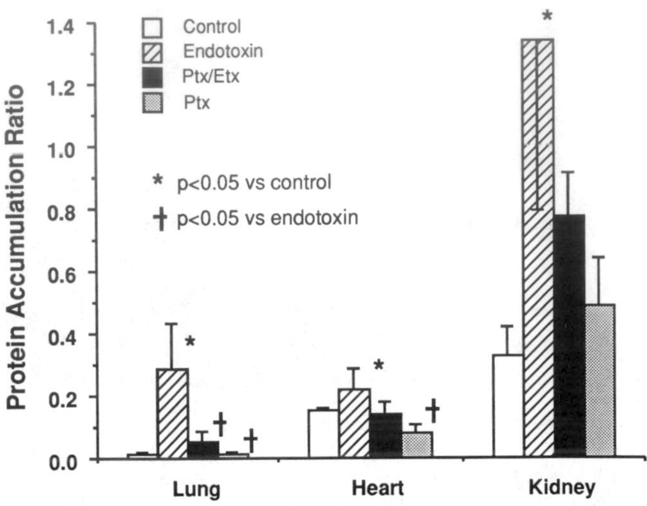


Fig 4–6.—Endotoxin increased extravascular accumulation of protein in lung, heart, and kidney. Trend toward reversal of protein in accumulation after pentoxifylline pretreatment was not significant. (Courtesy of Welsh CH, Lien D, Worthen GS, et al: *Am Rev Respir Dis* 138:1106–1114, November 1988.)

lung injury in dogs given *Salmonella enteriditis* endotoxin intravenously were examined. The animals were pretreated with either pentoxifylline, 20 mg/kg intravenously, followed by a continuous infusion of 0.1 mg/kg/min, or saline. Pulmonary vascular permeability to protein was determined after 2 hours by measuring extravascular accumulation of intravenously administered $^{113m}$In-transferrin.

Endotoxin increased the ratio of extravascular to intravascular protein activities, and this change was reversed by pentoxifylline (Fig 4–6). The effect of pentoxifylline on the heart and kidneys was in the same direction as its effect on the lungs. Pretreatment of neutrophils with pentoxifylline prevented the increase in lung retention of labeled neutrophils after administration of endotoxin.

It is not clear how pentoxifylline attenuates endotoxin-induced vascular injury, but an effect on the endothelium may be less important than changes in neutrophils. It is possible that pentoxifylline also can counter the development of multiorgan failure, as commonly occurs in the setting of sepsis or adult respiratory distress syndrome.

▶ A number of recent reports indicate that the methylxanthine pentoxifylline may have a therapeutic effect in animal models of sepsis. Pentoxifylline, for example, increases survival in rats with peritonitis (1). In Abstract 4–11, pentoxifylline pretreatment prevented the lung injury caused by tumor necrosis factor. In a subsequent publication, the authors have found that posttreatment with pentoxifylline or a cyclic adenosine monophosphate (AMP) analogue reduces the lung injury caused by the infusion of live *Escherichia coli*.

In Abstract 4–12, pentoxifylline was given to dogs infused with a low dose of *Salmonella enteriditis* endotoxin. This dose of endotoxin increases pulmonary and systemic vascular permeability, but does not increase extravascular lung water. Pentoxifylline prevented the increase in pulmonary vascular permeability and appeared to decrease the vascular injury in the heart and kidney. The mechanism responsible for this effect of pentoxifylline is not well defined. Pentoxifylline is a phosphodiesterase inhibitor and thus can increase intracellular cyclic AMP (2). An increase in cyclic AMP has been shown to reduce the permeability of pulmonary vascular endothelial cells (3) and to reduce superoxide anion production by neutrophils (4). Compounds that can increase intracellular cyclic AMP have also been shown to reduce acute lung injury (5–7). For a discussion of these articles see the 1987 YEAR BOOK OF PULMONARY DISEASE, pages 120–121, the 1988 YEAR BOOK OF PULMONARY DISEASE, pages 260–261, and the 1989 YEAR BOOK OF PULMONARY DISEASE, pages 127–129.—J.R. Michael, M.D.

*References*


1. Chalkiadakis GE, Kostakis A: Pentoxifylline in the treatment of experimental peritonitis in rats. *Arch Surg* 120:1141–1144, 1985.
2. Hill AR, Augustine NH, Newton JA, et al: Correction of a development defect in neutrophil activation and movement. *Am J Pathol* 128:307–314, 1987.
3. Stelzner TJ, Weil JV, OBrien RF: Role of cyclic adenosine monophosphate in the induction of endothelial barrier properties. *J Cell Physiol* 139:157–166, 1989.
4. Bessler H, Gilgal R, Djaldetti M, et al: Effect of pentoxifylline on the phagocytic activity, c-AMP levels and superoxide anion production by monocytes and polymorphonuclear cells. *J Leukocyte Biol* 40:747–754, 1986.
5. Minnear FL, Johnson A, Malik AB: β-Adrenergic modulation of pulmonary transvascular fluid and protein exchange. *J Appl Physiol* 60:266–274, 1986.
6. Farrukh IS, Gurtner GH, Michael JR: Pharmacological modification of pulmonary vascular injury: Possible role of cAMP. *J Appl Physiol* 62:47–54, 1987.
7. Kobayashi K, Kobayashi T, Fukushima M: Effects of dibutyryl cAMP on pulmonary air embolism-induced lung injury in awake sheep. *J Appl Physiol* 63:2201–2207, 1987.


## Treatment of Canine Aspiration Pneumonitis: Fluid Volume Reduction vs. Fluid Volume Expansion

Long R, Breen PH, Mayers I, Wood LDH (Univ of Chicago)
*J Appl Physiol* 65:1736–1744, October 1988 4–13

One approach to treating aspiration pneumonitis is to raise the cardiac output and oxygen delivery to insure adequate tissue oxygenation at the risk of increasing the pulmonary edema. Alternatively, edema may be reduced by lowering pulmonary microvascular pressure, at the risk of reducing oxygen delivery and tissue oxygenation. These 2 approaches were compared in 24 anesthetized ventilated dogs with a pulmonary wedge pressure of 12.5 mm Hg.

Before and 1 hour after endobronchial instillation of 0.1 N HCl cardiac output, oxygen delivery, tissue oxygenation, venous admixture, and in vivo extravascular lung fluid were measured. The dogs were then randomly divided into 4 equal groups: group 1 animals were maintained at a pulmonary wedge pressure of 12.5 mm Hg with high cardiac output,

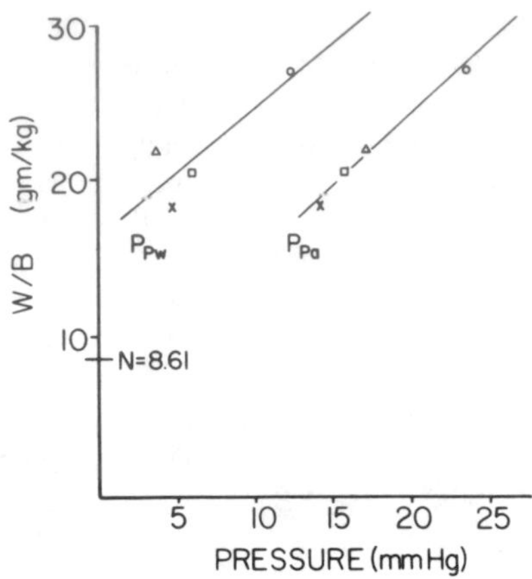


Fig 4–7.—Relationship between pulmonary vascular pressures and edema in this model. Pressure associated with each ratio of wet weight to body weight (W-B) in each of 4 groups is mean pressure over 4-hour treatment phase of experiment. *Ppw*, pulmonary wedge pressure; *Ppa*, pulmonary arterial pressure. *Circles*, group 1; *squares*, group 2; ×, group 3; *triangles*, group 4. (Courtesy of Long R, Breen PH, Mayers I, et al: *J Appl Physiol* 65:1736–1744, October 1988.)

group 2 animals were maintained at a pressure of 7.5 mm Hg with intermediate cardiac output, group 3 animals were maintained at a pressure of 4.5 mm Hg with low cardiac output, and group 4 animals were maintained at a pressure of 4.5 mm Hg plus dopamine with intermediate cardiac output. Measured values were followed for 4 more hours, after which the lungs were excised to compare wet weight-to-body weight ratios (W-B).

Edema did not increase after plasmapheresis lowered the pulmonary wedge pressure. The W-B of groups 2, 3, and 4 were significantly less than in group 1 (Fig 4–7). Although cardiac output decreased with the wedge pressure, increased hematocrit value and reduced venous admixture maintained oxygen delivery in group 2 but not in group 3. In group 4 an intermediate cardiac output maintained oxygen delivery even at a pulmonary wedge pressure of 4.5 mm Hg, but edema increased to the group 2 level, presumably because pulmonary microvascular pressure rose with cardiac output on dopamine. Tissue oxygenation remained constant over time in each group.

Canine HCl-induced pulmonary edema is sensitive to reductions in pulmonary microvascular pressure. Changes in edema can be clinically monitored by the indicator-dilution method. In the exudative phase a reduction in microvascular pressure that does not lower oxygen delivery below 20 mL/kg/min is unlikely to alter the normal independence of tissue oxygenation from oxygen delivery.

▶ One strategy used to reduce pulmonary edema in patients with adult respiratory distress syndrome (ARDS) is to decrease pulmonary microvascular pressure to the lowest level that is still compatible with adequate cardiac output, oxygen delivery, and oxygen consumption. This report and others by the authors support the concept that reducing pulmonary capillary wedge pressure from 12.5 mm Hg to 5 or 7.5 mm Hg significantly will reduce the amount of pulmonary edema that occurs in dogs after acute lung injury (1–3). (See the 1987 YEAR BOOK OF PULMONARY DISEASE, pp 133–135). Because dopamine may be used to maintain cardiac output when pulmonary vascular pressure is reduced, the authors compared the effects of treatment with a wedge pressure of 4.5 alone versus treatment with a wedge pressure of 4.5 mm Hg plus dopamine 10 μg/kg/min. The addition of dopamine in this model appeared to increase pulmonary edema perhaps because it raised pulmonary arterial pressure. As discussed by the authors, whether the amount of pulmonary edema is an important factor influencing mortality or eventual lung function in ARDS patients is an open question (4–6).—J.R. Michael, M.D.

*References*

1. Sznajder JI, Zucker AR, Wood LDH, et al: The effects of plasmapheresis and hemofiltration on canine acid aspiration pulmonary edema. *Am Rev Respir Dis* 134:222–228, 1986.
2. Gottlieb SS, Wood LDH, Hansen DE, et al: The effect of nitroprusside on pulmonary edema, oxygen exchange, and blood flow in hydrochloric acid aspiration. *Anesthesiology* 67:47–53, 1987.
3. Prewitt RM, McCarthy J, Wood LDH: Treatment of acute low pressure pulmonary edema in dogs: Relative effects of hydrostatic and oncotic pressure, nitroprusside, and positive end-expiratory pressure. *J Clin Invest* 67:409–418, 1981.
4. Brigham KL, Kariman K, Harris TR, et al: Correlation of oxygenation with vascular permeability surface area but not with lung water in humans with acute respiratory failure and pulmonary edema. *J Clin Invest* 72:330–349, 1983.
5. Eisenberg PR, Hansbrough JR, Anderson D, et al: A prospective study of lung water measurements during patient management in an intensive care unit. *Am Rev Respir Dis* 136:662–668, 1987.
6. Simmons RS, Berdine GG, Seidenfeld JJ, et al: Fluid balance and the adult respiratory distress syndrome. *Am Rev Respir Dis* 135:924–929, 1987.

---

**Relationship of Pleural Effusions to Increased Permeability Pulmonary Edema in Anesthetized Sheep**

Wionor Kronich JP, Broaddus VC, Albertine KH, Gropper MA, Matthay MA, Staub NC, Osorio O (Univ of California, San Francisco; Jefferson Med College, Philadelphia)

*J Clin Invest* 82:1422–1429, October 1988 4–14

---

A previous study demonstrated the presence of pleural effusions in rats given α-naphthyl-thiourea to produce an elevated permeability pulmonary edema. Recent radiographic studies documented the presence of pleural effusions in 36% of the patients with increased permeability pulmonary edema. Very little is known about the pathophysiology of these pleural effusions. Anesthesized sheep were studied to determine the relationship of increased permeability pulmonary edema and the development and mechanism of pleural effusion formation.

The time course of pleural liquid formation after intravenous administration of oleic acid, 0.12 mL/kg was studied in 12 sheep with intact, closed thoraces. There was no pleural effusion after 1 hour, even though extrasvascular lung water increased 50%. After 3 hours, pleural effusions had formed, reaching a maximum at 5 hours. At 8 hours, there was no additional accumulation of pleural liquid. Morphological examination showed subpleural edema, but no detectable injury to the visceral pleura, suggesting that the pleural liquid originated from the lung, and not the pleura. The rate of formation of pleural liquid was quantified in 9 sheep by enclosing 1 lung in a plastic bag. The rate of liquid absorption from the intact chest was estimated to be 0.32 mL/kg per hour. In normal sheep, the liquid absorption rate was 0.28 mL/kg per hour.

Pleural effusions develop in sheep after increased permeability pulmonary edema is produced. The effusions are moderate sized and have a total protein concentration comparable to lung lymph, suggesting that the pleural liquid originates primarily from the pulmonary interstitium. Normal pleural liquid is thought to be formed by the parietal and visceral pleural microcirculations. Because about 21% of the extravascular lung water accumulated as pleural fluid, the pleural space is an important pathway for removing lung edema.

▶ In contrast to patients with cardiogenic pulmonary edema, patients with noncardiogenic pulmonary edema (ARDS) generally are not thought to have pleural effusions. In a clinical study, the authors, however, have found that 36% of patients with ARDS have pleural effusions on routine chest radiographs (1). In an experimental model of acute lung injury in sheep, the authors found that approximately 20% of the extra lung water produced by the injury accumulated in the pleural space. The pleural fluid appears to arise from interstitial edema. Thus, drainage of pulmonary edema fluid into the pleural space and reabsorption of the fluid by the pleura may serve as another mechanism by which the lung can remove extra lung water.—J.R. Michael, M.D.

*Reference*

1. Aberle DR, Wiener-Kronish JP, Webb WR, et al: The diagnosis of hydrostatic versus increased permeability edema based on chest radiographic criteria in critically ill patients. *Radiology* 168:73–79, 1988.

---

**Impairment After Adult Respiratory Distress Syndrome: An Evaluation Based on American Thoracic Society Recommendations**

Ghio AJ, Elliott CG, Crapo RO, Berlin SL, Jensen RL (Univ of Utah)

*Am Rev Respir Dis* 139:1158–1162, May 1989 4–15

---

There is evidence that most survivors of adult respiratory distress syndrome (ARDS) recover nearly normal lung function within a year. Pulmonary function tests were carried out from 1 to 388 weeks after the onset of ARDS in 41 patients aged 7 to 61 years. In 27 of the patients impairment was evaluated 1 year or more after the onset of ARDS. Standards adopted by the American Thoracic Society in 1986 were used in the studies.

Impairment was present in 18 of the 27 patients, with the rate ranging from 33% when the ratio of forced expiratory volume in 1 second to forced vital capacity ($FEV_1$/FVC) was used to 82% when measurement of single-breath, carbon monoxide diffusing (DLCO) capacity was used. Impairment was mild in 13 cases, moderate in 4, and marked in 1. Physiologic indices of the severity of ARDS were predictive of impairment, but smoking status was not. There was no statistically significant association between impairment and symptoms.

Some degree of pulmonary impairment is common after recovery from ARDS. The degree of impairment appears not to change after the first year. Five of the present patients assessed more than a year after the onset (18.5%) had impairment severe enough to influence their employment status. Impairment was most frequent in patients whose ARDS was more severe.

▶ This is the most thorough study of patients status post ARDS. One year or longer after ARDS, two thirds of the patients met criteria of the American Thoracic Society for abnormal pulmonary function tests. The most common abnormality was a decreased DLCO (found in 82%), although a third of patients had abnormally low $FEV_1$/FVC ratios. Five of 27 patients followed longer than 1 year had enough pulmonary disability to affect their ability to work. The severity of the acute lung injury and the length of time they required positive pressure ventilation were associated with a greater risk of impairment.—J.R. Michael, M.D.

## Weaning From the Ventilator

▶ ↓ These 5 articles discuss various aspects of weaning. Abstract 4–16 investigates the factors that predict weaning and survival in patients with chronic obstructive pulmonary disease (COPD) that require intubation for acute respiratory failure. Abstract 4–17 represents a controlled trial comparing the success rate of weaning with intermittent mandatory ventilation or T-piece using defined protocols in medical and surgical patients. Abstract 4–18 describes a method to determine the optimal level of pressure support to be used in weaning. Abstract 4–19 illustrates the effectiveness of using inspiratory muscle resistive training as an adjunct in the weaning of patients who have failed multiple weaning trials. Abstract 4–20 suggests that dopamine may increase diaphragmatic strength in ventilated COPD patients.—J.R. Michael, M.D.

---

**Determinants of Weaning and Survival Among Patients With COPD Who Require Mechanical Ventilation for Acute Respiratory Failure**
Menzies R, Gibbons W, Goldberg P (Montreal Chest Hosp; McGill Univ)
*Chest* 95:398–405, February 1989 4–16

---

Mechanical ventilation (MV) in patients with chronic obstructive pulmonary disease (COPD) and acute respiratory failure (ARF) is associated with a high risk of complications and a poor long-term prognosis; thus, the decision to institute MV in such patients is difficult. A study was con-

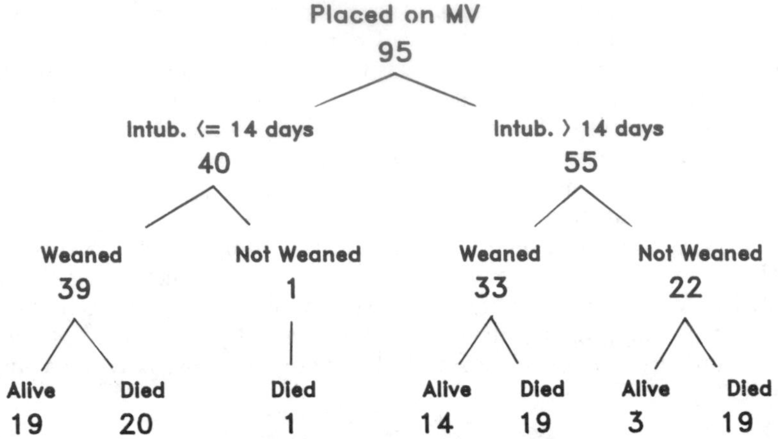


**Fig 4–8.**—Outcomes of the 95 study patients after institution of MV. (Courtesy of Menzies R, Gibbons W, Goldberg P: *Chest* 95:398–405, February 1989.)

ducted to determine the outcomes of patients with COPD and ARF requiring MV; to identify factors related to intubation duration, weaning, and survival; and to develop predictive models for outcomes.

The study included 95 patients with COPD and ARF who required MV; 55 patients needed MV for more than 2 weeks. Seventy-two patients were weaned successfully, and 59 died within 1 year (Figs 4–8 and 4–9). Factors associated with survival were premorbid activity level, forced expiratory volume in 1 second, serum albumin level, and severity of dyspnea (Fig 4–10). Cor pulmonale demonstrated on ECG, premorbid hypercarbia, and history of left ventricular failure were more common among nonsurvivors. Weaning of MV was associated with premorbid level of activity, forced expiratory volume in 1 second, albumin level, and negative inspiratory pressure and respiratory rate during T-piece

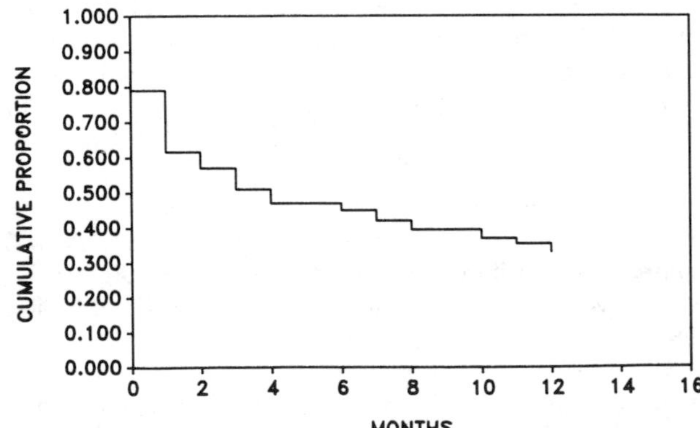


**Fig 4–9.**—Life-table of all 95 patients. Time 0 represents the time of weaning; 22% of patients died while receiving MV; thus, survival at time 0 is only 78%. (Courtesy of Menzies R, Gibbons W, Goldberg P: *Chest* 95:398–405, February 1989.)

| LIFESTYLE CATEGORY | FEV1 CATEGORY (% Predicted) <25% | 25–40% | >40% |
|---|---|---|---|
| 3+4 house-bound or worse | 9/19 | 12/15 | 8/8 |
| 2 somewhat restricted | 3/4 | 7/8 | 7/7 |
| 0+1 working or independent | 2/2 | 5/6 | 10/10 |

Fig 4–10.—Cross-tabulation demonstrating the combined influence of premorbid lung function and level of activity on the likelihood of being weaned from MV. (Courtesy of Menzies R, Gibbons W, Goldberg P: *Chest* 95:398–405, February 1989.)

trial. Intubation duration was associated only with premorbid activity level.

The decision to institute MV in patients with COPD and ARF is difficult because of the high rate of complications, the risk of long-term dependence, and uncertainties about long-term prognosis. Physicians can consider all significant factors using predictive models with a programmable pocket calculator or a simple software program to identify the patients most likely to benefit from MV.

▶ This article provides useful information about prognosis in COPD patients intubated because of acute respiratory failure. Overall, two thirds of the patients were dead within 1 year. The key prognostic factor was the premorbid activity level. Of patients working or living independently before becoming ill, 75% survived. Of patients living on their own, but severely exercise-limited, 50% survived 1 year. Only 22% survived who were house-, bed- or chair-bound.

Other studies emphasize that COPD patients with acute respiratory failure who require intubation have a substantially higher mortality than do patients who do not require intubation. The 1-year survival rate for COPD patients who do not need intubation is 74% (1); for patients who are intubated, the 1-year survival rate varies between 34% and 49% (2–5).—J.R. Michael, M.D.

*References*

1. Sukumalchantra Y, Dinakara P, Williams MH: Prognosis of patients with chronic obstructive pulmonary disease after hospitalization for acute ventilatory failure: A three year follow-up study. *Am Rev Respir Dis* 93:215–222, 1966.
2. Asmundsson T, Kilburn K: Survival of acute respiratory failure. *Ann Intern Med* 70:471–484, 1969.
3. Wessel-Aas T, Vale JR, Hauge HE: Artificial ventilation in chronic pulmonary insufficiency: Indications and prognosis. *Scand J Respir Dis Suppl* 72:36–41, 1970.
4. Sluiter HJ, Blokzijl EJ, van Dijl W, et al: Conservative and respirator treatment

of acute respiratory insufficiency in patients with chronic obstructive lung disease. *Am Rev Respir Dis* 105:932–943, 1972.
5. Gillespie DJ, Marsh HMM, Divertie MB, et al: Clinical outcome of respiratory failure in patients requiring prolonged (>24 hours) mechanical ventilation. *Chest* 90:364–369, 1986.

## A Prospective Comparison of IMV and T-Piece Weaning From Mechanical Ventilation

Tomlinson JR, Miller KS, Lorch DG, Smith L, Reines HD, Sahn SA (Med Univ of South Carolina)
*Chest* 96:348–352, August 1989 4–17

Two hundred consecutive medical and surgical patients who required mechanical ventilation were entered in a prospective randomized trial of weaning by either intermittent mandatory ventilation (IMV) or T-piece. Patients in these groups were of similar age and the same sex and had similar total ventilation times. Different weaning protocols were assigned to each of 3 study groups (table).

Of the 165 patients who continued in the study until the weaning phase began, 155 were successfully weaned by protocol, and 136 of them were weaned on the first attempt. Weaning time did not differ in the IMV and T-piece groups. Eleven of the 19 patients not weaned on the first trial were successfully weaned on the second or third trial. Two thirds of those who were weaned in 2 hours were postoperative patients who were ventilated for less than 72 hours.

Successful weaning can be achieved by either IMV or T-piece when simple bedside criteria for ventilation are met. Patients who do not meet criteria for weaning can receive a brief trial on IMV or T-piece under careful observation. Rapid weaning by protocol can be a significant cost-containment measure that reduces patient stays in the intensive care unit.

▶ The authors found the following weaning criteria useful for medical and surgical patients. The patients needed (1) a $Pao_2 > 55$ mm Hg on an $Fio_2 < 0.5$; (2) a minute ventilation < 12 L/min; (3) plus 2 of the following 4 items: maximal voluntary ventilation more than twice their minute ventilation; a tidal volume of > ml/kg; vital capacity > 10 ml/kg; or negative inspiratory force ≤ 20 cm $H_2O$. Ninety-four percent of patients who meet these criteria were successfully weaned. The weaning protocols using either IMV or T-piece are shown in the accompanying table. Most surgical patients were in group A; most medical patients fit into group B. The success rate was the same among patients weaned with either IMV or T-piece. Thus, for the vast majority of patients, it does not appear to matter which method is used. As the authors point out, the use of a well-defined weaning protocol can save time, speed extubation in stable patients, and insure uniform patient care.—J.R. Michael, M.D.

Summary of Weaning Steps for IMV and T-Piece Ventilation

| Group A (2-h wean) Stabilization (<72 h) | | Group B (7-h wean) Stabilization (>72 h) | | Group C (3-day wean) (Never Satisfied Weaning Parameter or failed 3 weaning attempts) | |
|---|---|---|---|---|---|
| IMV | T-Piece | IMV | T-Piece | IMV | T-Piece |
| Rate 6:30 min | T-Piece:30 min | Rate 8:2 h | T-Piece:30 min q 2 h × 3 | Day 1:Rate 8 | Day 1 T-Piece:15 min q 4 h × 2<br>T-Piece:30 min q 4 h × 2 |
| Rate 4:30 min | Mechanical vent:30 min | Rate 6:2 h | | Day 2:Rate 6 | Day 2 T-Piece:15 min q 2 h × 4<br>T-Piece:30 min q 2 h × 4 |
| Rate 0:1 h | T-Piece:1 h | Rate 4:2 h | T-Piece:1 h | Day 3:Rate 4 | Day 3 T-Piece:1 h q 2 h × 4<br>T-Piece:2 h q 4 h × 2 |
| | | Rate 0:1 h | | Day 4:Rate 0 | Day 4 T-Piece:1 h |

Courtesy of Tomlinson JR, Miller KS, Lorch DG, et al: *Chest* 96:348–352, August 1989.

## Inspiratory Pressure Support Prevents Diaphragmatic Fatigue During Weaning From Mechanical Ventilation

Brochard L, Harf A, Lorino H, Lemaire F (Hôpital Henri Mondor, Créteil, France)
*Am Rev Respir Dis* 139:513–521, February 1989 4–18

As many as 20% of mechanically ventilated patients are reported to be unable to tolerate weaning from ventilation. Diaphragmatic fatigue probably is a major factor in patients recovering from acute respiratory failure. Recently inspiratory pressure support was designed to maintain a constant preset positive airway pressure during spontaneous breathing so as to lower the work done by the inspiratory muscles, particularly the diaphragm.

The value of pressure support ventilation was examined in 8 patients recovering from acute respiratory failure after other attempts at weaning from mechanical ventilation had failed. Pressure support was provided at different levels up to 20 cm of water.

Seven of the 8 patients had electromyographic signs of incipient diaphragmatic fatigue during spontaneous breathing. The work of breathing declined with increasing levels of pressure support, as did oxygen consumption of the respiratory muscles. Electric signs suggestive of diaphragmatic fatigue disappeared. The intrinsic positive end-expiratory pressure fell progressively. In each case a certain pressure support level maintained diaphragmatic activity without occurrence of fatigue. Hyperinflation and apnea sometimes occurred at higher than optimal levels of support.

Pressure support ventilation can prevent diaphragmatic fatigue during weaning from mechanical ventilation while allowing spontaneous diaphragmatic activity. The proper level of support can be determined by monitoring the activity of the sternocleidomastoid muscle.

▶ The authors attempted to develop a clinical method to determine the optimal level of pressure support that should be used in weaning ventilated patients (1). They defined the optimal level as the amount at which diaphragmatic activity occurred without inducing respiratory muscle fatigue. If the level of pressure support is too low, diaphragmatic fatigue likely will develop. If the pressure support level is set too high, hyperinflation and apnea may occur (2). (See the 1989 YEAR BOOK OF PULMONARY DISEASE, pp 168–169). The optimal level for individual patients varied between 0 and 20 cm $H_2O$. In 3 of the 8 patients, levels of 15 or 20 cm $H_2O$ caused intermittent apnea. When pressure support is too low and diaphragmatic fatigue begins, the activity of the sternocleidomastoid muscle is increased. Consequently, the authors suggest picking a level of pressure support by palpating the activity of the sternocleidomastoid muscle. They recommend that pressure support be lowered to the point at which sternocleidomastoid activity increases, then pressure support should be increased until the sternocleidomastoid muscle is no longer active.—J.R. Michael, M.D.

*References*

1. MacIntyre NR: Respiratory function during pressure support ventilation. *Chest* 89:677–683, 1986.
2. Black JW, Grover BS: A hazard of pressure support ventilation. *Chest* 93:333–335, 1988.

**Weaning From Mechanical Ventilation: Adjunctive Use of Inspiratory Muscle Resistive Training**

Aldrich TK, Karpel JP, Uhrlass RM, Sparapani MA, Eramo D, Ferranti R (North Central Bronx Hosp; Albert Einstein College of Medicine, Bronx, NY; Gaylord Hosp, Wallingford, Conn)

*Crit Care Med* 17:143–147, February 1989 4–19

Most patients can be weaned easily from mechanical ventilators by T-piece trials or progressively decreasing intermittent mandatory ventilation, but some remain dependent on ventilators. The principles of endurance training may be used to wean some ventilator-dependent patients who fail repeated weaning attempts using T-piece trials. A group of 27 patients with stable chronic respiratory failure, as a result of moderate neuromuscular disease or primary lung disease, were tested using an inspiratory resistive training (IRT) apparatus. A mean of 5 training sessions per week of spontaneous breathing with increasing duration and resistance was provided, to a maximum of 30-minute duration. Mechanical ventilation continued between training sessions.

Of 27 patients, 12 were weaned after a mean of 21 sessions of IRT, 5 were weaned to nocturnal ventilation after 18 sessions, and 10 remained unweanable after 21 sessions. All 7 patients with neuromuscular disease were weaned completely (no. = 4) or to nocturnal ventilation (no. = 3) (Fig 4–11). The 6 unweanable patients had improvement during IRT. Of 10 unweanable patients, 8 died, whereas only 1 of 12 completely weaned patients and 1 of 5 patients weaned to nocturnal ventilation died. The only complication was severe, nonfatal bradycardia with syncope, which occurred in only 1 patient.

These findings suggest that IRT may be useful in weaning patients from mechanical ventilation who have failed weaning attempts by standard techniques. This technique is safe if arterial blood gases are monitored and if the duration of training sessions does not overcome the patient's abilities. If this technique can allow weaning of otherwise "unweanable" patients, obvious benefits can be reaped.

▶ The authors studied patients with chronic respiratory failure who could not be weaned after 3 weeks. Twelve of 27 patients for whom inspiratory muscle training was used were successfully weaned, and another 5 were weaned to nocturnal ventilation. These results are consistent with previous reports that inspiratory muscle training can increase respiratory muscle strength in with chronic obstructive pulmonary disease or in patients with neuromuscular dis-

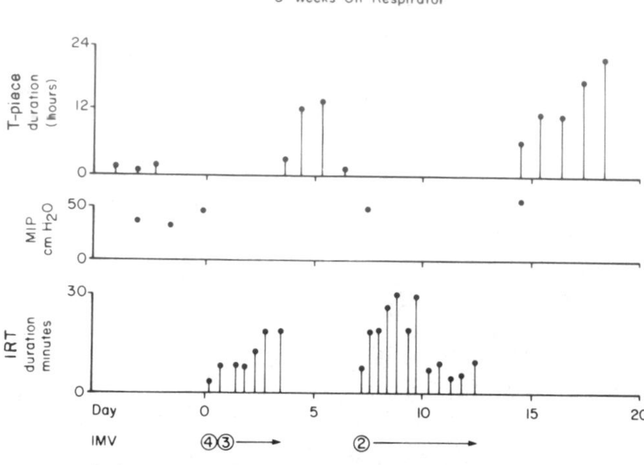


**Fig 4–11.**—Course of IRT and intermittent mandatory ventilation in 1 typical successfully treated patient. After 7 IRT sessions over 4 days, this patient had improved T-piece tolerance, but was not able to stay off the respirator for more than 13 hours. After another 12 sessions over 6 days, she was successfully weaned to spontaneous breathing. (Courtesy of Aldrich TK, Karpel JP, Uhrlass RM, et al: *Crit Care Med* 17:143–147, February 1989.)

ease (1–5). The reported results in this study with ventilated patients are impressive, but unfortunately this trial is uncontrolled. The authors are encouraged to perform a controlled trial.—J.R. Michael, M.D.

*References*


1. Aldrich TK, Karpel JP: Inspiratory muscle resistive training in respiratory failure. *Am Rev Respir Dis* 131:461–462, 1985.
2. Pardy RL, Rivington RN, Despas PJ, et al: The effects of respiratory muscle training on exercise performance in chronic airflow limitation. *Am Rev Respir Dis* 123:426–433, 1981.
3. Asher MI, Pardy RL, Coates AL, et al: The effect of inspiratory muscle training in patients with cystic fibrosis. *Am Rev Respir Dis* 126:855–859, 1982.
4. Gross D, Ladd HW, Reley EJ, et al: The effect of training on strength and endurance of the diaphragm in quadriplegia. *Am J Med* 68:27–35, 1980.
5. Estrup C, Lyager S, Noeraa N, et al: Effect of respiratory muscle training in patients with neuromuscular diseases and in normals. *Respiration* 50:36–43, 1986.


---

**Dopamine Effects on Diaphragmatic Strength During Acute Respiratory Failure in Chronic Obstructive Pulmonary Disease**

Aubier M, Murciano D, Menu Y, Boczkowski J, Mal H, Pariente R (Hôpital Beaujon, Clichy, France)

*Ann Intern Med* 110:17–23, Jan 1, 1989 4–20

---

Dopamine may increase diaphragmatic blood flow and therefore may improve diaphragmatic function in patients with chronic obstructive lung disease who have acute respiratory failure secondary to pulmonary infec-

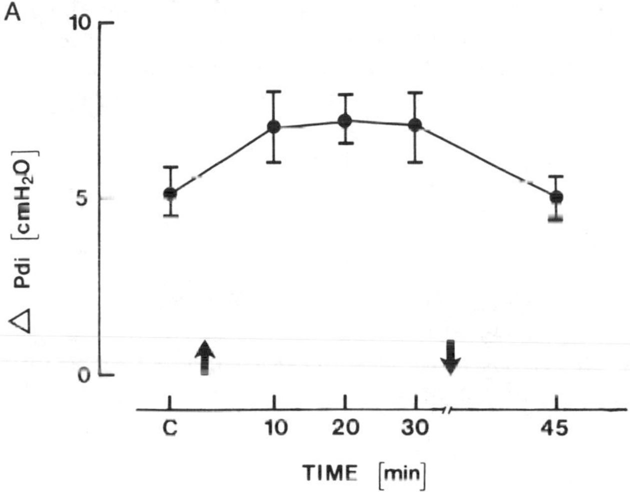


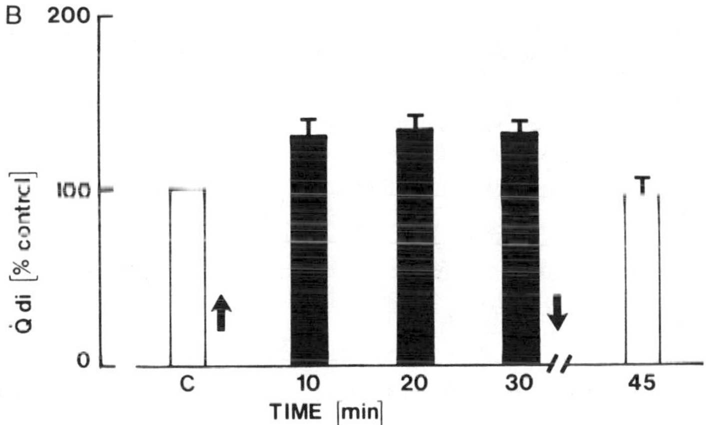


**Fig 4–12.**—**A,** time course of mean changes in transdiaphragmatic pressure *(Pdi)* generated during phrenic stimulation during control *(C),* throughout infusion of dopamine, and 15 minutes after end of infusion for 8 patients. *First arrow* indicates beginning of infusion, and second arrow indicates end. Bars represent 1 SE. *Open triangle,* variations in Pdi between control and dopamine. **B,** time course of mean changes in diaphragmatic blood flow *(Qdi)* during control *(C),* throughout infusion of dopamine, and 15 minutes after end of infusion for 3 patients. First arrow indicates beginning of infusion, and second arrow indicates end. Diaphragmatic blood flow is expressed in percentage of control values, that is, before infusion. *Bars,* 1 SE. (Courtesy of Aubier M, Murciano D, Menu Y, et al: *Ann Intern Med* 110:17–23, Jan 1, 1989.)

tion. Eight such patients were studied within 48 hours after admission for acute respiratory failure. The mean forced expiratory volume in 1 second averaged 24% of predicted value. Pulmonary infection caused respiratory failure in all instances. Dopamine, 10 μg/kg/min, was infused for 30 minutes.

On average, cardiac output rose 40% with the infusion of dopamine. Diaphragmatic blood flow increased 30% on average in the 3 patients studied (Fig 4–12). Diaphragmatic strength also increased significantly. Average transdiaphragmatic pressure on phrenic stimulation rose 30%. All values returned to baseline 15 minutes after infusion of dopamine ceased. Pulmonary capillary wedge pressure increased during the infusion but remained within the normal range.

Infusion of the vasoactive drug dopamine can improve diaphragmatic strength in patients with chronic obstructive lung disease in acute respiratory failure. It should be noted, however, that increased diaphragmatic strength does not necessarily mean increased minute ventilation.

▶ The investigators should perform a controlled trial investigating the clinical utility of dopamine on diaphragmatic function and weaning in COPD patients with acute respiratory failure. Does the slight increase in diaphragmatic strength caused by infusing 10 μg/kg/min of dopamine produce clinical benefits that justify the increase in heart rate, systemic blood pressure, and pulmonary arterial pressure?—J.R. Michael, M.D.

## Pulmonary Vascular Disease

▶ ↓ Abstract 4–21 elegantly demonstrates that hypoxic pulmonary hypertension is a reversible condition in dogs. Abstract 4–22 suggests that hypoxia causes vasoconstriction by decreasing the production of the vasodilator cyclic guanosine 5′-monophosphate. Abstract 4–23 emphasizes the frequent neurologic manifestations of pulmonary arteriovenous malformations and reviews the long-term effectiveness of embolization therapy. Abstract 4–24 demonstrates the reliability of ultrasonography as a noninvasive test to diagnose thrombosis of the femoral and popliteal veins. Abstract 4–25 suggests that patients with multiple sclerosis are protected from deep vein thrombosis. Abstract 4–26 raises questions about the value of volume loading in the treatment of pulmonary emboli.—J.R. Michael, M.D.

---

### Pulmonary Hypertension and Pulmonary Vascular Reactivity in Beagles at High Altitude

Grover RF, Johnson RL Jr, McCullough RG, McCullough RE, Hofmeister SE, Campbell WB, Reynolds RC (Univ of Colorado; Univ of Texas, Dallas)
*J Appl Physiol* 65:2632–2640, December 1988 4–21

---

Although most species experience pulmonary hypertension at high altitudes, dogs may be hyporesponders. The response of the canine pulmonary vascular bed to chronic hypoxia was measured in beagle dogs from sea level that were exposed to an altitude of 3,100 m for 12–19 months. Age-matched controls remained at an altitude of 130 m (Fig 4–13). The respective barometric pressures were 525 and 750 torr.

Beagles taken to high altitude as adults had a mean pulmonary artery pressure (PAP) at high altitude of 21.6 torr, compared with 13.2 torr for controls. When dogs were taken to high altitude at age 2.5 months, the mean PAP was 23.2 torr, compared with 13.8 torr in controls (Fig 4–14). A doubling of pulmonary vascular resistance occurred, but there was

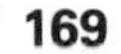

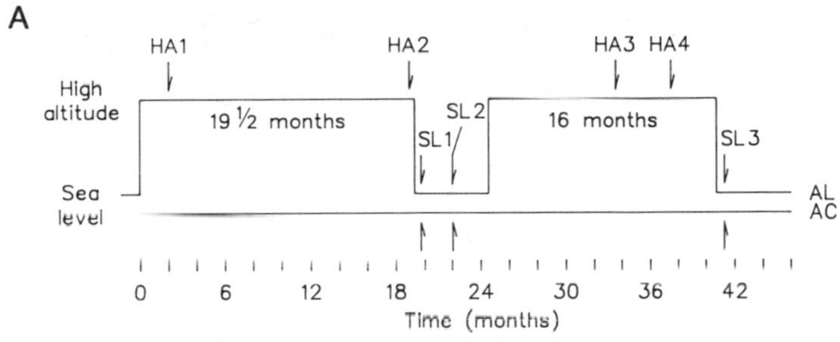


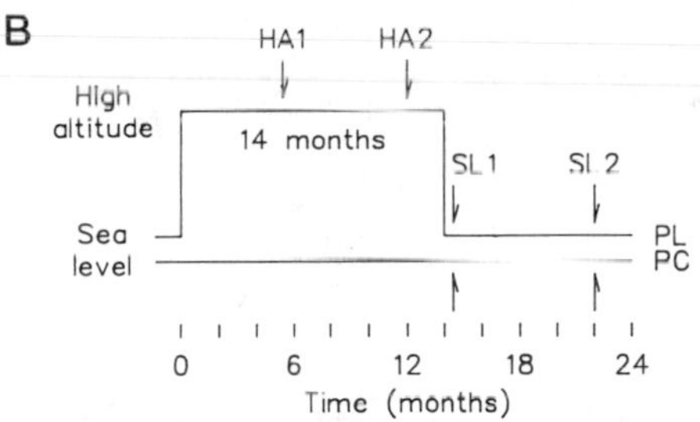


Fig 4–13.—Chronology of studies in adult dogs (A) and puppies (B). Five adult beagles had 2 sojourns at high altitude *(AL)* and 5 adult controls *(AC)* remained at sea level. Five beagle puppies had a single sojourn at high altitude (PL), and 5 puppy controls (PC) remained at sea level. Time in months is indicated, starting with ascent to high altitude. ↓, times of hemodynamic studies at high altitude *(HA)* for AL and PL at sea level *(SL)* for AL and AC, PL and PC. (Courtesy of Grover RF, Johnson RL Jr, McCullough RG, et al: *J Appl Physiol* 65:2632–2640, December 1988.)

no progression with increasing time at altitude. Pulmonary vascular reactivity to acute hypoxia was enhanced at high altitude. Inhibition of prostaglandin synthesis by indomethacin did not attenuate the pulmonary hypertension or counter the enhanced vascular reactivity. Pulmonary hypertension, once established, was only partly reversed by relieving chronic hypoxia, but nearly complete reversal followed a return to low altitude.

At an altitude of 3,100 m beagles have pulmonary hypertension comparable in severity to that in human beings at similar altitudes.

▶ This carefully conducted study indicates that long-term exposure to high altitude leads to hypoxic pulmonary hypertension in beagles and that these pathophysiologic changes are reversible upon continuous relief of hypoxia by moving the animals to sea level. These results and the findings from a study of humans (1) support the concept that many of the pathophysiologic changes in the pulmonary circulation that occur in patients with COPD or cystic fibrosis with hypoxic pulmonary hypertension may be potentially reversible.—J.R. Michael, M.D.

*Reference*

1. Sime F, Penaloza D, Ruiz L: Bradycardia, increased cardiac output, and reversal of pulmonary hypertension in altitude natives living at sea level. *Br Heart J* 33:647–657, 1971.

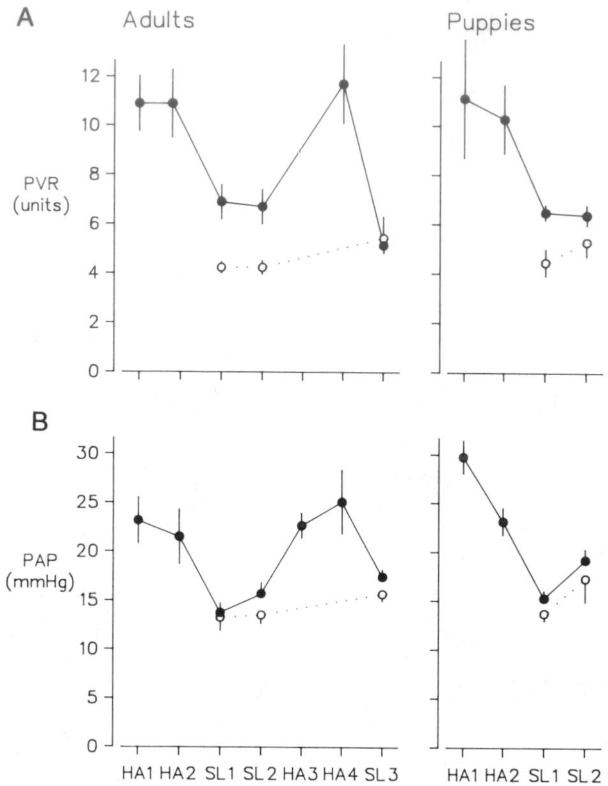


**Fig 4–14.**—**A,** Pulmonary vascular resistance (PVR), and **B,** PAP in adult dogs (**left**) and puppies (**right**). Data were obtained at high altitude *(HA)* and at sea level *(SL)* at times shown by arrows in Figure 4–13. Beagles taken to high altitude *(shaded circles)* are compared with control beagles remaining at sea level *(open circles)*. Values are means ± standard error. (Courtesy of Grover RF, Johnson RL Jr, McCullough RG, et al: *J Appl Physiol* 65:2632–2640, December 1988.)

---

## $H_2O_2$ and cGMP May Function as an $O_2$ Sensor in the Pulmonary Artery

Burke-Wolin T, Wolin MS (New York Med College, Valhalla)
*J Appl Physiol* 66:167–170, January 1989 4–22

---

Oxygen tension is the chief regulator of blood flow in the lungs, but the mechanisms involved are not understood. Activation of guanylate cyclase apparently is mediated by the metabolism of hydrogen peroxide ($H_2O_2$) by catalase associated with formation of the oxidized intermediate of catalase, compound I. To determine whether $H_2O_2$-dependent modulation of guanylate cyclase has a role in $O_2$ tension-dependent changes in force in the isolated bovine pulmonary artery, precontracted arteries 4 to 6 mm in diameter were studied.

The arteries exhibited a decrease in force with increasing $O_2$ tension that was antagonized when activation of soluble guanylate cyclase was inhibited by methylene blue or when catalase was inactivated by pretreatment with 3-amino-1,2,4,-triazole. Oxygen tension-dependent relaxation was associated with an increase in intracellular metabolism of $H_2O_2$ through catalase and cyclic guanosine 5'-monophosphate (cGMP).

There is good evidence of the involvement of cGMP and $H_2O_2$ in oxygen-elicited arterial relaxation. This mechanism of oxygen tension-elicited relaxation may contribute to the maintenance of low resistance in ventilated regions of the lungs.

▶ Whether hypoxic vasoconstriction occurs because hypoxia releases a vasoconstrictor or because hypoxia decreases the production of a dilator is unclear. The authors propose that hypoxia decreases the production of a dilator (1). They suggest that at normal oxygen tensions hydrogen peroxide is produced, which interacts with catalase to form compound I. Compound I stimulates the soluble guanyl cyclase leading to production of the dilator cGMP. They propose that a decrease in oxygen tension reduces cGMP production, which contributes to the increase in tone produced by hypoxia.—J.R. Michael, M.D.

*Reference*

1. Burke TM, Wolin MS: Hydrogen peroxide elicits pulmonary arterial relaxation and guanylate cyclase activation. *Am J Physiol* 252:H721–H732, 1987.

---

**Pulmonary Arteriovenous Malformations: Techniques and Long-Term Outcome of Embolotherapy**

White RI Jr, Lynch-Nyhan A, Terry P, Duescher PC, Fermlett EJ, Charnas L, Shuman K, Kim W, Kinnison M, Mitchell SE (Johns Hopkins Med Institutions, Baltimore)

*Radiology* 169:663–669, December 1988 4–23

---

Until 1977, pulmonary arteriovenous malformations (PAVMs) were treated strictly by surgical intervention. Since then, PAVMs have been treated with embolotherapy using stainless steel coils and detachable balloons. The development of better catheterization techniques has led to improved techniques for embolotherapy of PAVMs.

During a 9.5-year study period, 76 patients aged 5 to 76 years (mean,

TABLE 1.—Pulmonary Symptoms in 76 Patients With PAVM

| Symptoms | No. of Patients |
|---|---|
| Epistaxis | 60 (79) |
| Dyspnea | 54 (71) |
| Hemoptysis | 10 (13) |
| Hemothorax | 7 (9) |

*Note:* Numbers in parentheses are percentages.
(Courtesy of White RI Jr, Lynch-Nyhan A, Terry P, et al: *Radiology* 169:663–669, December 1988.)

TABLE 2.—Neurologic Symptoms in 76 Patients With PAVM

| Symptoms | No. of Patients |
|---|---|
| Stroke | 14 (18) |
| Transient ischemic attack | 28 (37) |
| Abscess | 7 (9) |
| Migraine | 33 (43) |
| Seizure | 6 (8) |

*Note:* Numbers in parentheses are percentages.
(Courtesy of White RI Jr, Lynch-Nyhan A, Terry P, et al: *Radiology* 169:663–669, December 1988.)

36 years), underwent occlusion of 276 PAVMs with balloon embolotherapy. Pulmonary symptoms included epistaxis in 60 patients, dyspnea in 54, hemoptysis in 10, and hemothorax in 7 (Table 1). Neurologic symptoms included a history of stroke in 14 patients, transient ischemic attack in 28, abscess in 7, migraine in 33, and seizure in 6 (Table 2). Computed tomography performed in 59 patients showed stroke in 21 patients (36%). In addition to a comprehensive diagnostic work-up of the patient undergoing embolotherapy, family members with a history of epistaxis or telangiectasia were screened by the measurement of arterial blood gases and chest radiography.

Hereditary hemorrhagic telangiectasia (HHT) was present in 67 (88%) of the 76 patients; 11 were discovered by family screening. Of the 276 PAVMs treated with balloon embolotherapy, 222 (80%) were simple, and 54 were complex. PAVMs located in the lower lobes were found in 65%, a finding that correlated with the presence of hypoxemia in the sitting or upright position. None of the patients required surgical intervention because of failure to occlude a PAVMs with embolotherapy. Complications were only minor; 8 patients had self-limited pleurisy which occurred 12 to 48 hours after embolization and lasted 3 to 5 days. Paradoxical embolization occurred in 2 PAVMs (0.7%). Operator error accounted for the complication in both cases. Follow-up studies have indicated persistent relief of hypoxemia and demonstrated only minimal growth of small remaining PAVMs. Because of the significant association of embolic stroke in patients with multiple PAVMs and HHT, the screening of family members with HHT should be pursued vigorously.

▶ This report indicates the high incidence of neurologic complications in patients with pulmonary arteriovenous malformations. Eighteen percent had a clinical history of stroke, 37% had a history of a transient ischemic attack, 43% had migraine headaches, and 8% had seizures. Thirty-six percent of patients had evidence of a stroke on head CT scans. The possibility of a PAVM should be considered for young patients with stroke, hypoxemia, hemoptysis, severe epistaxis, or hemothorax. Embolization of the malformations significantly increases arterial oxygen pressure and markedly reduces the incidence of paradoxical emboli and neurologic symptoms.—J.R. Michael, M.D.

**Detection of Deep-Vein Thrombosis by Real-Time B-Mode Ultrasonography**

Lensing AWA, Prandoni P, Brandjes D, Huisman PM, Vigo M, Tomasella G, Krekt J, ten Cate JW, Huisman MV, Büller HR (Academic Med Ctr, Amsterdam; Univ of Padua, Italy; Onze Lieve Vrouwe Gasthuis, Amsterdam; Second Hosp Service of Radiology, Padua, Italy)

*N Engl J Med* 320:342–345, Feb 9, 1989 4–24

Diagnosing deep-vein thrombosis on the basis of clinical signs and symptoms in outpatients is unreliable. In a prospective study of 220 consecutive outpatients with clinically suspected deep-vein thrombosis, the use of real-time B-mode ultrasonography in which vein compressibility was the sole criterion was compared with the use of contrast venography. The common femoral and popliteal veins were assessed for full compressibility, indicating no thrombosis, and noncompressibility, indicating thrombosis.

In 142 of 143 patients with normal findings on venograms, both veins were fully compressible. All 66 patients with proximal vein thrombosis had noncompressible femoral/or popliteal veins, or both. Overall, the sensitivity and specificity of real-time B-mode ultrasonography when using this criterion were 91% and 99%, respectively. For isolated thrombosis of the calf veins, the sensitivity was only 36%.

Ultrasonography with the single criterion of vein compressibility is an accurate, simple, objective, and reproducible noninvasive method for detecting proximal vein thrombosis in outpatients with clinically suspected deepvenous thrombosis.

▶ Ultrasonography has proven to be a reliable noninvasive technique to identify thrombosis of the femoral and popliteal veins. In this and other studies (1), its sensitivity is 91% (false negative rate of 9%) and its specificity is 99% (1% false positive rate). It should be borne in mind, however, that this technique is unable to detect isolated thrombi in the iliac vein or the segment of the superficial femoral vein that is within the adductor canal. This technique is also poor at detecting isolated thrombi in calf veins (sensitivity of 36% with a 64% false negative rate).—J.R. Michael, M.D.

*Reference*

1. White RH, McGahan JP, Daschbach MM, et al: Diagnosis of deep-vein thrombosis using duplex ultrasound. *Ann Intern Med* 111:297–304, 1989.

**Are Patients With Multiple Sclerosis Protected From Thrombophlebitis and Pulmonary Embolism?**

Kaufman J, Khatri BO, Riendl P (Med College of Wisconsin, Milwaukee)

*Chest* 94:998–1001, November 1988 4–25

Incidence of Deep Venous Thrombosis and Pulmonary Embolism

| | No. of Multiple Sclerosis Admissions | No. of Nonmultiple Sclerosis Admissions |
|---|---|---|
| Admissions classified only as pulmonary embolism | 0 | 158 |
| Admissions classified as only deep venous thrombophlebitis | 0 | 258 |
| Admissions where both deep venous thrombophlebitis pulmonary embolism were diagnosed | 0 | 17 |
| Total admissions for deep venous & pulmonary thromboembolic events | 0 | 433 |
| Admissions for causes other than deep venous thrombosis and pulmonary embolism | 1,986 (p<0.001) | 57,416 |

(Courtesy of Kaufman J, Khatri BO, Riendl P: *Chest* 94:998–1001, November 1988.)

Multiple sclerosis (MS) is a demyelinating disorder that results in debility with reduced activity and immobilization. Although there have been several excellent reviews of activity status, morbidity, and mortality in patients with MS, none has mentioned an association of MS with pulmonary embolism (PE) or deep venous thrombophlebitis (DVT). To study the incidence of DVT and PE in patients with MS, the charts of 228 patients with MS who were admitted in 1986 to a single institution in a 3.5 year period were reviewed.

The records were analyzed for any other hospitalization for DVT and PE. These patients had no admissions for either condition (table). Of the more than 57,412 non-MS-related admissions in the same period, 175 were for PE and 258 were for DVT.

No DVT or PE was found among these patients. This low incidence of thromboembolic events in patients with MS is less than expected in the general population. The presence of lower extremity spastic disease might prevent clotting. Further studies are needed to investigate this phenomenon.

▶ Patients with multiple sclerosis appear to be protected against developing deep vein thrombosis. Patients with spinal cord paralysis also appear to have an unexpectedly low incidence of deep vein thrombosis (1). Patients with spinal cord injury and paraplegia for less than 2 months have a high incidence of deep vein thrombosis (6 of 28 patients), but patients paraplegic for more than 2 months have a very low incidence of deep vein thrombosis (0 of 122 patients) (1).—J.R. Michael, M.D.

*Reference*

1. Tribe CR: Causes of death in the early and late stages of paraplegia. *Paraplegia* 1:19–47, 1963.

**Effects of Volume Loading During Experimental Acute Pulmonary Embolism**

Belenkie I, Dani R, Smith ER, Tyberg JV (Univ of Calgary, Alta)

*Circulation* 80:178–188, July 1989 4–26

Volume loading has been proposed in acute pulmonary embolism to raise the right ventricular (RV) end-diastolic volume, and thereby the cardiac output. However, a leftward shift in the ventricular septum could decrease left ventricular (LV) end-diastolic volume and stroke work. The effects of volume loading were examined in dogs with increased RV afterload caused by pulmonary embolization from injected clot fragments. Studies were performed in anesthetized closed-chest, ventilated animals.

The LV area index, reflecting LV volume, increased during baseline volume loading and decreased after repeated embolizations. Left ventricular stroke work increased on volume loading and decreased markedly after repeated embolizations. The decrease in LV area index correlated with an increased septum-to-RV free wall diameter and a decreased septum-to-LV free wall diameter. Left ventricular transmural pressure decreased in response to volume loading after repeated embolizations, indicating a marked increase in pericardial pressure.

Volume loading can cause hemodynamic deterioration after pulmonary embolism in this model, through both a leftward septal shift and increased pericardial pressure. In addition, LV transmural pressure (preload) is reduced. Stroke work declines by the Frank-Starling mechanism. It should not be assumed that volume loading will help patients who are hemodynamically impaired after acute pulmonary embolism. If it is attempted, it might be worthwhile to monitor the estimated transmural LV end-diastolic pressure.

▶ The investigators have previously shown in previously healthy animals that pulmonary emboli do not decrease LV compliance or contractility and that the primary mechanism for a decrease in LV function is reduced preload (1). One traditional approach to improving preload in patients with pulmonary emboli and hemodynamic compromise is to infuse large amounts of volume in an attempt to increase LV preload. This and other studies (2, 3) suggest that excessive volume loading may worsen LV preload by overdistending the right ventricle leading to a leftward shift of the intraventricular septum and to an increase in pericardial pressure. The net effect can be a decrease in LV transmural pressure, a decrease in LV preload, and a fall in stroke volume. The authors found that the change in right atrial pressure relative to the change in pulmonary capillary wedge pressure caused by volume loading correlates with the change in the transeptal pressure gradient. They suggest that this can be used clinically to assess whether too much volume has been given. For example, if the increase in right atrial pressure exceeds the increase in pulmonary capillary wedge pressure, this suggests that further volume loading may be counterproductive.—J.R. Michael, M.D.

*References*

1. Belenkie I, Dani R, Smith ER, et al: Ventricular interaction during experimental acute pulmonary embolism. *Circulation* 78:761–768, 1988.
2. Jardin F, Dubourg O, Gueret P, et al: Quantitative two-dimensional echocardiography in massive pulmonary embolism: Emphasis on ventricular interdependence and leftward septal displacement. *J Am Coll Cardiol* 10:1201–1206, 1987.
3. Ozier Y, Dubourg O, Farcot JC, et al: Circulatory failure in acute pulmonary embolism. *Intens Care Med* 10:91–97, 1984.

## General Critical Care

▶ ↓ Abstract 4–27 proposes that invasive monitoring and deliberately attempting to increase cardiac output improves survival in high-risk surgical patients. Abstract 4–28 investigates the mechanism by which shock leads to apnea. Abstract 4–29 studies the cardiac dysfunction that occurs with *Escherichia coli* and *Staphylococcus aureus* bacteremia. Abstracts 4–30 and 4–31 compare the utility of standard pulmonary artery catheters and fiberoptic catheters that measure mixed venous oxygen tension. Abstract 4–32 represents a controlled trial of normobaric or hyperbaric oxygen in patients with acute carbon monoxide poisoning. Abstract 4–33 demonstrates that *Clostridium difficile* may be a frequent nosocomial infection. Abstract 4–34 investigates the adequacy of manual ventilation of critically ill patients during transport. Abstract 4–35 questions the marked difference in the frequency of "do not resuscitate" orders for patients with different diseases but similar prognoses.—J.R. Michael, M.D.

---

### Prospective Trial of Supranormal Values of Survivors as Therapeutic Goals in High-Risk Surgical Patients

Shoemaker WC, Appel PL, Kram HB, Waxman K, Lee T-S (Harbor–UCLA Med Ctr, Torrance, Calif; King-Drew Med Ctr, Los Angeles)
*Chest* 94:1176–1186, December 1988 4–27

---

Patients surviving high-risk surgery have higher cardiac indices and oxygen consumption values than nonsurvivors, and higher values of $\dot{D}O_2$. It may be that an increased cardiac index and $\dot{D}O_2$ reflect circulatory circulatory compensation for increased postoperative metabolism. This hypothesis was tested in a prospective series of 252 high-risk general surgical patients and in 146 other high-risk patients assigned to central venous pressure or pulmonary arterial monitoring. The patients had an estimated mortality risk close to 30% (table).

Summary of Mortality of the Prospective Series

| Series | Date | Control Number | Control Deaths | Protocol Number | Protocol Deaths, % |
|---|---|---|---|---|---|
| Series 1 | 1/78-6/80 | 168 | 57 (34%) | 108 | 21 (19%) |
| Control period between trials | 6/80-5/83 | 239 | 66 (28%) | ... | ... |
| Series 2 | 5/83-5/84 | 105 | 34 (32%) | 28 | 1 (4%) |
| Control period after trials | 5/84-5/85 | 160 | 40 (25%) | ... | ... |
| Total | | 672 | 197 (29%) | 136 | 22 (16%) |

(Courtesy of Shoemaker WC, Appel PL, Kram HB, et al: *Chest* 94:1176–1186, December 1988.)

When the goal was to achieve the supranormal values observed in postoperative survivors, survival was greater than when the goal was merely to maintain normal hemodynamic values. Mortality was lowest in the former patients when pulmonary artery monitoring was used. These patients had the fewest complications and the shortest stays in intensive care and in hospital. In addition, costs were lower when a pulmonary artery catheter was placed preoperatively.

Pulmonary artery catheterization is quite cost-effective when used to augment physiologic circulatory function perioperatively in high-risk patients. "Normal" hemodynamic values are appropriate only for relatively unstressed patients. Otherwise it is best to attempt to achieve the values characteristic of patients who survive critical illness.

▶ This article suggests that increasing cardiac output and oxygen delivery in critically ill surgical patients improves survival. Unfortunately, the authors do not provide the reader with enough information to convince them that the study was well designed and executed. For example, protocols used to increase cardiac output and not spelled out, and thus it is unclear whether the protocols were actually followed in this study. Carefully performed clinical trials are needed to test this important hypothesis.—J.R. Michael, M.D.

**Cardiovascular Failure and Apnea in Shock**

Nava S, Bellemare F (McGill Univ)

*J Appl Physiol* 66:184–189, January 1989 4–28

Shock was produced in anesthetized dogs by limiting venous return with a balloon inflated in the right atrium. This rapidly reversible form of cardiogenic shock was used to determine whether arterial pressure can recover when respiration ceases and whether this is accompanied by recovery of inspiratory muscle function. Change in ventilation in response to lowering diastolic blood pressure to 50 torr was estimated by recording transdiaphragmatic pressure and electric activity in the diaphragm and parasternal intercostal muscles.

Although ventilation was initially increased, it declined progressively until apnea occurred after a mean of 103 minutes. The changes included 60% reductions in breathing frequency, transdiaphragmatic pressure, and intercostal electric activity and a 30% decrease in diaphragmatic electric activity. Diaphragmatic contractility did not decrease in response to artificial stimulation of the phrenic nerve.

Cardiocirculatory function deteriorated and the change became irreversible at the time of apnea. Recovery from apnea did not occur without recovery of arterial pressure.

It appears that, in this model, the fall in ventilation and ensuing apnea result from a decrease in central respiratory neural output associated with progressively declining cardiocirculatory function. The cause of the cardiovascular decline is not known, but failure of both the heart and systemic vascular control may be involved. Whether the apparent association of cardiovascular failure with apnea is real or merely coincidental remains to be learned.

▶ The investigators produced shock by inflating a balloon in the right atrium until diastolic blood pressure decreased to 50 mm Hg. The inflation of the balloon then was adjusted to maintain diastolic pressure at this level. When apnea developed, diaphragmatic contractility was measured to determine whether apnea occurred primarily because of a decrease in neurologic drive or a decrease in contractility. The results of this study suggest that when apnea occurred the major abnormality was in neurologic drive, because, if the diaphragm was electrically paced, diaphragmatic contractility was normal. Deflation of the balloon when apnea developed did not lead to cardiovascular recovery. Thus, once cardiovascular function has deteriorated to the point that apnea develops, shock may be irreversible.—J.R. Michael, M.D.

---

**Role of Endotoxemia in Cardiovascular Dysfunction and Mortality: *Escherichia coli* and *Staphylococcus aureus* Challenges in a Canine Model of Human Septic Shock**

Natanson C, Danner RL, Elin RJ, Hosseini JM, Peart KW, Banks SM, MacVittie TJ, Walker RI, Parrillo JE (NIH; Armed Forces Radiobiology Research Inst, Bethesda, Md)

*J Clin Invest* 83:243–251, January 1989 4–29

---

There is some evidence that organisms without endotoxin can cause septic shock by disrupting the gastrointestinal mucosal barrier so that gram-negative bacteria or endotoxin can enter the circulation. The cardiovascular changes produced by *Escherichia coli* and *Staphylococcus aureus* were compared in a canine model designed to simulate human septic shock. The organisms were placed in an intraperitoneal clot, sometimes after being killed by formalin, and cardiovascular function was assessed in conscious animals by radionuclide scanning and measurement of thermodilution cardiac output.

All dogs infected with viable bacteria had species-specific positive blood cultures. They were more ill than dogs given formalin-killed bacteria, but most infected dogs recovered completely within 7 to 10 days. All groups of animals showed strongly concordant hemodynamic changes. Mortality was greater in dogs given *S. aureus* than in those infected with *E. coli*. Greater myocardial depression occurred in the former group. Significant endotoxemia occurred only with *E. coli*.

Microorganisms that lack endotoxins can produce the same myocardial depression and hemodynamic changes as those that produce endotoxin. Multiple bacterial substances apparently can trigger a common pathway that leads to cardiovascular injury and death.

▶ Although we usually associate gram-negative infections with septic shock, some patients with staphylococcal bacteremia also present with the clinical picture of septic shock. The authors have made major contributions to defining the cardiac dysfunction that can occur with sepsis (1–4). In both dogs and human beings, they have found that gram negative sepsis leads to a reversible decrease in left ventricular function within the first few days. This dysfunction is manifest by a decrease in ejection fraction. Cardiac index and stroke volume, however, usually are maintained by dilation of the heart and an increase in both left ventricular end-diastolic and end-systolic volumes (1–3). In human beings the decrease in myocardial function does not appear secondary to a decrease in coronary blood flow (4). In this report, the investigators addressed whether endotoxin itself was required to produce this hemodynamic pattern. The same hemodynamic pattern was produced by live or formalin killed *E. coli,* which produces endotoxin, and by *S. aureus,* which does not make endotoxin. These results suggest that gram-positive organisms, such as *S. aureus,* as well as gram-negative organisms can produce significant myocardial depression. In fact, *S. aureus* infection produced greater mortality and greater myocardial depression than did *E. coli* infection. For related articles please see the 1987 YEAR BOOK OF PULMONARY DISEASE, pages 158–159.—J.R. Michael, M.D.

*References*


1. Parker MM, Shelhamer JH, Bacharach SL, et al: Profound but reversible myocardial depression in patients with septic shock. *Ann Intern Med* 100:483–490, 1984.
2. Natanson C, Fink MP, Ballantyne HK, et al: Gram-negative bacteremia produces both severe systolic and diastolic cardiac dysfunction in a canine model that stimulates human septic shock. *J Clin Invest* 78:259–270, 1986.
3. Natanson C, Danner RL, Fink MP, et al: Cardiovascular performance with *E. coli* challenges in a canine model of human sepsis. *Am J Physiol* 254:H558–H569, 1988.
4. Cunnion RE, Schaer GL, Parker MM, et al: The coronary circulation in human septic shock. *Circulation* 73:637–643, 1986.

**Analysis of the Effects of Continuous On-Line Monitoring of Mixed Venous Oxygen Saturation on Patient Outcome and Cost-Effectiveness**

Jastremski MS, Chelluri L, Beney KM, Bailly RT (State Univ of New York, Syracuse)

*Crit Care Med* 17:148–153, February 1989 4–30

The continuous on-line measurement of mixed venous oxygen saturation ($S\bar{v}O_2$) is a new technique for monitoring tissue oxygen balance in critically ill patients. The technique involves the use of a pulmonary artery (PA) catheter that utilizes reflective fiberoptic oximetry for continuous $S\bar{v}O_2$ monitoring. Although the accuracy and reliability of this new technique have been confirmed in earlier studies, its clinical significance and cost-effectiveness are being questioned. This technique was assessed in 99 patients admitted to an intensive care unit (ICU) who required PA catheters either for hemodynamic stabilization or in preparation for major surgery. A total of 49 patients received standard quadruple-lumen flow-directed thermodilution PA catheters, and 50 patients were given the new flow-directed thermodilution PA Opticath catheter designed for the continuous measurement of $S\bar{v}O_2$. Both groups were followed throughout their ICU stay. Data recorded included admission Acute Physiology and Chronic Health Evaluation (APACHE) score, daily Therapeutic Intervention Scoring System (TISS) scores, duration of ICU stay, number of blood gases, and ICU mortality.

Statistical analysis of the collected data demonstrated that the use of the Opticath did not decrease the number of potentially adverse hemodynamic events, length of ICU stay, or ICU mortality. Although the use of continuous oximetry is a valuable educational tool for medical students as it illustrates important concepts, the Opticath has no impact on patient outcome.

**A Comparison Between a Conventional and a Fiberoptic Flow-Directed Thermal Dilution Pulmonary Artery Catheter in Critically Ill Patients**

Rajput MA, Richey HM, Bush BA, Glendening DL, Matthews JI (Brooke Army Med Ctr, San Antonio, Tex)

*Arch Intern Med* 149:83–85, January 1989 4–31

The clinical usefulness and cost-effectiveness of the recently introduced fiberoptic flow-directed thermal dilution pulmonary artery (PA) catheter for the continuous measurement of mixed venous oxygen saturation were evaluated in 51 critically ill patients who required hemodynamic monitoring in an intensive care unit (ICU). 26 patients (mean age, 63 years) were given a standard balloon-tipped PA catheter and 25 patients (mean age, 68 years) received the new fiberoptic PA catheter. The 2 study groups were well randomized with respect to age and illness severity.

There were no statistically significant differences between the 2 groups in monitoring time, arterial blood gas measurements per 24 hours, hours of mechanical ventilator support, vasopressor therapy, time in the ICU, or mortality. The only statistically significant differences between the 2 groups were in the insertion time and in the number of defective catheters. The mean insertion times were 4.5 minutes for the standard PA catheter and 7.1 minutes for the fiberoptic PA catheter. One standard catheter and 4 fiberoptic catheters had defective balloons. No trends or unexpected adverse events were predicted by the use of the fiberoptic PA catheter. There were also more technical problems in consistently obtaining wedge pressures in patients with fiberoptic catheters.

Considering that the fiberoptic PA catheter costs $175 compared with $75 for a standard PA catheter, coupled with the fact that using the new fiberoptic catheter did not result in any benefit for the patients as to morbidity or mortality, the routine use of a fiberoptic PA catheter is not clinically useful nor cost-effective, and is therefore not indicated.

▶ These 2 studies (Abstracts 4–30 and 4–31) compared a regular pulmonary artery catheter with a fiberoptic catheter that monitors mixed venous oxygen saturation. The fiberoptic catheters are more expensive, and their use has been promoted because of the potential ability to quickly identify adverse hemodynamic changes. These controlled trials did not find that the fiberoptic catheter offered any objective benefit in terms of identifying adverse hemodynamic changes. A previous prospective study has found a similar result (1). The authors also mention that nurses and house staff did not like the fiberoptic catheter because it was more time-consuming to set up, harder to wedge, more difficult to calibrate, and associated with frequent problems in obtaining reliable pulmonary arterial tracings. The real value of monitoring mixed venous oxygen tension is also questionable because other clinical studies have shown that mixed venous oxygen tension or saturation may be a poor indicator of tissue oxygenation in critically ill patients (2, 3).—J.R. Michael, M.D.

*References*

1. Boutros AR, Lee C: Value of continuous monitoring of mixed venous blood oxygen saturation in the management of critically ill patients. *Crit Care Med* 14:132–134, 1986.
2. Danek SJ, Lynch JP, Weg JG, et al: The dependence of oxygen uptake on oxygen delivery in the adult respiratory distress syndrome. *Am Rev Respir Dis* 122:387–395, 1980.
3. Abraham E, Bland RD, Cobo JC, et al: Sequential cardiorespiratory patterns associated with outcome in septic shock. *Chest* 85:75–80, 1984.

---

### Trial of Normobaric and Hyperbaric Oxygen for Acute Carbon Monoxide Intoxication

Raphael J-C, Elkharrat D, Jars-Guincestre M-C, Chastang C, Chasles V, Vercken J-B, Gajdos P (Hôpital Raymond Poincaré, Garches, France; Hôpital St Louis, Paris)

*Lancet* 2:414–418, Aug 19, 1989 4–32

---

Acute carbon monoxide intoxication remains a frequent occurrence in the home. Although oxygen is the usual treatment, the indications for hyperbaric oxygen (HBO) remain uncertain. In 629 adults who were poisoned at home within 12 hours of hospital admission, the value of HBO was studied.

When consciousness was intact, 6 hours of normobaric oxygen (NBO) were compared with 2 hours of HBO at 2 atm absolute plus 4 hours of NBO. In those with initially impaired consciousness, the effect of 1 and 2 sessions of HBO were compared. The 2 sessions were 2 to 12 hours apart.

In patients with intact consciousness treatment with NBO alone and combined HBO-NBO was similarly successful. About two thirds of the patients had recovered at 1 month. In those with impaired consciousness, the use of 1 and 2 sessions of HBO had similar effects. All these patients also received NBO. Slightly more than half of these patients had recovered at 1 month. All 7 patients with neuropsychiatric sequelae and all 4 who died had been admitted in coma. The type of treatment still made no difference when the outcome was stratified by the presenting concentration of carboxyhemoglobin.

Normobaric oxygen is adequate for carbon monoxide-intoxicated patients whose consciousness is unimpaired. Those with brief loss of consciousness may receive 1 session of HBO. It is not likely that 2 sessions of HBO have significant value, but whether more than 2 sessions are indicated remains uncertain.

▶ Uncontrolled trials have suggested that hyperbaric oxygen therapy may be more effective than normobaric oxygen in treating carbon monoxide poisoning. Abstract 4–32 reports the results of a large-scale, controlled trial in which hyperbaric oxygen therapy was not helpful in patients who initially did not lose consciousness. One month later, regardless of the type of oxygen therapy, 97% of these patients had resumed their normal occupations and social activities, and 66% had no symptoms or signs.

For patients with initial loss of consciousness, one 2-hour treatment period with hyperbaric oxygen was as effective as 2 hyperbaric treatments. The authors did not compare normobaric and hyperbaric oxygen in these patients, so the need for hyperbaric oxygen in this group is uncertain. Death or neurologic sequelae occurred in only 7 of 629 patients, and all these patients were comatose upon presentation at the hospital.—J.R. Michael, M.D.

---

**Nosocomial Acquisition of *Clostridium difficile* Infection**

McFarland LV, Mulligan ME, Kwok RYY, Stamm WE (Univ of Washington; West Los Angeles VA Med Ctr; Univ of California, Los Angeles)

*N Engl J Med* 320:204–210, Jan 26, 1989 4–33

---

Previous studies have failed to distinguish between nosocomial acquisition of *Clostridium difficile* and preexisting endogenous colonization that causes disease when antibiotics are given in the hospital. The acquisition

Environmental Isolation of *Clostridium difficile*

| Culture Source | Rooms With Culture-Negative Patients* | Rooms With Asymptomatic Carriers | Rooms With Patients With C. Difficile Diarrhea | Total Positive/ Total Tested (%) |
|---|---|---|---|---|
| | no. of positive cultures (%) | | | |
| Bedrail | 0 | 2 | 10 | 12/31 (39) |
| Commode | 1 | 3 | 1 | 5/13 (38) |
| Floor | 5 | 3 | 18 | 26/72 (36) |
| Call button | 1 | 2 | 6 | 9/30 (30) |
| Windowsill | 0 | 1 | 2 | 3/10 (30) |
| Toilet | 0 | 0 | 3 | 3/17 (18) |
| Other† | 0 | 0 | 4 | 4/43 (9) |
| Total positive cultures | 7 (8) | 11 (29) | 44 (49) | 62 (29) |
| No. of cultures | 88 | 38 | 90 | 216 |

*Rooms in which no patients with positive cultures for *C. difficile* were in residence for more than 48 hours.
†Other sources included dialysis machine (1), sink (1), nasogastric alimentation preparation (1), and slipper bottoms (1).
(Courtesy of McFarland LV, Mulligan ME, Kwok RYY, et al: *N Engl J Med* 320:204–210, Jan 26, 1989.)

and transmission of C. *difficile* was studied on a general hospital ward by serially culturing rectal swab specimens obtained prospectively at admission and subsequently from 428 patients over an 11-month period. Strains of C. *difficile* were differentiated by immunoblot typing.

Twenty-nine patients (7%) had positive cultures when admitted. Another 83 (21%) acquired C. *difficile* while in the hospital. Thirty-one of these patients (37%) had diarrhea, but none had colitis.

Time-space clustering of incident cases with identical strains was observed, and patients exposed to culture-positive patients acquired C. *difficile* earlier and more often. Most of those who cared for culture-positive patients themselves had positive hand cultures. Nearly 30% of the environmental sites sampled were positive (table). More than 80% of incident cases still had positive cultures at discharge.

Asymptomatic hospital patients are an important reservoir of C. *difficile*. Person-to-person transmission by both patients and hospital personnel is the chief means of spread; environmental reservoirs also may be important. Nosocomial transmission of C. *difficile* can be limited by hand washing, routine use of body-substance precautions for all patients, and frequent environmental disinfection.

▶ Infection with *C. difficile* is a frequent problem in hospitalized patients and in intensive care units. This article clearly demonstrates the potential for nosocomial infection of patients and hospital workers with *C. difficile*. Seven percent of patients admitted to hospitals were carriers. Of patients without *C. difficile* on admission, 21% acquired it during their hospital stays. Only a third of these patients had diarrhea; the other two thirds were asymptomatic. Despite antibiotic treatment, 80% of the patients nosocomially infected still had positive cultures at discharge. Hospital personnel caring for these patients had a high incidence of positive hand cultures (60%). The 2 techniques that appeared to reduce the frequency of positive hand cultures were to wear gloves and to wash with disinfectant soap.—J.R. Michael, M.D.

**Safe Intrahospital Transport of Critically Ill Ventilator-Dependent Patients**

Weg JG, Haas CF (Univ of Michigan)

*Chest* 96:631–635, September 1989 4–34

Recent studies suggest that ventilatory complications during patient transport are more frequent than formerly thought. A prospective single-blind study was carried out on 20 mechanically ventilated patients to determine whether manual ventilation (MAN) leads to hemodynamic or blood gas abnormalities. The study protocol is illustrated in Figure 4–15.

A volume ventilator was used in an intensive care unit and at a study-treatment center; during transport patients were manually ventilated by a respiratory therapist.

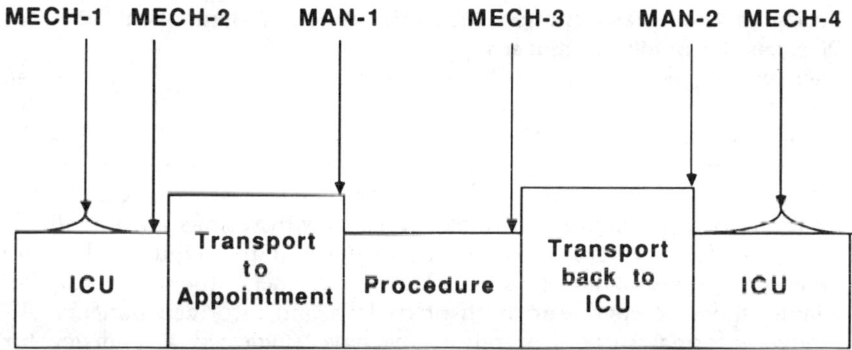


Fig 4–15.—Protocol for 20 mechanically ventilated *(MECH)* patients who required intrahospital transport with ventilation by a respiratory therapist who used MAN with a resuscitation bag. *MECH-1,* nearest arterial blood gases (ABG) during 8-hour period just prior to transport. *MECH-2,* ABG, heart rate (HR), and blood pressure (BP) just before transport. *MAN-1,* ABG, HR, BP on arrival at study area manually ventilated. *MECH-3,* ABG, HR, BP in study area mechanically ventilated. *MAN-2,* ABG, HR, BP on return to intensive care unit manually ventilated. *MECH-4,* nearest ABG in 8 hours after transport. (Courtesy of Weg JG, Haas CF: *Chest* 96:631–635, September 1989.)

No hemodynamic abnormalities were noted, and with 2 exceptions, arterial blood gases did not vary to a clinically significant degree. One patient had a reduced $PaO_2$ and an elevated $PaCO_2$ after an accidental oxygen disconnection. Another had an increase in pH of 0.13 unit with a 9-mm Hg fall in $PaCO_2$. The mean $PaO_2$ was significantly higher during MAN than with mechanical ventilation. Mean transport time to or from the appointment was 15 minutes.

Manual ventilation during in-hospital transport of mechanically ventilated patients is safe as long as a trained person can approximate the prevailing inspired oxygen fraction and minute ventilation. The routine use of portable transport ventilators and monitors is not necessary.

▶ A previous report has suggested that manual ventilation of critically ill patients during transportation results in a high incidence of potentially serious hemodynamic or blood gas abnormalities (1). This previous study recommends the use of a portable ventilator during transport of critically ill patients. The current study indicates that most ventilated patients can be transported safely using manual ventilation. There are several important caveats. First, the patients were ventilated during transport by a respiratory therapist. Second, the study did not include patients on high levels of PEEP (>10 cm $H_2O$), high $FiO_2$ (>0.7), or requiring a minute ventilation >25 L/min. Such patients may need special attention and special monitoring with, for example, pulse oximeters.—J.R. Michael, M.D.

*Reference*

1. Braman SS, Dunn SM, Amico CA, et al: Complications of intrahospital transport in critically ill patients. *Ann Intern Med* 107:469–473, 1987.

**Decisions About Resuscitation: Inequities Among Patients With Different Diseases But Similar Prognoses**

Wachter RM, Luce JM, Hearst N, Lo B (Stanford Univ; Univ of California, San Francisco)

*Ann Intern Med* 111:525–532, Sept 15, 1989 4–35

Studies that have documented the poor outcome of cardiopulmonary resuscitation and intensive care for patients with serious chronic illness have promoted the acceptance of "do-not-resuscitate" (DNR) orders and other limitations of life-sustaining treatment. Such orders are now becoming more acceptable to both physicians and informed patients. Although informal surveys of physicians have suggested a tendency for fewer interventions in the care of patients with metastatic cancer or AIDS than for other seriously ill patients, there are as yet no published data on how DNR orders are made for patients with different diagnoses but similar long-term prognoses.

To determine whether decisions on resuscitation are in fact made equitably, the medical records in 3 teaching hospitals were used to identify 1,200 patients with the following discharge diagnoses: AIDS, unresectable non–small-cell lung cancer, cirrhosis with esophageal varices, or severe congestive heart failure (CHF) with coronary disease. A review of the literature had shown that these 4 diagnoses have similar estimated 1- and 5-year survival rates.

A total of 317 patients met the study inclusion criteria; 100 had AIDS, 51 had lung cancer, 51 had cirrhosis, and 115 had CHF.

Eighty-nine of the 317 received DNR orders. Ten of the 89 had obvious in-hospital clinical events that prompted writing the order. Overall, DNR orders were written for 52% of the AIDS patients, 47% of those with lung cancer, 16% of those with cirrhosis, and 4% of those with CHF. After adjustment by multiple logistic regression for the potential confounding factors of functional status, mental status, reason for admission, and severity of illness, there still remained a strong association between DNR orders and disease category.

In a survey the medical house staff were asked to estimate how often they discussed DNR status with patients in each of the 4 disease categories and to estimate survival of patients in each category. Analysis of the completed questionnaires revealed that DNR orders were discussed more often with patients who had AIDS or lung cancer than with those who had cirrhosis or CHF, despite all clinicians being familiar with the similar prognoses. For as yet unexplained reasons, physicians approach the issue of DNR status unequally in patients with different diseases but similar prognoses.

▶ Previous studies indicate that physicians are hesitant to discuss cardiopulmonary resuscitation with their patients and do not accurately predict their patients' attitudes about terminal care (1, 2). Physicians consistently overestimate the percentage of patients who want resuscitation. Patients generally appreciate discussions about DNR status, and such discussions rarely create severe anxiety in patients (2–5).—J.R. Michael, M.D.

*References*


1. Bedell SE, Delbanco TL: Choices about cardiopulmonary resuscitation in the hospital: When do physicians talk with patients? *N Engl J Med* 310:1089–1093, 1984.
2. Shmerling RH, Bedell SE, Lilliefeld A, et al: Discussing cardiopulmonary resuscitation: A study of elderly outpatients. *J Gen Intern Med* 3:317–321, 1988.
3. Finucane TE, Shumway JM, Powers RL, et al: Planning with elderly outpatients for contingencies of severe illness: A survey and clinical trial. *J Gen Intern Med* 3:322–325, 1988.
4. Steinbrook R, Lo B, Moulton J, et al: Preferences of homosexual men with AIDS for life-sustaining treatment. *N Engl J Med* 314:457–460, 1986.
5. Lo B, McLeod GA, Saika G: Patient attitudes to discussing life-sustaining treatment. *Arch Intern Med* 146:1613–1615, 1986.

# 5 Pediatric Lung Disease

## Introduction

One has only to look at the number and diversity of articles received for this year's edition to realize that creative energy and interest in pulmonary disorders in children abounds. The spectrum of articles ranges from the fetus to the mature child and includes some rethinking of our understanding of common clinical problems or therapies as well as some "hot science." What is most exciting is the quality of both the basic and clinical research and the growth of the collaborations between these groups of investigators. Also, it is interesting that in pediatrics there is still room for basic physiology research, even in the age of the gene.

**Gerald M. Loughlin, M.D.**

## Asthma

▶ ↓ This section is devoted to current concerns in asthma management ranging from issues of acute care to asthma mortality. Asthma continues to be a pesky clinical problem despite advances in pharmacologic therapy. Our understanding of the pathogenesis of exercise-induced and viral-induced wheezing is incomplete. In addition, emergency room and intensive care management is in a state of flux, and the gospel regarding early intervention with steroids has not been widely disseminated.—G.M. Loughlin, M.D.

### An Investigation of the Effects of Heat and Water Exchange in the Recovery Period After Exercise in Children With Asthma

Smith CM, Anderson SD, Walsh S, McElrea MS (Royal Prince Alfred Hosp, Camperdown, Australia)
*Am Rev Respir Dis* 140:598–605, September 1989 5–1

The fall in forced expiratory volume in 1 second ($FEV_1$) that follows inhalation of cold, dry air during exercise has been reported to be worsened by increasing the heat content of inspired air during the recovery period. A sudden reduction in osmolarity within the airways, caused by further condensation of water as air at body temperature and ambient pressure, and saturated with water vapor, makes contact with the cooled respiratory mucosa, could be responsible.

To compare changes in $FEV_1$ in asthmatic boys after exercise, with and without the potential for condensation, 17 boys aged 12–17 years were studied. After a cycle exercise challenge with breathing of cold, dry air and rewarming, the boys were challenged with ultrasonically nebulized water.

Conditions designed to cause rapid rewarming of airways did not enhance the response, whether or not inspired air had the potential of causing additional condensation in the airway. The boys were relatively unresponsive to nebulized water.

This study neither proves nor disproves that condensation of water is responsible for an enhanced asthmatic response after exercise with inhalation of cold, dry air. The findings are, however, inconsistent with the hypothesis that rapid rewarming of airways causes exercise-induced asthma.

▶ The pathogenesis of exercise-induced asthma remains unclear. However, it would seem that, at least in children, rapid rewarming of the airways after exercise does not appear to be an important contributing factor. The role of hypo-osmolarity induced by condensation remains unequivocal. It may turn out to be a dose-dependent phenomenon influenced by how much and how rapidly water is condensed. This study suggests that small amounts of condensation probably are not a factor. Additional studies are needed because the hypothesis of temperature shifts is still attractive. However, observations in this study (patients with symptoms before the end of exercise), as well as the variety of ambient conditions in which exercise symptoms can occur, suggest that the triggers may be multifactorial, and the airway rewarming and condensation may be operational in a subset of patients. As was demonstrated in the original studies on cold-air-induced asthma, rigorous control over experimental conditions is essential if we are to compare results from exercise challenges performed in different populations.—G.M. Loughlin, M.D.

*Additional Reading*

1. McFadden ER: Exercise and asthma, *New Engl J Med* 317:502–504, 1987.
2. McFadden ER et al: Postexertional airway rewarming and thermally induced asthma. *J Clin Invest* 78:18–25, 1986.

---

**Diminished Lung Function as a Presdisposing Factor for Wheezing Respiratory Illness in Infants**

Martinez FD, Morgan WJ, Wright AL, Holberg CJ, Taussig LM, Group Health Medical Associates' Personnel (Arizona Health Sciences Ctr, Tucson)

*N Engl J Med* 319:1112–1117, Oct 27, 1988 5–2

---

Several studies have shown that schoolchildren with histories of lower respiratory tract illness (LRTI) during infancy have both poorer lung function at spirometric testing and a higher prevalence of bronchial hyperresponsiveness than children without such histories. Likewise, adults with chronic asthmatic bronchitis more often report childhood respiratory problems than do normal adults or those with smoking-related chronic obstructive lung disease.

Pulmonary Function Before the Occurrence of Lower Respiratory Tract Illness (LRI) According to the Type of Illness (With or Without Wheezing) Reported at Follow-Up*

| INDEX | NO LRI | LRI WITHOUT WHEEZING | LRI WITH WHEEZING | F | P VALUE |
|---|---|---|---|---|---|
| $T_{me}/T_E$ (%) | | | | | |
| Boys | 30.8±8.7 (39) | 34.8±7.6 (8) | 23.3±7.3† (11) | 5.1 | 0.009 |
| Girls | 31.6±9.7 (49) | 24.4±5.7 (4) | 27.1±6.3 (13) | 2.2 | 0.12 |
| Total | 31.2±9.2 (88) | 31.4±8.5 (12) | 25.4±6.9‡ (24) | 4.4 | 0.01 |
| Respiratory conductance (liter/sec/cm $H_2O$) | | | | | |
| Boys | 0.038±0.010 (17) | 0.037±0.007 (3) | 0.028±0.004 (4) | 1.8 | 0.2 |
| Girls | 0.033±0.005 (13) | 0.036±0.014 (3) | 0.028±0.007 (7) | 1.5 | 0.2 |
| Total | 0.035±0.009 (30) | 0.036±0.010 (6) | 0.028±0.006† (11) | 3.4 | 0.04 |
| Functional residual capacity (ml) | | | | | |
| Boys | 107.3±19.8 (30) | 95.2±9.0 (5) | 107.2±22.3 (8) | 0.9 | 0.43 |
| Girls | 100.3±13.5 (41) | 114.7±18.1 (3) | 85.5±11.8† (7) | 5.7 | 0.006 |
| Total | 103.2±16.7 (71) | 102.5±15.6 (8) | 97.1±20.8 (15) | 0.5 | 0.63 |
| $\dot{V}_{max}FRC$ (ml/sec) | | | | | |
| Boys | 112.5±39.0 (35) | 111.6±43.9 (8) | 105.7±59.2 (9) | 0.08 | 0.9 |
| Girls | 146.7±49.4 (42) | 139.3±45.5 (3) | 128.3±44.4 (12) | 0.7 | 0.5 |
| Total | 131.2±47.9 (77) | 119.1±44.0 (11) | 118.6±51.2 (21) | 0.7 | 0.5 |

*Plus-minus values are means ± SD. The numbers of patients tested are shown in parentheses; $T_{me}/T_E$ denotes the percentage of expiratory time necessary to reach peak tidal expiratory flow (calculated at age 8.4 weeks); and $\dot{V}_{max}$ *FRC*, the maximal flow at the end-tidal expiratory point (calculated at length 57.4 cm, age 8.4 weeks, and weight 5.1 kg). Respiratory conductance, the inverse of respiratory resistance, was calculated at length 57.4 cm; functional residual capacity was calculated at age 8.4 weeks, weight 5.1 kg, and length 57.4 cm.

†$P \leq .05$ for the comparison with the group with no LRI, by Duncan's multiple-comparison test.

‡$P \leq .01$ for the comparison with the group with no LRI, by Duncan's multiple-comparison test.

(Courtesy of Martinez FD, Morgan WJ, Wright AL, et al: *N Engl J Med* 319:1112–1117, Oct 27, 1988.)

To determine whether early differences in lung function predispose to LRTI, 124 healthy infants were enrolled at birth as part of a long-term longitudinal assessment of acute and chronic lung diseases in infants and children. All infants underwent lung function testing shortly after birth. At follow-up, the incidence of LRTI during their first year of life was correlated with their early lung function test results. During the first year of life, 36 (29%) infants had at least 1 LRTI, but none were admitted to a hospital for LRTI. Twelve (10%) infants had a LRTI without wheezing, and 24 (19%) had a LRTI with wheezing. Infants who subsequently had a LRTI without wheezing did not consistently or significantly differ from those who did not have a LRTI with respect to lung function measurements taken shortly after birth (table). In contrast, the risk of having LRTI with wheezing was 3.7 times greater among infants whose lung function measurements shortly after birth had placed them in the lowest third.

These findings suggest that an additional diminished lung function as determined shortly after birth predisposes infants for the development of LRTI with wheezing in association with common viral respiratory infections.

▶ Evidence is accumulating that infants with recurrent respiratory illness are predisposed to these conditions by preexisting alteration in lung growth and development. This predisposition can arise from events that occur either prenatally or early in life and result in an impaired ability to tolerate the natural consequences of viral infections that localize to the lower respiratory tract. It appears that, because the airways start out smaller, these infants are more likely to wheeze when airway caliber is reduced by edema or smooth muscle constriction induced by infection. These data also shed light on what has been presumed to be viral-induced reductions in pulmonary function in infants who have had infections such as croup or bronchiolitis. It seems that a proportion of the decline in lung function is due not to the effects of the acute infection, but to other genetic or prenatal factors that affect airway growth. This information requires reconsideration of previous thinking on the relationship between viral lower respiratory infections in infants and the development of chronic pulmonary disease—G.M. Loughlin, M.D.

*Additional Reading*

1. Burrows B, Taussig LM: "As the twig is bent, the tree inclines" (perhaps). *Am Rev Respir Dis* 122:813–816, 1980.
2. Samet JM et al: The relationship between respiratory illness in childhood and chronic airflow obstruction in adulthood. *Am Rev Respir Dis* 127:508–523, 1983.

---

**High- vs. Low-Dose, Frequently Administered, Nebulized Albuterol in Children With Severe, Acute Asthma**

Schuh S, Parkin P, Rajan A, Canny G, Healy R, Rieder M, Tan YK, Levison H, Soldin SJ (Hosp for Sick Children, Toronto)

*Pediatrics* 83:513-518, April 1989 5–3

---

Nebulized albuterol is an established treatment for severe childhood asthma. However, its optimal safe dose is not known. The efficacy and safety of high and low doses of albuterol therapy frequently given to children with acute severe asthma in an emergency department were studied.

A total of 32 children, aged 5–17 years, were randomly assigned to receive nebulized albuterol, 0.15 mg/kg or 0.05 mg/kg, every 20 minutes for 6 doses. The high-dose regimen produced significantly greater improvement in forced expiratory volume in 1 second than the low-dose regimen did. The high-dose regimen also resulted in greater improvements in forced vital capacity and wheeze score and a lower rate of hospitalization. Changes in heart rate, respiratory rate, blood pressure, white blood cell count, and serum potassium concentration were comparable in both treatment groups, as was the incidence of adverse effects. Side effects included tremor, hyperactivity, and vomiting. Serum albuterol levels were highly variable and unrelated to increases in heart rate or other side effects.

Frequent high doses of nebulized albuterol seem to be safe and effective in treating severe acute asthma in otherwise healthy children. The side effects are mild, temporary, and negligible compared with the risk of prolonging patient distress. This regimen is not recommended for home use.

▶ This paper is included for a variety of reasons. First, it demonstrates the dramatic improvements in pulmonary function that can be seen with inhaled bronchodilators administered in a carefully controlled repetitive fashion. These data add support to the notion that either continuous or high-frequency β-agonist therapy is an excellent approach to an episode of acute severe asthma. This work demonstrates that these medications can be given safely, provided that persons giving these medications are knowledgeable in asthma care and that careful monitoring is in place. Several cautions must be raised. Many patients have home nebulizers, but this level of therapy should not be undertaken in the home.

Furthermore, although not discussed by these investigators, caution must be observed when using this protocol for severely ill children and adolescents. β-Agonists have been shown to produce transient drops in oxygen saturation after inhalation therapy. Increased heart rate occurs because of the effects of these agents on cardiac output. Venous return may be reduced by hyperinflation and peripheral vasodilation from β-agonists. This combination can compromise myocardial oxygen supply. In addition to careful monitoring of patients enrolled in this type of asthma management protocol, it is essential that all nebulized medications be given with oxygen as the diving gas and that oxygen saturation be monitored in addition to heart rate.—G.M. Loughlin, M.D.

*Additional Reading*

1. Robertson CF et al: Response to frequent low doses of nebulized salbutamol in acute asthma. *J Pediatr* 106:672–674, 1985.
2. Becker AB et al: Inhaled salbutamol versus injected epinephrine in the treatment of acute asthma in children. *J Pediatr* 102:465–469, 1983.

▶ ↓ The following 2 articles are presented together because the take-home message from both the emergency room and intensive care unit experience with asthma management reported in these articles is very similar. Therapy of an acute asthma attack must be initiated early. It should be aggressive and should include not only adjustment or addition of bronchodilators, or both, but also use of oral steroids at home. Both papers highlight the dangers of delay or inconsistency in outpatient management. Emergency room physicians, in addition to controlling symptoms, must also attempt to help patients identify a person who can provide follow-up and continuity of care. Patients who use an emergency room for their asthma care tend to have more emergency room visits and hospitalizations. Similarly, admissions to pulmonary intensive care units (PICU) for asthma, which in many instances are tantamount to episodes of respiratory failure, are a marker for increased morbidity and mortality. A child who requires admission to a PICU should not just be treated and released. It is incumbent upon the part of the pediatric intensivist to arrange for follow-up of these patients by persons with special expertise in asthma management.—G.M. Loughlin, M.D.

---

**Acute Asthma: Observations Regarding the Management of a Pediatric Emergency Room**

Canny GJ, Reisman J, Healy R, Schwartz C, Petrou C, Rebuck AS, Levison H (Hosp for Sick Children; Toronto Western Hosp, Toronto)

*Pediatrics* 83:507–512, April 1989 5–4

---

Inadequate evaluation and inappropriate treatment of acute asthma have been implicated in morbidity and even deaths. The records of all children with acute asthma who visited an emergency department in a 16-month period were reviewed to determine how these children were being evaluated and treated.

The study included 1,864 children with a mean age of 5.6 years who were seen at an emergency room on 3,358 occasions with acute asthma. Visits were more common in winter and in the evening; 93% of the families were self-referred and the mean duration of symptoms was 41 hours. Infection was associated with most of the acute episodes. Although chest auscultation, heart rate, and respiratory rate were recorded during most visits, evidence that pulsus paradoxus had been measured was found for only 1% of the visits. Chest radiographs were obtained in 18% of visits, but lung function and blood gas values rarely were recorded. Drugs used in the emergency room included $\beta_2$-agonists, theophylline, and systemically administered steroids. None of the children received anticholinergic treatment. Hospitalization was the result of 26% of visits and 1 child died.

The emergency room management of acute asthma at this hospital was concluded to be below generally accepted standards. The severity of asthma apparently was assessed in an erratic fashion, and physicians often failed to document whether lung function was measured. The high rate of hospitalization might have been avoided had bronchodilators and corticosteroids not been underused.

---

**Severe Acute Asthma in a Pediatric Intensive Care Unit: Six Years' Experience**

Stein R, Canny GJ, Bohn DJ, Reisman JJ, Levison H (Hosp for Sick Children, Toronto)

*Pediatrics* 83:1023–1028, June 1989 5–5

---

Rates of admission to intensive care units (ICUs) and rates of death among patients with severe asthma have been increasing. A recent editorial suggested that the increased use of ICUs for the treatment of patients with severe acute asthma may subject those patients to diagnostic and treatment hazards whose risk-benefit balance is not clear. The management and outcome of severe acute asthma in children at 1 ICU were reviewed.

Eighty-nine children were admitted 125 times between 1982 and 1988 for the treatment of severe acute asthma. Twenty-four percent were admitted to the ICU more than once. Before hospitalization, the children had been symptomatic for a mean 48 hours. All patients were treated with bronchodilators before hospitalization, but only 23% had received oral corticosteroids. Seventy-seven percent of the children had hypercapnia according to initial blood gas values. Nebulized $\beta_2$-agonists, theophylline, steroids, nebulized ipratropium bromide, and intravenously administered albuterol and isoproterenol were used in the ICU. Thirty-three percent of the children needed mechanical ventilation, with a mean duration of 32 hours. There were 10 cases of pneumothorax, 6 of which were related to mechanical ventilation. Three patients who were given mechanical ventilation died. In each case, sudden severe asthma episodes began at home and resulted in respiratory arrest.

The need for ICU admission may result partly from delays in seeking medical care and underuse of oral corticosteroids at home. In this series, the mortality of children placed in the ICU for severe asthma was 7.5%. Thus, when bronchodilators and systemic steroids are used optimally and patients needing ventilation are carefully selected, outcomes for children requiring ICU admission for severe acute asthma are excellent.

---

**Respiratory Failure From Asthma: A Marker for Children With High Morbidity and Mortality**

Newcomb RW, Akhter J (Univ of Chicago; La Rabida Children's Hosp and Research Ctr, Chicago)

*Am J Dis Child* 142:1041–1044, October 1988 5–6

---

Most episodes of asthma do not involve respiratory failure. It is thought that most deaths from asthma occur from respiratory failure that was untreated or undertreated because its severity was underestimated by the treating physician. However, these catastrophes are rare, and treating all patients as if they were in equal danger of respiratory failure from asthma would strain medical resources. The ability to distinguish prognostic categories of patients who are at risk of respiratory failure would be useful.

It is believed that the danger of having the disease is in fact related to the maximum severity of asthma episodes, and children who have had initial episodes of respiratory failure may be again at high risk for respiratory failure. To support this hypothesis, the records of all 78 children who had been admitted during a 7-year period with documented episodes of respiratory failure from asthma were reviewed. During 407 patient-years of follow-up, the 78 children had 227 episodes of respiratory failure (2.9 episodes per patient). Fifty-three (68%) of the 78 children had been treated for 2 or more episodes of respiratory failure during the study period. In most children, a second episode developed within 2 years of the initial episode, but some had a delay between episodes of more than 6 years. Seven children died of respiratory failure; 2 other children sustained hypoxic brain damage. In contrast, only 2 deaths from respiratory failure from asthma occurred among 2,892 other children who were admitted during the study period, but who had not had previous episodes of respiratory failure.

Children whose asthma has caused even 1 episode of respiratory failure constitute a special group of asthmatic patients who are at high risk for repeated episodes of respiratory failure and its catastrophic complications.

▶ It is not clear why morbidity and mortality associated with childhood asthma is on the rise. Regardless, it is important for clinicians to be aware of the markers that place a child at high risk. In addition to a prior episode of respiratory failure, as described by Newcomb and Akhter, other signs of severe disease include onset of asthma early in life, continuous or poorly controlled symptoms, frequent exacerbations requiring steroid bursts or ER visits, and a pattern of early morning decline in peak expiratory flow rate. Other factors that may contribute to life-threatening asthma episodes include a delay in diagnosis of a severe condition, a delay or inconsistent response to increased symptoms, and failure to monitor a patient closely during an acute attack. A number of factors undoubtedly contribute to increased morbidity and mortality, some of which are impossible to control at this time; however, others can be controlled, especially those related to the quality of asthma care delivered to patients. Despite advances in pharmacologic management, asthma should not be taken lightly. It must be seen as a chronic condition that, even in apparently asymptomatic patients, is associated with airway inflammation and residual pulmonary function abnormalities that may contribute to acute exacerbations and respiratory failure.—G.M. Loughlin, M.D.

*Additional Reading*

1. Strunk RC et al: Physiologic and psychological characteristics associated with deaths due to asthma in childhood: A case controlled study. *JAMA* 254:1193–1198, 1985.

## Cystic Fibrosis

▶ ↓ The advances in cystic fibrosis (CF) throughout the 80s represent a stunning example of the potential for progress when persons with sound clinical experience are linked with interested and creative basic scientists. Watching the progress made in our understanding of the molecular and cellular biology of the respiratory epithelium in CF has been exciting. However, it is sobering to note that important clinical questions, such as the role of chest physiotherapy, antibiotics, and screening programs, remain unanswered. This area will bear close watching in the future.—G.M. Loughlin, M.D.

**Role of Conventional Physiotherapy in Cystic Fibrosis**

Reisman JJ, Rivington-Law B, Corey M, Marcotte J, Wannamaker E, Harcourt D, Levison H (Hosp for Sick Children, Toronto)

*J Pediatr* 113:632–636, October 1988 5–7

Chest physiotherapy (CPT) consisting of postural drainage with mechanical percussion is a traditional component of the daily therapy of patients with cystic fibrosis (CF). Although CPT facilitates expectoration of mucus from the respiratory tract, its effect on the rate of pulmonary deterioration is not known. Because the cost of daily home CPT is significant in terms of time and emotional involvement, a 3-year prospective study compared the long-term effects of daily therapy using CPT plus the forced expiratory technique (FET) with those of using FET alone.

The study included 63 patients with CF with mild to moderate pulmonary impairment; 33 children (mean age, 11.8 years) were treated with FET alone, and 30 children (mean age, 12.6 years) were treated with both CPT and FET. Patients were examined every 3 months to monitor their health status. When acute exacerbations developed, patients were treated in the hospital with vigorous physiotherapy and intravenously administered antibiotics. Pulmonary function testing was performed twice a year. Results were expressed as a percentage of predicted value for sex and height. Chest roentgenograms were also obtained twice a year. Patients enrolled in the FET-alone group had a significantly greater degree of decline in their forced expiratory flow between 25% and 75% of vital capacity than did the group that performed conventional CPT daily. The rates of decline in the CPT group were similar to those reported in previous studies.

These results strongly suggest that the long-term course of pulmonary function is adversely affected when conventional CPT is abandoned. It is recommended that the routine daily use of CPT consisting of percussion and postural drainage remain a standard part of the daily therapeutic regimen in the treatment of children with CF.

▶ It is fascinating to me that, in the age of the discovery of the CF gene, we are still arguing about the role of CPT in the management of the pulmonary disease associated with cystic fibrosis. The authors correctly point out that this is one of many clinical questions in need of study. Chest physiotherapy consumes time and energy and poses a logistic problem for adults with CF who live alone or who would like to break away from parental dependency. This 3-year study supports the notion that CPT (compared with a simple forced expiratory maneuver) does have some positive effect in terms of a slower rate of decline in pulmonary function tests. However, the differences are small. Curiously, no statistical differences in the forced vital capacity or clinical scores were noted. More important, regular CPT did not reduce dramatically the number of hospitalizations. Unfortunately, this study was unable to generate a profile of who really needs CPT. It is likely that this therapy benefits some patients substantially and others not at all or so minimally as to make the investment in time and energy not worthwhile.

An important point not evaluated in this study is the role of coughing and the potential adverse effects of forced expirations on airway smooth muscle tone. The amount of coughing was not controlled for. Perhaps the difference between CPT and FET simply is related to the amount of coughing. It would be interesting to know whether CPT currently may be the most effective way to induce coughing and, if so, perhaps other less time- and energy-consuming methods could be identified. Another concern is the effects of FET maneuver on airway tone. Rapid inhalation and exhalation have been shown to increase airway smooth muscle tone and reduce expiratory flow rates. This could adversely affect coughing, which is so dependent on achieving high flow rates.

The authors conclude that CPT should remain a part of routine care of patients with CF. Unfortunately, they are probably correct in this recommendation for now. However, there is room for further study to identify which patients with CF really need CPT and to define better what it is about CPT that really makes it work.—G.M. Loughlin, M.D.

---

**Survival and Clinical Outcome in Patients With Cystic Fibrosis, With or Without Neonatal Screening**

Dankert-Roelse JE, te Meerman GJ, Martijn A, ten Kate LP, Knol K (Univ Hosp; Univ of Groningen, The Netherlands)

*J Pediatr* 114:362–367, March 1989 5–8

---

Neonatal screening for cystic fibrosis (CF) is controversial. A follow-up study of patients involved in an experimental neonatal screening program was conducted to assess the possible positive and negative influences of neonatal screening for CF.

The screening program was carried out in The Netherlands in 1973–1979. Before the beginning of the 1980 follow-up study, patients with CF were partly treated in different local hospitals; after the follow-up program was started, all patients in the study received similar care. A cumulative survival rate was calculated, excluding patients with meconium ileus. At the age of 11 years, the 19 patients from the screened population had a significantly better survival rate than the 25 patients from the nonscreened population. At study entry, the screened patients had significantly better chest radiograph scores; there were no other significant differences. At age 9 years, after several years of similar treatment for all patients, the screened patients had significantly better clinical and chest radiograph scores, lower IgG levels, and higher vitamin A levels.

Neonatal screening programs probably improve survival rates and clinical outcomes in patients with CF. Early diagnosis may be important for the prevention of early irreversible lung damage. A neonatal screening program should not be initiated, however, unless optimal patient treatment also is provided.

▶ It is quite likely that the actual screening technique used will change in response to advances in molecular genetics and that the controversies surrounding the impact of false positive and false negative test results will continue, but it appears that the principles, supporting early detection and intervention in cystic fibrosis, are secure. However, as is demonstrated in this study from The Netherlands, simply to screen a population for a chronic disease is insufficient. A successful screening program with easy access to a state-of-the-art treatment program must be designed. This recommendation is not intended to replace primary care physicians. Clearly, they are part of the care team. However, the data accumulated from a number of studies demonstrate that care in CF centers improves survival and quality of daily life. One may argue about the pros and cons of screening programs per se, but there can be no argument that early attention to the pulmonary function and care of young children with CF is essential if we are to continue to push back on the life tables.—G.M. Loughlin, M.D.

▶ ↓ The following 2 studies extend our understanding of the chloride transport defect in patients with cystic fibrosis (CF). Advances in our understanding of chloride transport mechanisms, coupled with the recent identification of the CF gene on chromosome 7 and its proposed gene product—a transmembrane regulatory protein—hold great promise for improving our ability to regulate or perhaps correct the defect in C1-transport that is involved in the clinical manifestations of CF. The paper by Willumsen and co-workers (Abstract 5–9) is important because it localizes the defect to the apical portion of epithelial cell membrane. It confirms that basolateral membrane function is normal in terms of C1-transport. The work by Li and co-workers from Iowa (Abstract 5–10) demonstrate that, depending on physiologic state of the cell, protein kinase C (an important secretory regulatory protein) can activate or inactivate a C1-channel in healthy persons, but in cells from patients with CF, the activation of the C1-channel was defective. Similarly, defective activation by protein-kinase A has been observed in CF. These observations suggest a defect in CF involving an inability of the apical chloride channel to be phosphorylated or a defect in the mechanism by which phosphorylation causes activation of the channel. Needless to say, these exciting observations have opened new vistas for collaborative research in the areas of cellular and molecular biology.—G.M. Loughlin, M.D.

*Additional Reading*

1. Tsui L-C et al: Cystic fibrosis locus defined by a genetically linked polymorphic DNA marker. *Science* 230:1054–1057, 1985.

---

**Cellular C1$^-$ Transport in Cultured Cystic Fibrosis Airway Epithelium**

Willumsen NJ, Davis CW, Boucher RC (Univ of North Carolina, Chapel Hill)

*Am J Physiol* 256:C1045–C1053, 1989 5–9

---

In cystic fibrosis the C1$^-$ permeability of the apical epithelial-cell membrane is reduced. Whether this is the only C1$^-$ transport defect in cystic fibrosis epithelium is not clear. In this study, cystic fibrosis nasal specimens from 15 patients with cystic fibrosis diagnosed with typical clinical criteria (including an elevated sweat $C1^-$ concentration) were examined with double-barreled $C1^-$-selective microelectrodes to measure membrane potential and intracellular $C1^-$ activity.

The intracellular $C1^-$ activity of cystic fibrosis cultures did not differ significantly from that of normal human nasal epithelial cells. A reduced luminal $C1^-$ concentration failed to unmask any apical $C1^-$ permeability in cystic fibrosis cultures. Bumetanide decreased $C1^-$ activity without altering the electrical parameters of the cells. Lowering the serosal $C1^-$ concentration led to a marked decrease in intracellular $C1^-$ activity; the effect was partly blocked by bumetanide. The fall in serosal $C1^-$ concentration led to rapid depolarization of the basolateral membrane potential, a decrease in fractional apical membrane resistance, and increased transepithelial resistance.

In contrast to the apical membrane of cystic fibrosis airway epithelium, which is impermeable to $C1^-$, paths for $C1^-$ translocation are operative in the basolateral membrane. Transport there occurs chiefly via a bumetanide-inhibitable cotransport system, but also through $C1^-$ conductance. Neither of those mechanisms is affected by cystic fibrosis.

---

**Regulation of Chloride Channels by Protein Kinase C in Normal and Cystic Fibrosis Airway Epithelia**

Li M, McCann JD, Anderson MP, Clancy JP, Liedtke CM, Nairn AC, Greengard P, Welsh MJ (Univ of Iowa; Case Western Reserve Univ; Rockefeller Univ)
*Science* 244:1353–1356, June 16, 1989 5–10

---

Defective regulation of chloride channels in epithelium may contribute to the pathophysiology of cystic fibrosis (CF). Because protein kinase C (PKC) controls ion channels in several types of cells, the effects of PKC on chloride channels were examined in the intact cell by using phorbol 12-myristate 13-acetate to activate PKC. Efflux of $^{125}I$ was measured as an index of activation of chloride channels.

In normal intact cells activation of PKC by phorbol ester stimulated or inhibited secretion of chloride, depending on the physiologic state of the cell. At a high calcium concentration in cell-free membrane patches PKC inactivated chloride channels. At a low calcium level it activated chloride channels. In CF cells PKC-dependent inactivation of chloride channels was normal, but activation was defective.

It appears that PKC phosphorylates and regulates 2 different sites on the chloride channel or an associated membrane protein, 1 of which is defective in CF. The defect likely is either in the ability of the channel to be phosphorylated or in the mechanism by which phosphorylation activates the channel.

## Infant Lung Infection

▶ ↓ This continues to be a hot area in pediatric pulmonary disease. Much can be learned about the growth and development of the lung as well as responses to injury from these studies. Work in this area should be encouraged, but attention to the details of the methods is vital.—G.M. Loughlin, M.D.

**Effect of Chloral Hydrate on Arterial Oxygen Saturation in Wheezy Infants**

Mallol J, Sly PD (Royal Children's Hosp, Melbourne)

*Pediatr Pulmonol* 5:96–99, 1988 5–11

Chloral hydrate is a widely used sedative for infants during pulmonary function testing. Because sedation generally is not recommended for infants with acute wheezing illnesses, a study was conducted to assess the effects of administering commonly used doses of chloral hydrate on arterial $O_2$ saturation ($SaO_2$) in wheezy infants undergoing pulmonary function testing. Ten infants recovering from acute viral bronchiolitis and 5 infants with clinically stable cystic fibrosis were studied.

Chloral hydrate, at doses of 70 to 100 mg/kg, caused a significant fall in oxygen saturation ($SaO_2$) and a significant reduction in clinical score in infants recovering from acute viral bronchiolitis but not in clinically stable infants with cystic fibrosis. Infants whose baseline $SaO_2$ was no more than 94% exhibited the lowest $SaO_2$ levels after sedation with chloral hydrate. The arterial desaturation seen with chloral hydrate was not the effect of sleep.

These findings raise serious questions about the advisability of sedating wheezy infants with chloral hydrate in doses currently used to facilitate pulmonary function testing.

▶ This paper leads off the section on infant testing as a caveat to the legions of "baby testers" forming in the nation and around the world. Sedation is an important component of obtaining reproducible data on pulmonary function in infants and young children. In healthy infants or patients with stable pulmonary conditions, sedation for testing appears to be without risk. However, caution must be advised when sedating infants either recovering from acute pulmonary disease or who may be unstable because significant drops in oxygen saturation can be seen in this group.

The study involves infants with bronchiolitis, but this warning may well apply to infants recovering from a variety of conditions, such as hyaline membrane disease. Additional data on other populations are needed. On the other hand, the observations of Mallol and Sly should not prevent investigators from studying these conditions. Valuable and clinically necessary information about the pathophysiology of acute lung disease in children can be obtained from these studies. It seems that, as long as investigators are aware of this potential side effect of chloral hydrate sedation, problems should be minimal. This study also raises questions regarding the safety of chloral hydrate sedation for other procedures in patients recovering from acute lung disease and, as indicated by the authors, demonstrates the importance of standardizing clinical scoring protocols for the respiratory system in terms of sleep and wake states.—G.M. Loughlin, M.D.

**Effect of Spironolactone-Hydrochlorothiazide on Lung Function in Infants With Chronic Bronchopulmonary Dysplasia**

Engelhardt B, Blalock WA, DonLevy S, Rush M, Hazinski TA (Vanderbilt Univ)

*J Pediatr* 114:619–624, April 1989 5–12

Long-term diuretic therapy has been advocated for the treatment of infants with bronchopulmonary dysplasia (BPD). If diuresis per se accounts for the improved lung function during diuretic therapy, diuresis induced by spironolactone-hydrochlorothiazide should also improve urine output and lung function. To test this hypothesis, 21 hospitalized, spontaneously breathing, oxygen-dependent infants with chronic BPD were evaluated in a randomized, controlled study. Infants received either a 1:1 mixture of spironolactone and hydrochlorothiazide orally (no. = 12), 3 mg/kg/day of both compounds, or no treatment (no. = 9) for 6 to 8 days. Dynamic lung compliance, total pulmonary resistance, and hemoglobin oxygen saturation were measured on the first and last days of each study period, and fluid intake and urine output were measured daily.

Spironolactone-hydrochlorothiazide significantly increased urine output, but improved neither lung function nor oxygenation. The increase in urine output was comparable to that achieved in a previous study of furosemide therapy. Further, doubling the oral dose in 3 additional patients did not improve lung mechanics or oxygenation. Statistical analysis indicated that a type II error could not explain the failure to detect a beneficial effect.

These data provide indirect evidence that diuresis per se does not explain the improved lung function during diuretic therapy for BPD.

▶ Furosemide has been shown to improve a variety of pulmonary function parameters in infants with BPD. Clinical improvement in respiratory status generally has paralleled the diuretic effect. Consequently, it is tempting to implicate the effects of diuresis on intravascular volume and oncotic pressure as the factors contributing to this effect. However, this study, which supports previous work in anephric dogs, suggests otherwise. It indicates that the potent nonrenal effects of furosemide on water and ion transport most likely is responsible for the beneficial effects on lung function that have been observed. This study also brings into question the rationale for the common clinical practice of switching from furosemide to a spironolactone-hydrochlorothiazide combination. The switch may be beneficial in reducing complications from furosemide, but no benefit in terms of improved lung function is apparent.

This work also demonstrates the important effects of lung function in infants of lung fluid balance and shifts of fluid out of interstitial and peribronchial spaces. Improvement is seen not only in quasi-measurements of lung compliance but also in measures of airway function. Clinicians may need to reconsider the switch from furosemide to the spironolactone-thiazide combination if improvement in lung function is the therapeutic goal.—G.M. Loughlin, M.D.

*Additional Reading*

1. Engelhardt B et al: Short- and long-term effects of furosemide on lung function in infants with bronchopulmonary dysplasia *J Pediatr* 109:1034–1039, 1986.

**Comparison of Dynamic and Static Measurements of Respiratory Mechanics in Infants**

Gerhardt T, Reifenberg L, Duara S, Bancalari E (Univ of Miami)

*J Pediatr* 114:120–125, January 1989 5–13

Conventional measurement of respiratory mechanics with an esophageal tube was compared with the less invasive occlusion technique in 39 preterm infants requiring mechanical ventilation on the first day of life. The infants were assessed before discharge at a mean postnatal age of 67 days, and 27 were reevaluated at 1 year. Flow was measured by pneumotachometry through a nose piece; airway pressure, directly at the nasal piece; and esophageal pressure, through a water-filled tube.

Dynamic and static measurements did not differ significantly in the younger infants. In older infants, static compliance was 80% of dynamic lung compliance, and static resistance was 24% higher than dynamically measured expiratory resistance. Correlation of the resistance values was 0.91. The lower static compliance value and higher resistance value are explained by inclusion of the very compliant chest wall in static determinations.

The occlusion method of measuring respiratory mechanics gives accurate and reproducible results for young infants, and is well tolerated. The method must be evaluated further in smaller infants with endotracheal tubes or those in acute respiratory failure.

▶ The methodologies and theory underlying infant testing still are being developed and discussed. Many questions exist about comparability of techniques and factors that may influence results. This study is important then for several reasons. First, it compares dynamic and passive measurements in the same subjects at 3 different ages. Furthermore, the data come from a group with excellent credentials in infant testing. This work, however, demonstrates that these very different techniques give consistent results. It also demonstrates the significant influence changes in chest wall compliance can have on the dynamic measurements. In the very young premature infant, the very compliant chest wall minimizes the contribution of the chest wall to the total respiratory system compliance measurement (CRS) as well as reduces lung compliance because greater chest wall compliance may result in uneven distribution of tidal volumes. At the higher respiratory frequency of these smaller infants, dynamic lung compliance will be underestimated (frequency dependence of compliance). The stiffer chest wall of the older infant minimizes these influences.

Effects similar to those on compliance by the changing chest wall compliance can be theorized regarding the resistance measurements. The authors suggest that the passive relaxation technique will be influenced less by these differences. Passive relaxation techniques offer an additional advantage over dynamic measurements in that they can be obtained without passing an esophageal balloon, which carries its own set of problems and artifacts. As suggested, more studies are needed to improve understanding of the advantages and limitations of this technique, with particular attention paid to the effects of age.—G.M. Loughlin, M.D.

---

**Response of Normal Infants to Inhaled Histamine**

Lesouëf PN, Geelhoed GC, Turner DJ, Morgan SEG, Landau LI (Princess Margaret Hosp for Children, Perth, Australia)

*Am Rev Respir Dis* 139:62–66, January 1989 5–14

---

The age at which nonspecific bronchial hyperresponsiveness (BHR) first occurs is not known, but both genetic and environmental variables have been implicated in its etiology. The response of healthy infants to inhaled histamine was investigated.

Respiratory function in 12 infants, aged 3–18 months, with no history of significant respiratory disease, was monitored. The maximal flow at function residual capacity ($\dot{V}$maxFRC) was obtained using the forced expiratory flow-volume method. The infants inhaled histamines in doubling concentrations from 0.125 to 8 g/L. A response was defined as a drop of more than 30% in $\dot{V}$maxFRC. All the infants had responses to histamine, with the geometric mean concentration for their response being 1.4 g/L. The infants also had transient rises in respiratory rate and falls in $SaO_2$. After the last dose of histamine, forced expiratory flow-volume curves were concave in all cases.

Because healthy infants respond to relatively low concentrations of inhaled histamine, it is possible that such infants have "hyperresponsive" airways compared with older healthy children and adults. Genetic or environmental factors may then cause some infants not to lose it later in life.

▶ Studies such as this by Lesouëf and colleagues are vital to our understanding of the pathogenesis and natural history of airway hyperactivity. The conventional wisdom has been that airway hyperactivity arises in healthy infants as a consequence of acquired airway injury (viral infections, aspiration, passive smoking). The role of a genetic predisposition is unclear, but it may contribute to sustaining the effects of the initial injury or may be what separates simple hyperactivity from clinical disease, that is, asthma. Before recent advances in infant lung function testing capabilities, it was not possible to test this hypothesis. These data, even with methodologic limitations well reviewed by these authors, provide important preliminary data that strongly suggest that airway hyperresponsiveness may be a normal physiologic occurrence in infancy. The role of genetic factors and acquired airway injury may be in escalating the intensity of the basal responsiveness or in altering the slope of the natural decline in reactivity seen with aging. It is also important that investigators be aware of the limitations of the methodologies of the tests used and the physiologic differences between adults and infants that affect delivery and distribution of challenge agents.—G.M. Loughlin, M.D.

## Neonatology

**Shallow Versus Deep Endotracheal Suctioning in Young Rabbits: Pathologic Effects on the Tracheobronchial Wall**

Bailey C, Kattwinkel J, Teja K, Buckley T (Children's Med Ctr, Charlottesville, Va; Univ of Virginia)

*Pediatrics* 82:746–751, November 1988 5–15

The technique of endotracheal tube suctioning traditionally has involved inserting a catheter until resistance is met, withdrawing slightly, and applying suction (deep technique). Because the purpose of endotracheal tube suctioning is to remove secretions that are not accessible to bypassed cilia, insertion of the catheter as far as the end of the tube (shallow technique) has been recommended.

The extent of tracheobronchial tissue damage by the deep technique was compared with that of shallow suctioning in 6 intubated 3-week-old rabbits. Suction was performed by experienced nurses in a neonatal intensive care unit. Light and scanning electron microscopy of tracheobronchial tissues from deeply suctioned animals showed disruption of mucosal epithelium (increased necrosis), near total loss of cilia, inflammatory reaction in the mucosa and submucosa, and markedly increased mu-

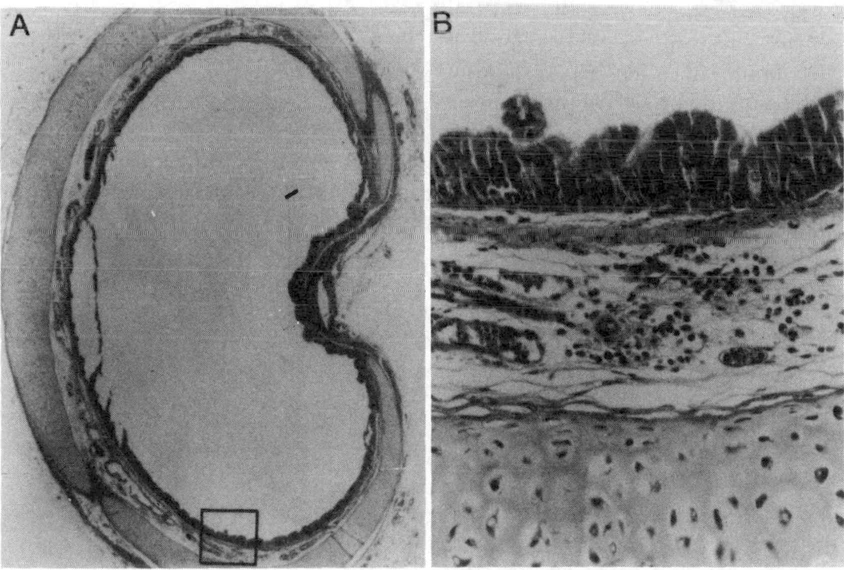


Fig 5–1.—A, cross section of trachea after shallow suctioning. Mucosal bleb at 9 o'clock position is artifact. B, closer view of inset shows intact mucosa, few polymorphonuclear cells, and mild submucosal edema. (Courtesy of Bailey C, Kattwinkel J, Teja K, et al: *Pediatrics* 82:746–751, November 1988.)

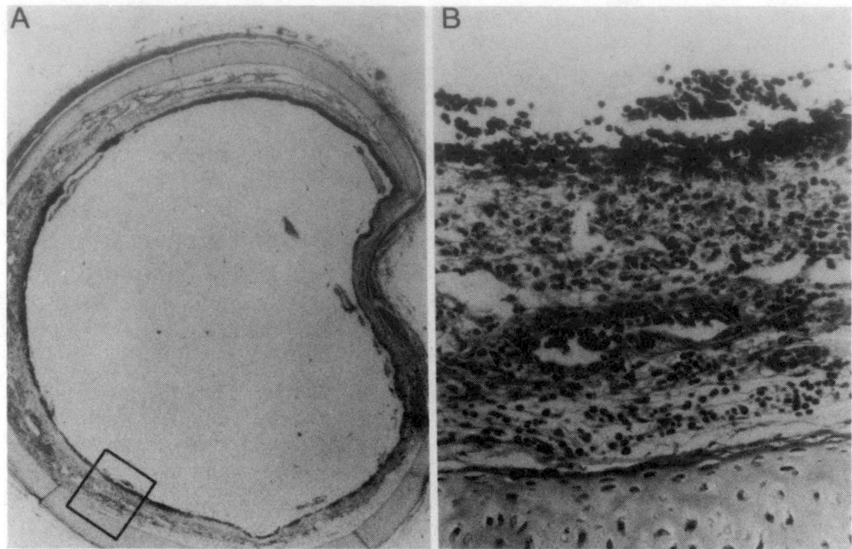


**Fig 5–2.**—**A,** cross section of trachea after deep suctioning. **B,** closer view of inset shows necrosis and complete loss of mucosal cells. Note intense polymorphonuclear cell infiltration of mucosa and submucosa obscuring underlying edema. Few polymorphonuclear cells have spilled into lumen. Leukostasis in submucosal vessel is also present. (Courtesy of Bailey C, Kattwinkel J, Teja K, et al: *Pediatrics* 82:746–751, November 1988.)

cus production (Figs 5–1 and 5–2). In addition, recovery of secretions was significantly less with the deep technique.

The prevalence of each technique for routine suctioning in neonatal intensive care units was determined with a nationwide mail survey. Of the 405 neonatal intensive care unit physicians who responded, 82% reported frequent or exclusive use of the deep technique for routine suctioning.

Deep endotracheal suctioning is associated with significantly more tracheobronchial pathology than the shallow, premeasured technique. The shallow technique should be adopted for routine suctioning of intubated neonates.

▶ Since Northway's original description of bronchopulmonary dysplasia, considerable attention has been focused on factors that result in the lung parenchymal characteristic of bronchopulmonary dysplasia. On the contrary, far less attention has been paid to injury to the major airways that occur commonly in intubated infants. Airway complications include subglottic stenosis, tracheobronchial malacia, stenosis, and granuloma formation. The presence of an endotracheal tube is by no means the sole contributor to these complications. The trauma induced by vigorous suctioning clearly plays a role. This study by Bailey and co-workers demonstrates the adverse consequences of the time-honored intensive care unit nursing technique of deep endotracheal tube suctioning (see Figs 5–1 and 5–2). There is no evidence that passing a suction catheter through an endotracheal tube until it meets resistance and then initiating suctioning offers any advantage in improving clearance of airway secretions. In fact, it probably does more harm than good.

These recommendations may be viewed with consternation by many NICU and PICU nurses, but it seems prudent for intensive care units to initiate and enforce a suctioning technique based on passing the catheter tip just beyond the predetermined length of the endotracheal tube. In-service educational programs supported by demonstration of tho damage caused by suctioning to medical and nursing staff (fiberoptic bronchoscopy can provide proof in color) may be necessary to replace sacred suctioning dogma.—G.M. Loughlin, M.D.

*Additional Reading*

1. Nagarai HS et al: Recurrent lobar atelectasis due to acquired bronchial stenosis in neonates. *J Pediatr Surg* 15:411–415, 1980.

**In Vitro Morphological Changes Induced by 4-(Methylnitrosamino)-1-(3-Pyridyl)-1-(Butanone) in Fetal Hamster Respiratory Tract Tissue**

Joshi PA, Schuller HM, Rossignol G, Castonguay A (Univ of Tennessee, Knoxville; Laval Univ, Quebec City)

*Cancer Lett* 44:173–178, March 1989 5–16

The tobacco-specific nitrosamine 4-(methylnitrosoamino)-1-(3-pyridyl) 1 butanone (NNK) is metabolized by fetal hamster respiratory tissue to form DNA-alkylating and clastogenic intermediates. Whether those biochemical changes are reflected in morphological alterations in respiratory tract tissues cultured with NNK in vitro was investigated. Explants of fetal hamster trachea and lung were exposed to varying concentrations of NNK and examined with light and electron microscopy.

The tracheal explants exposed to NNK had dose-dependent preneoplastic lesions, such as squamous metaplasia and the formation of mature keratin. Lung explants showed changes consistent with disordered production or release of surfactant. The alveolar type II cells exhibited concentric-type lamellae, which are typical of simian lung.

The fetal trachea may be a potential target for a transplacental carcinogenic effect of NNK. The findings in fetal hamster lung indicate that NNK can adversely affect surfactant synthesis, which could then lead to infant respiratory distress syndrome.

▶ Another adverse effect to be added to the list of reasons why women shouldn't smoke during pregnancy or, for that matter, ever. There always is a concern about drawing conclusions from animal data and extending them to humans, but these findings give one pause, particularly in light of the strong epidemiologic data that has implicated fetal exposure to the by-products of cigarette smoke as contributing to decreased birth weight and increased prenatal mortality. Complications of pregnancy lead to an increased number of stillbirths and deaths from hyaline membrane disease, asphyxia, and immaturity.

The observed changes in the hamster respiratory tract may well contribute to a number of problems identified in infants born to mothers who smoke during pregnancy because there appears to be morphological evidence of disruption of the surfactant system. The long-term implications of the preneoplastic changes have yet to be defined, but this population of children exposed to cigarette smoke in utero bear watching. If not already a part of the program, an aggressive approach to smoking cessation should be incorporated into any prenatal care program, especially for populations among whom smoking is more common.—G.M. Loughlin, M.D.

*Additional Reading*

1. *Health Effects of Smoking on Children. Statement of the American Thoracic Society,* 1985.
2. Tager I: "Passive smoking" and respiratory health in children: Sophistry or cause for concern? *Am Rev Respir Dis* 133:959–961, 1986.
3. Weiss ST et al: The health effects of involuntary smoking. *Am Rev Respir Dis* 129:933–942, 1983.

**Postnatal Undernutrition Slows Development of Bronchiolar Epithelium in Rats**

Massaro GD, McCoy L, Massaro D (Univ of Miami; VA Med Ctr, Miami)
*Am J Physiol* 255:R521–R526, October 1988. 5–17

The small conducting airways of the lung are sites of abnormal function early in the course of chronic lung diseases. Evidence suggests that some environment aspects during childhood may play a role in the increased prevalence of chronic airway disease during adulthood. Encouraged by these considerations and the significant postnatal anatomical development of bronchiolar epithelium, researchers attempted to determine the effects of early postnatal undernutrition on the anatomical development of the bronchiolar epithelium in rats. Undernutrition was produced by increasing litter size shortly after birth.

Undernutrition delayed development of the mitochondria and rough endoplasmic reticulum of bronchiolar Clara cells. Particularly interesting is that underfeeding rat pups resulted in considerably diminished mitosis by Clara cells, decreased nuclear numerical density of bronchiolar ciliated cells, evidence of diminished conversion of Clara cells to ciliated cells, and an abnormal cellular composition of the small-airway epithelium that persisted well beyond the period of underfeeding.

Early neonatal events can have long-term effects on the bronchiolar epithelium, perhaps increasing the predisposition to small airway diseases.

▶ Studies such as this serve to remind us that sometimes it is the little things we don't do in the course of managing acute lung injury in young infants that may influence the long-term consequences. The development of chronic lung disease in infants after acute neonatal lung injury undoubtedly is multifactorial, with supplemental oxygen and positive pressure ventilation being major players. Allowing for differences in species, this study of rat pups raises important concerns about the role of early nutrition in postnatal lung growth. Malnutrition in these neonates primarily affected airway cell growth and maturation. Because lung growth is presumed to be dysynaptic, the consequences of malnutrition may vary from species to species depending on the timing of the injury relevant to the part of the lung (airways vs. parenchyma) that is undergoing the more active growth and differentiation. Also of concern is that, in this model, malnutrition may have compromised the potential for lung growth as well as the ability of the airway epithelium to heal itself. This could have important implications for the management of acute lung injury in neonates with hyaline membrane disease. Because these infants may be quite ill in the first week of life, adequate nutrition may be compromised, thus inadvertently contributing to the pathogenesis of chronic lung disease.—G.M. Loughlin, M.D.

*Additional Reading*

1. Frank L et al: Undernutrition as a major contributing factor in the pathogenesis of bronchopulmonary dysplasia. *Am Rev Respir Dis* 138:725–729, 1988.
2. O'Brodovich H et al: Bronchopulmonary dysplasia. *Am Rev Respir Dis* 132:694–709, 1985.

---

**Surfactant Replacement Therapy: Impact on Hospital Charges for Premature Infants With Respiratory Distress Syndrome**

Maniscalco WM, Kendig JW, Shapiro DL (Univ of Rochester; Strong Mem Hosp, Rochester, NY)

*Pediatrics* 83:1–6, January 1989 5–18

---

Surfactant replacement therapy for neonatal respiratory distress syndrome potentially can reduce morbidity and mortality in very premature infants. To determine whether surfactant replacement therapy also can reduce hospital charges for these infants, such charges incurred by 38 premature infants with respiratory distress syndrome who received surfactant replacement therapy were compared with charges of 31 control infants who received standard ventilatory treatment.

Mortality in the surfactant-treated group (8%) was significantly less than that in the control group (29%). Average daily hospital charges for all surfactant-treated infants were 25% less than those for the controls, mostly because of the 52% reduction in daily ancillary charges for laboratory, radiograph, respiratory therapy, and other ancillary services. During the first full week of hospitalization, ancillary charges were significantly less by $1,883 in surfactant-treated patients. The average total hospital charges for the 2 groups were similar, but the total hospital charges to produce a survivor were reduced by as much as 22%, or $18,500, in the surfactant-treated group than in the control group.

Surfactant replacement therapy for neonatal respiratory distress syndrome significantly improves survival and reduces hospital charges for ancillary services among survivors. Surfactant replacement may be cost-effective by improving survival without increasing overall hospital costs.

► As with neurodevelopmental outcome, beneficial effects of surfactant therapy can be identified, but one must look closely at the data to find them. This rule also applies to cost-effectiveness. In this study from Rochester, New York, surfactant was shown to reduce the morbidity and mortality associated with hyaline membrane disease (HMD) in premature infants. However, the margin of effectiveness is not as wide as one would have guessed. The reasons for this minimizing effect are complex and well discussed by these investigators. By looking at the costs to produce a survivor, we see that surfactant therapy clearly works. The savings most likely would still be significant even after the costs of 1 or 2 doses of surfactant are included. However, it seems that surfactant brings to the party its own set of problems. More premature infants will survive, but not without problems or extended care costs.

In fact, the increased availability and acceptance of surfactant therapy will permit treatment of even more immature infants who, although possibly benefiting from a reduction in the severity of the HMD, certainly will have many other clinical problems that contribute not only to morbidity but also to cost of care. As for the other advances in therapy discussed, we must look at the big picture before we start celebrating.—G.M. Loughlin, M.D.

**Survival of Infants With Persistent Pulmonary Hypertension Without Extracorporeal Membrane Oxygenation**

Dworetz AR, Moya FR, Sabo B, Gladstone I, Gross I (Yale Univ)

*Pediatrics* 84:1–6, July 1989 5–19

A conservative approach to persistent pulmonary hypertension (PPH) was evaluated in infants who met published criteria of Bartlett and associates or Short and associates for extracorporeal membrane oxygenation (ECMO) therapy. Mortality of 80% to 90% can be predicted with these criteria, which are based on historical data, if ECMO is not used.

Hyperventilation was the mainstay of management in 1980 through 1981, when 23 infants weighing more than 2 kg at birth were treated; however, because of concern that this therapy was contributing to the high morbidity and mortality, hyperventilation was avoided in 17 infants treated in 1986 through 1988. Aklaline pH was achieved with bicarbonate infusion rather than hyperventilation in this period. Values for the partial pressure of oxygen in arterial blood between 45 and 50 mm Hg and for the partial pressure of $CO_2$ in arterial blood between 45 and 50 mm HG were acceptable.

In the earlier period, 1 of 6 infants eligible for ECMO according to the Bartlett criteria survived. In the later period, 9 of 10 infants eligible for ECMO lived. When the alveolar-arterial oxygen tension difference criteria of Short and colleagues were used, the corresponding survival figures were none of 5 earlier infants but 8 of 9 in the later series.

About 90% of infants with PPH who are candidates for ECMO now survive without the use of this therapy. A conservative approach may well provide an effective, less expensive, and possibly safer alternative to ECMO for most infants with severe PPH. A randomized trial to compare conservative ventilation with hyperventilation and ECMO should be undertaken before committing further efforts to ECMO centers.

▶ The controversy surrounding the use of ECMO therapy continues. The reader is referred to 2 excellent editorial reviews (1, 2) that focus on how "high-tech" therapies such as ECMO can become incorporated into the mainstream of medical practice without undergoing rigorous randomized, controlled clinical trials. Several factors inherent in the way we as physicians approach life-threatening clinical situations prevent investigators from initiating randomized clinical trials. First, investigators are reluctant to go head to head with conventional therapy because early comparison with new technologies, which frequently require tinkering to get them finely tuned, might prevent use of what eventually could be an effective form of therapy. A second factor is the double standard of ethics and peer review when to use these trials. Recommending randomization is difficult when the risk that the new procedure will not work early in its application may be quite high. Parents are unlikely to agree to randomizing their children to the more dangerous therapy group. Finally, human nature being what it is, the investigators hope that the efficacy of the new treatment will be so great that comparison with historical controls will suffice to prove their point. The article by Dworetz and associates clearly demonstrates the fallacy of this logic. We forget that, fortunately, the learning curve also applies to conventional therapy.

Considering the costs and risks to the patient from ECMO therapy, it would seem that "improved" conventional management is the way to go in 1990. Readers should be cautioned to review with a jaundiced eye studies reporting success with new high-tech therapies. Close attention must be paid to what is being compared. The study of O'Rourke and co workers (3) seems like a vote of confidence for ECMO therapy. However, a close look at what was being used as conventional therapy indicates this it was out of date. Using the approach outlined by Dworetz and associates it is likely that the survival numbers would be quite similar. As recommended by Chalmers, there is a role for randomized clinical trials in modern medicine, and nowhere is this role more vital than in the area of high-tech advances in therapy.—G.M. Loughlin, M.D.

*Additional Reading*


1. Meinert CL: Extracorporeal membrane oxygenation trials. *Pediatrics* 85:365–366, 1990.
2. Chalmers TC: Belated randomized control trial. *Pediatrics* 85:366–368, 1990.
3. O'Rourke PP et al: Extracorporeal membrane oxygenation and conventional medical therapy for neonates with persistent pulmonary hypertension of the newborn. *Pediatrics* 84:957–963, 1989.


---

**Failure of Postnatal Adaptation of the Pulmonary Circulation After Chronic Intrauterine Pulmonary Hypertension in Fetal Lambs**

Abman SH, Shanley PF, Accurso FJ (Univ of Colorado, Denver)

*J Clin Invest* 83:1849–1858, June 1989 5–20

---

Normal infants undergo dramatic transitions within minutes of birth from dependence on the placenta for gas exchange to establishment of adequate ventilation and perfusion of the lungs. The mechanisms contributing to this transition are not completely understood. Increased oxygen tension, ventilation, development of an air-liquid interface, and possibly the release of vasoactive mediators seem to have important roles in this process. The chronic effects of partial compression of the ductus arteriosus in fetal sheep were studied to determine whether intrauterine events can change fetal pulmonary vascular structure, reactivity, and adaptation to postnatal conditions.

Chronic increases in pulmonary artery pressure were induced in 24 late-gestation fetal lambs. Partial compression of the ductus arteriosus was maintained with an inflatable vascular occluder. Pulmonary artery pressure was elevated from a mean of 44 mm Hg to 62 mm Hg for 3 to 14 days. Blood flow in the left pulmonary artery initially rose, but the increase in flow was not sustained during chronic ductus compression, despite persistent increases in pulmonary artery pressure. Chronic hypertension lowered the slope of the pressure-flow relationship and blunted the pulmonary vascular response to small elevations in the partial pressure of oxygen. Pulmonary hypertension sustained for more than 8 days increased the wall thickness of small pulmonary arteries. Hypertensive lambs had higher pulmonary artery pressure, lower pulmonary blood flow, and predominant right-to-left ductus shunting after cesarean delivery when compared with control animals.

Chronic intrauterine pulmonary hypertension caused by partial compression of the ductus arteriosus appears to result in abnormal fetal and neonatal pulmonary vascular reactivity, structural remodeling of small pulmonary arteries, and the failure of the pulmonary circulation to adapt after birth. The fetal lamb model used in this study has several striking parallels with the clinical characteristics of persistent pulmonary hypertension of the human newborn.

▶ This important study demonstrates the long-term consequences of a prenatal event in determining both the fetal and neonatal responses to stress. Blunting of pulmonary vasoreactivity can have important clinical consequences both in terms of contributing to the persistence of increased pulmonary vascular resistance after birth (persistent fetal circulation, PFC) and in interfering with the therapeutic benefits of increasing inspired oxygen concentration, a key component of therapy. It would be of some interest to know how long this effect persists after birth. Does it correlate with the severity of PFC? Are the morphological changes reversible over time, and do they contribute to chronic pulmonary hypertension? As the authors suggest, this model has important scientific implications in terms of improving our ability to understand factors that influence the transition from fetal to postnatal pulmonary circulation.—G.M. Loughlin, M.D.

---

**High-Frequency Oscillatory Ventilation Compared With Conventional Mechanical Ventilation in the Treatment of Respiratory Failure in Preterm Infants**

The HIFI Study Group (Univ of Manitoba, Winnipeg; Tufts Univ, Boston; Univ of California, San Diego; Case Western Reserve Univ, Cleveland; Univ of Miami; et al)
*N Engl J Med* 320:88–93, Jan 12, 1989 5–21

A multicenter, randomized clinical trial was conducted to compare the efficacy and safety of high-frequency ventilation with conventional mechanical ventilation in the treatment of respiratory failure in preterm infants.

Of 673 infants weighing between 750 and 2,000 g, 346 were assigned to receive conventional mechanical ventilation and 327 to receive high-frequency oscillatory ventilation.

The frequency of bronchopulmonary dysplasia was similar in the 2 groups (41% in the conventional mechanical group and 40% in the high-frequency ventilation group). During the first 28 days, high-frequency ventilation did not reduce mortality or the level of ventilatory support. The crossover rate from high-frequency ventilation to conventional mechanical ventilation was greater than from mechanical to high-frequency ventilation (26% vs. 17%). High-frequency ventilation was associated with an increased incidence of pneumoperitoneum of pulmonary origin, grades 3 and 4 intracranial hemorrhage, and periventricular leukomalacia.

High-frequency oscillatory ventilation offers no advantage over conventional mechanical ventilation in the treatment of respiratory failure in preterm infants and appears to be associated with undesirable side effects.

▶ In light of the above comments on ECMO therapy it is rewarding to see how a randomized clinical trial can provide perspective on the effectiveness of new high-tech therapy. This study also demonstrates another benefit of these trials, that is, detection of potential adverse outcomes. Not only is high-frequency oscillatory ventilation not advantageous in managing neonatal lung disease, but it may do more harm in terms of extrapulmonary complications. The randomized trial facilitates acquisition of this important information. What is curious about the results of this study is the benefit to some severely affected infants of the crossover to the other form of ventilation. Perhaps a closer look at these patients may provide a clinical or physiologic profile that can be used prospectively to identify candidates for a particular ventilatory strategy.—G.M. Loughlin, M.D.

## Control of Respiration and SIDS

▶ ↓ The final section is devoted to several important papers focused on factors that regulate respiration and upper airway function in infants and to a potentially related perplexing clinical problem: sudden infant death syndrome (SIDS). These topics are presented as a unit because it is our belief that creative studies of basic science such as these will pave the way for better understanding of the pathophysiology of SIDS. Considering the complexities of both of these areas, I have asked John Carroll, M.D., Assistant Professor of Pediatrics and Director of the Pediatric Polysomnography Laboratory at The Johns Hopkins Children's Center, to provide his perspective on this year's selections in these areas. I am most grateful to him for this thoughtful and insightful analysis.—G.M. Loughlin, M.D.

**Pharyngeal Fluid Clearance and Aspiration Preventive Mechanisms in Sleeping Infants**

Pickens DL, Scheffl GL, Thach BT (Children's Hosp, St Louis; Washington Univ)

*J Appl Physiol* 66:1164–1171, March 1989 5–22

During sleep various respiratory and upper airway motor responses function to prevent intrapulmonary aspiration of fluids that collect in the

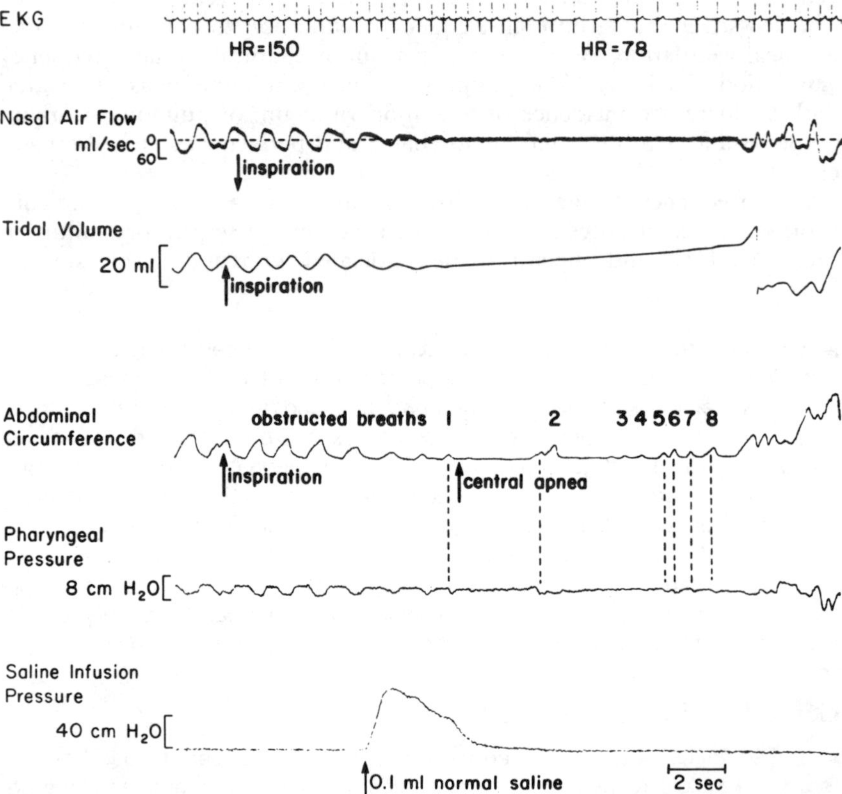


Fig 5–3.—Polygraphic tracings of infant's responses to 0.1-mL saline bolus. Responses include central apnea and obstructed breaths, but swallows are absent. Obstructed breaths are associated with negative pressure deflections recorded in pharynx and, therefore, level of obstructed breaths is presumed to be above catheter tip. There is bradycardia with onset 6 seconds after stimulus. Bradycardia is brief and resolves rapidly with sudden reopening of airway. *HR*, heart rate. (Courtesy of Pickens DL, Scheffl GL, Thach BT: *J Appl Physiol* 66:1164–1171, March 1989.)

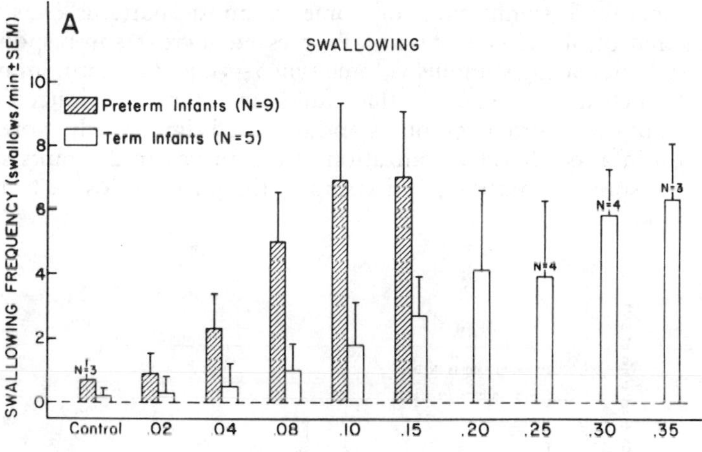


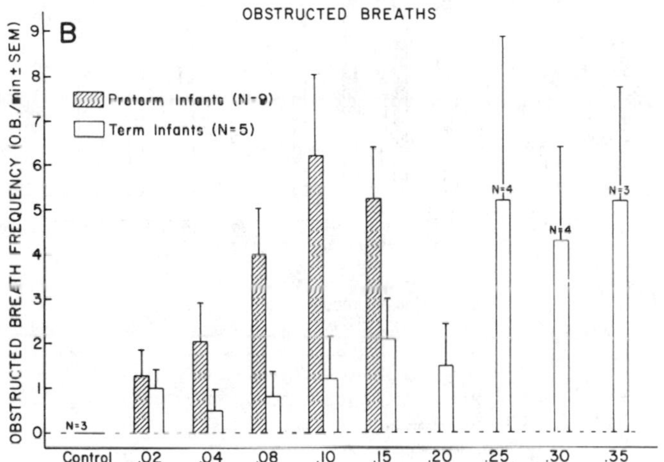


Fig 5–4.—A, through D, response frequencies for different bolus volumes. Results are shown for swallows, obstructed breaths, apnea, and arousal as function of stimulus volume for 2 infant groups. *(Continued.)*

pharynx. Ventilatory and airway protective responses to pharyngeal stimulation during sleep were characterized in 5 healthy full-term infants and 9 preterm infants with histories of prolonged apnea. The frequency of the responses, the effect of increased stimulus intensity, and the relation of stimulus fluid to laryngeal structures were studied. A nasopharyngeal catheter was used to deliver small boluses of warm saline to the oropharynx.

Swallows, obstructed respiratory efforts, brief apnea, prolonged apnea, and cough were repeatedly observed in both fullterm and preterm infants shortly after the saline stimulus. Swallowing was the most frequent response, and cough, the rarest. Swallowing was usually present when other responses occurred, but central apnea and obstructed breaths could and did occur independently of swallowing (Fig 5–3).

The functional significance of some response patterns was clear, whereas that of others was obscure. Progressive increases in response occurred with increasing stimulus volume (Fig 5–4), and preterm infants responded much more frequently than full-term infants. Prolonged apnea was a composite of other responses and occurred significantly more often in preterm infants. Direct visualization of the airway in 2 infants shortly after death showed that the relationship of the piriform fossae to the in-

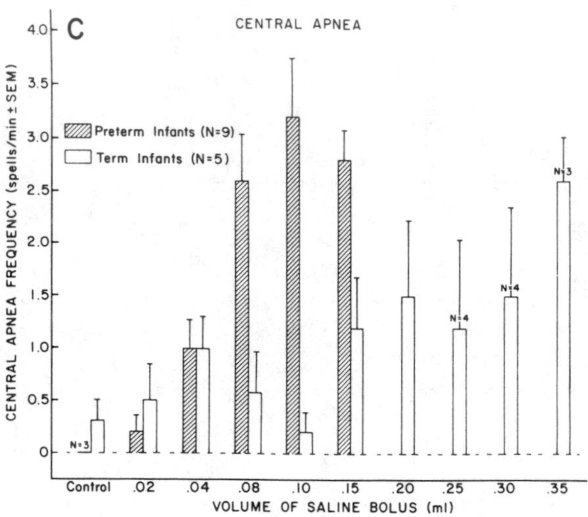


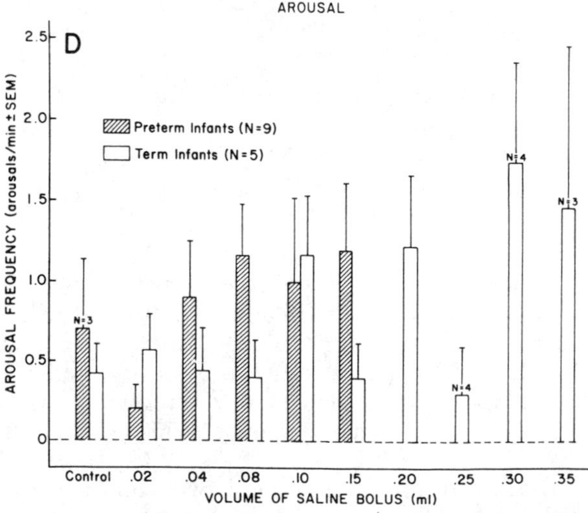


**Fig 5–4, cont.**—Three of 9 preterm infants received sham (control) stimuli, and not all full-term infants received stimuli of greater than 0.20 mL. Response frequency was significantly correlated with increasing bolus volume for all responses except for arousal. (Courtesy of Pickens DL, Schefft GL, Thach BT: *J Appl Physiol* 66:1164–1171, March 1989.)

terarytenoid notch was important in determining the frequency of the response.

Airway chemoreceptors in the interarytenoid space may play a prominent role in the normal removal of airway secretions during sleep. Receptors for swallowing in the interarytenoid space can provide the stimulus for swallowing when secretions that accumulate in the piriform fossae reach a critical volume.

This unique location for the receptors is functionally significant: the space between the arytenoid cartilages provides access for pharyngeal fluids to the swallow receptors, and the narrowness of the interarytenoid channel reduces the risk of a large volume of fluid being aspirated into the larynx.

---

**Characteristics of Upper Airway Chemoreflex Prolonged Apnea in Human Infants**

Davies AM, Koenig JS, Thach BT (Washington Univ; St Louis Children's Hosp)
*Am Rev Respir Dis* 139:668–673, March 1989 5–23

---

Water instilled into the pharynx of sleeping infants produces a variety of chemoreflex responses, which sometimes include prolonged apnea: the absence of ventilation for 20 seconds or more, or shorter if accompanied by bradycardia of less than or equal to 100 beats/min or cyanosis. To learn more about airway receptors that mediate prolonged apneic responses and factors that determine their occurrence, the importance of stimulus location and associations among prolonged apnea, bradycardia, and upper airway responses were studied in 12 infants.

Water stimulation in these infants produced 29 episodes of prolonged apnea. Although bradycardia followed the stimulus, it always was preceded by apnea and did not appear as an independent chemoreflex response. Behavioral arousal and prolonged apnea were not mutually exclusive. Recovery from prolonged apnea was not always closely associated with arousal. Prolonged apnea occurred more often after pharyngeal stimulation than after nasal stimulation and was commonly associated with coughing but not sneezing.

These observations suggest that prolonged apnea is elicited from a sensory site that is close to or the same as one mediating cough. This may have clinical importance because cough and prolonged apnea are prominent symptoms of several infectious infantile diseases, such as respiratory syncytial viral, chlamydia, and pertussis infection. The predominant receptors for chemoreflex-prolonged apnea were concluded to be in the pharynx or larynx instead of in the nose.

▶ Abstracts 5–22 and 5–23 illustrate the complexity of interactions involved in defense of the airway. Although it may seem like stating the obvious, they also remind us that the respiratory and gastrointestinal tracts share a common pathway as far as the larynx. Complicated and intricate reflex mechanisms have evolved to keep these 2 systems out of each other's way, and these reflexes must function effectively both during wakefulness and sleep. As if the opportunity for error were not already great enough, airway protective reflexes (like anything else) undergo functional changes with maturation.

Abstract 5–22 presents us with yet another argument on the downside for being prematurely born ("preemie"). As if the poor preemie doesn't have enough problems, he is lying around with an airway full of receptors prepared to halt respiration if fluid is "perceived" to be in the wrong place. Add to this problem immature swallowing coordination and some degree of "normal" gastroesophageal reflux, and it is not surprising that premature infants frequently stop breathing. Preemies generally are viewed as having poor airway protective reflexes. This dogma will have to be refined as more data such as these become available. In fact, it appears that chemoreflex apnea responses are not only active but increased in preemies.

Abstract 5–23 raises another interesting point. It is fairly well established that airway chemical receptors ("chemoreceptors," not to be confused with arterial chemoreceptors) are located in the area around the epiglottis. Cough receptors are located in the larynx on vocal folds and farther down the airway. Stimulation of cough receptors produces cough, whereas stimulation of epiglottal chemoreceptors causes apnea. If respiratory infections trigger the cough reflex, then one would expect that they also could trigger the apnea reflex. What is interesting is that apnea associated with viral respiratory infections is dependent on the age of the patient and the specific infectious agent. Respiratory syncytial virus infection produces apnea frequently before clinical respiratory disease is evident. On the other hand, apnea associated with pertussis and chlamydia infections occurs in association with coughing paroxysms. One would presume from the proximity of these different receptors that apnea should occur fairly often in young children with upper respiratory infections. Fortunately, it is not frequent, although the presence of a mild respiratory infection is noted commonly in epidemiologic studies of sudden infant death syndrome.—J.L. Carroll, M.D., and G.M. Loughlin, M.D.

---

**Effect of Maturation on Spontaneous Recovery From Hypoxic Apnea by Gasping**

Jacobi MS, Thach BT (Washington Univ, St Louis)

*J Appl Physiol* 66:2384–2390, May 1989 5–24

---

Very young animals can withstand anoxia through gasping, or "autoresuscitation," a capacity that may be lacking in adults. The effects of maturation on recovery from hypoxic apnea by gasping were examined in 2 strains of Swiss Webster mice. The effects of movement also were examined, with barometric plethysmography. Apnea was induced with a mixture of 97% nitrogen and 3% $CO_2$.

In both strains of mice, the survival rate was significantly lower among animals aged 17–23 days than among those younger and older. The interstrain difference in survival also was significant at this age. Gasping was absent from or lasted less than 5 seconds in animals that failed to recover. Seizurelike activity was not significantly more frequent in mice that died. Limb movement did not interfere with gasping.

Autoresuscitation is a useful mechanism of recovery from hypoxia in very young mice and in adult animals, but at an intermediate age it often fails.

---

**Effects of Negative Upper Airway Pressure on Pattern of Breathing in Sleeping Infants**

Thach BT, Menon AP, Schefft GL (Washington Univ, St Louis; St Louis Children's Hosp)

*J Appl Physiol* 66:1599–1605, April 1989 5–25

---

Negative upper airway (UAW) pressure has been found to hinder diaphragm inspiratory activity in animals. The effects of UAW negative pressure on inspiratory airflow and respiratory timing were studied in tracheostomized infants during quiet sleep.

Seven babies were studied. A face mask and syringe were used to produce UAW suction without altering lower airway pressure. During the 2- to 3-second UAW suction trials, mean and peak inspiratory airflow and tidal volume were greatly decreased, irrespective of whether stimulation occurred in inspiration or expiration. The mean reflex latency was 42 ms. Suction applied during inspiration or late expiration produces shorter inspirations and shorter succeeding expirations. Suction applied in midexpiration, however, prolonged expiration and often prolonged inspiration.

Sudden onset of suction pressure within the upper airway affects respiratory timing. The effect is dependent on the time of stimulus delivery. The observed changes in flow, tidal volume, and timing indicate that UAW suction has a marked inhibitory effect on thoracic inspiratory muscles. This reflex may prevent pharyngeal collapse by inspiratory suction pressure.

▶ It seems that, even in the most general terms, it has not been possible to reach a consensus on the mechanism of obstructive sleep apnea. On one side it is argued that, during inspiration, UAW patency depends on a balance of forces between negative intraluminal pressure generated by the diaphragm and dilating forces generated by UAW muscles (1). The other camp says no. They propose that the upper airway behaves like a Starling resistor: a tube that is rigid on both ends with a collapsible segment in the middle. The pressure surrounding the collapsible segment is called the collapsible closing pressure or Pcrit', which has been shown in normal adults to be −13 $cmH_2O$. This side argues that, under conditions of airflow limitation, inspiratory airflow is determined by upstream (nasal) pressure, upstream resistance, and airway closing pressure (Pcrit). During flow limitation, inspiratory airflow would be independent of downstream (tracheal) pressure (2).

This article proposed, within the framework of the first hypothesis (balance of forces), that the "UAW suction reflex" would be protective of airway patency. Perhaps more important, this reflex was found to be extremely fast, on the order of 42 ms (total latency, neural latency 10–20 ms). This would allow such a reflex to operate within a breath, sensing UAW negative pressure and fine tuning UAW collapsibility and inspiratory driving pressure.

The "UAW suction reflex" has been found to be greater in infant than adult animals (3, 4). Although this work was not a study of maturation, it has documented the presence of this reflex in human newborns. If it turns out to be as important in maintaining UAW patency as proposed, then absence or maldevelopment of this reflex could be an important mechanism of obstructive sleep apnea in this age group. This important work should be followed by investigations of the maturation of such reflexes during postnatal development and the determinants of airway collapse in infants and children.—J.L. Carroll, M.D.

*References*

1. Remmers JE, WJ DeGroot, EK Sauerland, et al: Pathogenesis of upper airway occlusion during sleep. *J Appl Physiol* 44:931–938, 1978.
2. Smith PL, Wise RA, Gold AR, et al: Upper airway pressure-flow relationships in obstructive sleep apnea. *J Appl Physiol* 64:789–795, 1988.
3. Fisher JT, Mathew OP, Sant'Ambrogio FB, et al: Reflex effects and receptor responses to upper airway pressure and flow stimuli in developing puppies. *J Appl Physiol* 58:258–264, 1985.
4. Fisher JT, Sant'Ambrogio G: Airway and lung receptors and their reflex effects in the newborn. *Pediatr Pulmonol* 1:112–126, 1985.

---

**Effects of Sleep Deprivation on Respiratory Events During Sleep in Healthy Infants**

Canet E, Gaultier C, A'Allest A-M, Dehan M (Hôp Antoine Beclere, Clamart, France)

*J Appl Physiol* 66:1158–1163, March 1989 5–26

---

The interaction between sleep deprivation and breathing has never been studied with infants. The effects of short-term deprivation of sleep on respiratory events during sleep (e.g., central apnea, obstructive apnea, hypopnea, and periodic breathing) were studied in 10 unsedated full-term healthy infants aged 1 to 6 months. The infants were monitored polygraphically during "afternoon naps" on a control day and on the day after sleep deprivation. Results for respiratory events were expressed as (1) indexes of the total number of respiratory events and of specific respiratory events per hour of total sleep time (TST), "quiet" sleep (QS) time, and "active" sleep (AS) time; (2) total duration of total and specific respiratory events, expressed as a percentage of TST and QS and AS times.

After sleep deprivation, a significant increase in the number of short respiratory pauses during sleep was noted. Significant increases also were observed for respiratory event, central apnea, and obstructive respiratory event indexes. Respiratory event time as a percentage of TST and AS time also was significantly increased, as well as obstructive respiratory event time as a percentage of TST, QS, and AS times. The number of times the transcutaneous carbon dioxide tension fell by 5 Torr per recording was greater after sleep deprivation and correlated with the increase in respiratory events.

Short-term sleep deprivation in healthy infants increases the number and timing of respiratory events, mostly obstructive respiratory events in AS. These adverse effects of sleep deprivation may have implications for infants with craniomandibular malformation, upper airway narrowings, or respiratory difficulties during sleep.

▶ Another potential for a "vicious cycle" in infants aged 1 to 6 months, sleep deprivation results in more respiratory events (especially obstructive), which may lead to worse sleep disruption, which may worsen respiratory events, and so on and so forth. It should be kept in mind that these were healthy infants. In sick infants, such as those with bronchopulmonary dysplasia, sleep-related hypoxemia often leads to very disturbed sleep. If increases in central apnea and obstructive respiratory events also result from sleep deprivation in these infants, their hypoxemia could be worsened substantially and the vicious cycle exaggerated. A maxim in our clinic for infant apnea and chronic lung disease is, "Agitation during sleep is due to hypoxemia until proven otherwise."

This work adds to a growing body of evidence that we should be mindful of the potential respiratory causes and effects of sleep deprivation in infants and children. In fact, nowhere is this potential problem more evident than in modern neonatal intensive care units. Sleep disruption and deprivation are widespread: the lights are always on, the noise level is quite high, and nurses and physician must be about their work, which frequently disturbs these infants. It is interesting and perhaps no coincidence that apnea is endemic in these centers.—J.L. Carroll, M.D., G.M. Loughlin, M.D.

*Additional Reading*

1. Bowers GG et al: Effect of sleep fragmentation on ventilatory and arousal responses of sleeping dogs to respiratory stimuli. *Am Rev Resp Dis* 122:899–908, 1980.

---

**Hypoxia Reinforces Laryngeal Reflex Bradycardia in Infants**

Wennergren G, Hertzberg T, Milerad J, Bjure J, Lagercrantz H (Gothenburg Univ, Gothenburg, Sweden; Karolinska Inst; Sachs' Children's Hosp; Karolinska Hosp, Stockholm)

*Acta Paediatr Scand* 78:11–17, January 1989 5–27

---

The laryngeal chemoreflex involves bradycardia, apnea, swallowing, and peripheral vasoconstriction. This reflex may be involved in the pathogenesis of apnea in prematurity. The laryngeal chemoreflex was studied in 12 infants, aged 5 days to 28 weeks, who had sustained an apparent life-threatening event or were siblings of infants who died of sudden infant death syndrome (SIDS). The laryngeal reflex was activated by pharyngeal water instillation during normoxia and hypoxia (transcutaneous $PO_2$ [$tcPO_2$] = 4.6 to 8.3 kPa).

When the laryngeal reflex was triggered during normoxia, heart rate did not change significantly and a transient cessation of breathing occurred in all infants (Fig 5–5). In contrast, during acute, mild hypoxia,

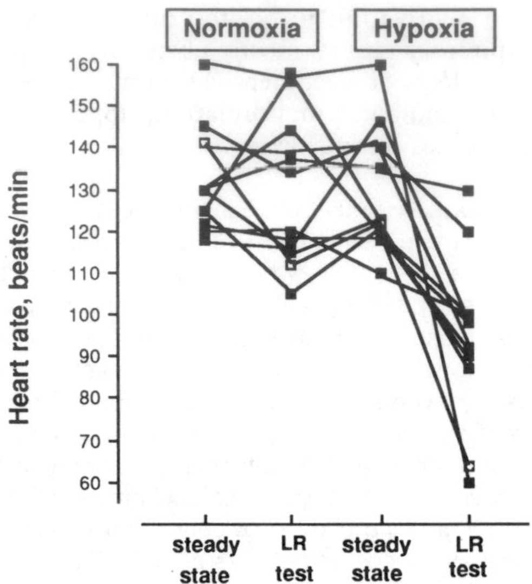


Fig 5–5.— Steady state values and values attained upon laryngeal receptor stimulation (LR test) for heart rate when performing the test during normoxia and hypoxia, respectively. Twelve infants, aged 5 days to 28 weeks. (Courtesy of Wennergren G, Hertzberg T, Milerad J, et al: *Acta Paediatr Scand* 78:11–17, January 1989.)

the bradycardia and apneic components of the reflex were significantly, and sometimes powerfully, reinforced (Fig 5–6). The percentage change in heart rate ranged from +26.4% to −21.0% during normoxia, as compared with −3.7% to −62.5% during hypoxia. Median apnea duration was 2.6 seconds (range, 0.7 to 15 seconds during normoxia and 5.3 seconds (range, 2 to 30 seconds) during hypoxia. The degree of bradycardia correlated inversely with the $tcPO_2$ level prevailing when the reflex was elicited. One infant who showed a particularly strong reinforcement of the cardiorespiratory response to laryngeal receptor stimulation later died of SIDS.

During hypoxia, the cardiorespiratory response to laryngeal stimulation significantly reinforced, probably because of the simultaneous activation of the peripheral arterial chemoreceptors. Reflex bradycardia induced by laryngeal stimulation may be involved in some patients with apparent life-threatening event or even SIDS.

▶ This excellent paper is a beautiful example of effectively bridging the gap between physiologic studies with animal models and those of human beings. Since the 1950s, Daly and Angell-James have published more than 40 papers on the cardiovascular effects of hypoxia. Largely from their work, it is now well known that stimulation of the carotid chemoreceptors causes bradycardia and peripheral vasoconstriction. Peripheral chemoreflex bradycardia normally is opposed by input from stretch receptors in the lungs and other inputs tending to increase heart rate. Thus, in spontaneously breathing subjects the heart rate response to hypoxia is variable and depends on the relative balance of heart rate

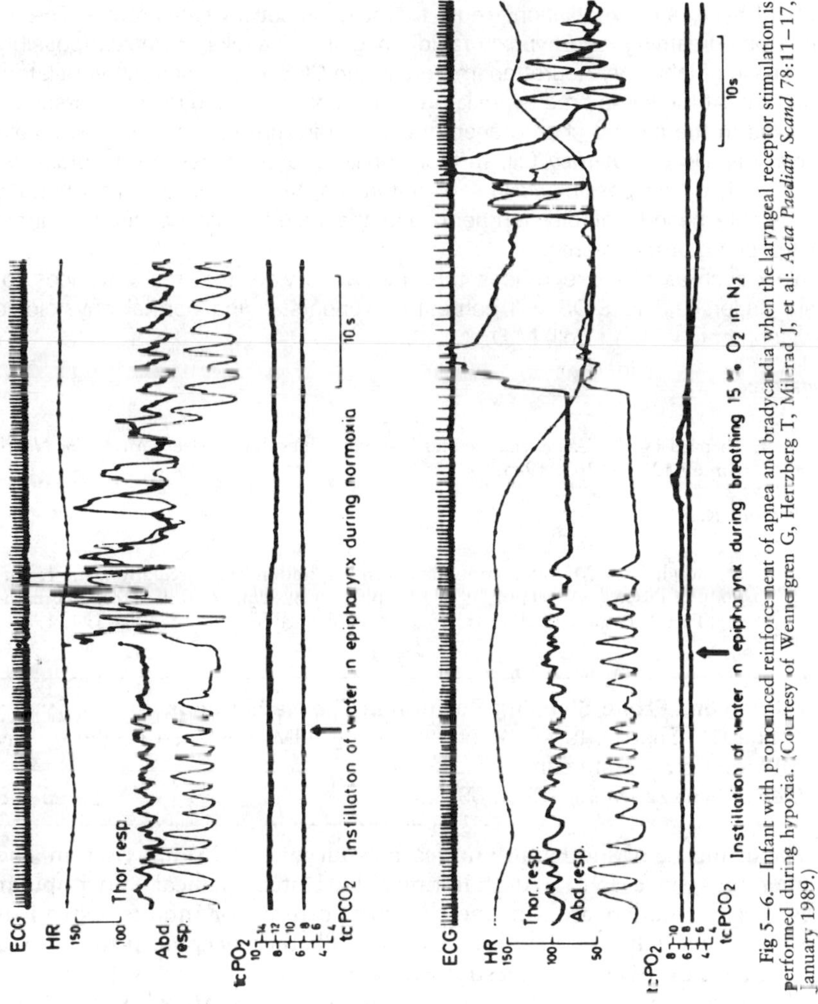


Fig 5–6.—Infant with pronounced reinforcement of apnea and bradycardia when the laryngeal receptor stimulation is performed during hypoxia. (Courtesy of Wennergren G, Hertzberg T, Milerad J, et al: *Acta Paediatr Scand* 78:11–17, January 1989.)

accelerating vs. slowing influences. However, if hypoxia occurs during apnea the power reflex bradycardia and peripheral vasoconstrictive effects from the peripheral chemoreceptors are unopposed. In other words, in the absence of stretch receptor feedback from the lungs (during apnea), hypoxia is likely to cause profound bradycardia and vasoconstriction.

In dogs, after 30 seconds of apnea $Pa_{O_2}$ falls from 92 to 60 mm Hg and $Pa_{CO_2}$ rises from 38 to 48 mm Hg (1). In infants, these changes are likely to be even greater because lung $O_2$ stores are smaller and metabolic rate is relatively greater (per unit of body surface area) than in adults. For a given duration of apnea, the infant is likely to become more hypoxic and do so more rapidly than an adult is.

Infants also appear to be more prone to centrally mediated depressant effects of hypoxia on ventilation. Thus, the stage is set for catastrophe. The infant stops breathing, and hypoxia rapidly begins to develop. Hypoxia (possibly by release of inhibitory neurotransmitters in the CNS) depresses the ventilatory response. At the same time hypoxia presents a powerful and rapidly worsening stimulus to the carotid chemoreceptors, which in turn cause profound bradycardia. Cardiac output may fall, further impairing oxygen delivery to brain tissues. Add to this possible failure of autoresuscitative mechanisms during a "vulnerable period" of development, and the result could be sudden unexpected death of the infant.

Work such as this strengthens this reviewer's view that real advances toward understanding SIDS will come from understanding normal physiologic development.—J.L. Carroll, M.D.

*Reference*

1. Shepard JW Jr: Gas exchange and hemodynamics during sleep. *Med Clin North Am* 69:1243–1263, 1985.

*Additional Reading*

1. De Burgh Daly M: Interactions between respiration and circulation, in: *Handbook of Physiology,* section 3: The Respiratory System, vol II, Control of Breathing, Part 2. Bethesda, MD, American Physiological Society, pp 529–594, 1986.

---

**Cot Death and Prone Sleeping Position in The Netherlands**

de Jonge GA, Engelberts AC, Koomen-Liefting AJM, Kostense PJ (Free Univ Hosp; Free Univ, Amsterdam)

*Br Med J* 298:722, March 19, 1989 5–28

---

The incidence of sudden infant death syndrome (SIDS) has risen in The Netherlands since 1971. At that time, the Dutch medical and popular press began to advocate a prone sleeping position for infants instead of the traditional lateral or supine position. Whether sleeping position is a determinant of SIDS was investigated.

The parents of 142 infants, aged 1 month to 1 year, who died from SIDS, were asked about the usual sleeping position of the child in the last weeks of his or her life. All the parents were able to recall their child's sleeping habits. Data on 320 unmatched and 254 matched controls were used for comparison. Eighty-eight percent of the infants who died were found prone. The incidence of SIDS among infants who usually slept prone was nearly 5 times higher than among infants who did not. The relative risk for SIDS among babies habitually sleeping prone was still significantly increased after correction for prematurity, age, socioeconomic class, and local traditions.

In this series, infants who usually slept in the prone position had a greater risk of dying of SIDS than those who usually did not sleep prone. A lateral or supine sleeping position for infants should be recommended unless medical conditions contraindicate it.

▶ Does sleeping prone increase the risk of SIDS, or are infants predisposed to SIDS more likely to adopt or be placed in a prone sleeping position? This study doesn't answer that question, but it raises some interesting ones and points out several research directions. Past studies have not found sleeping position to be an important factor in SIDS, underscoring the need to confirm the findings of de Jonge and associates. The prone sleeping position affects head position, which may affect airway patency and collapsibility. This knowledge may be particularly important in light of mounting evidence that upper airway obstruction plays a role in the death of these infants. Functional residual capacity is different in the prone position, a potentially important point because the infant's lung $O_2$ stores are smaller (especially during rapid eye movement sleep) and metabolic rate is greater relative to body size. If the association of prone sleeping position and SIDS is confirmed by other studies, then physiologic effects of body position during sleep among infants at risk will deserve more attention.—J.L. Carroll, M.D.

**Sudden Infant Death Syndrome in Hong Kong: Confirmation of Low Incidence**

Lee NNY, Chan YF, Davies DP, Lau E, Yip DCP (Chinese Univ of Hong Kong, Shatin; Princess Margaret Hosp, Kowloon; Med and Health Dept, Hong Kong)
*Br Med J* 298:721, March 18, 1989 5–29

Because previous retrospective study had reported a low incidence of sudden infant death syndrome (SIDS) in Hong Kong, a prospective investigation was done to verify that finding.

Fifty-one infants aged 1–12 months who were found dead at home unexpectedly and for whom there was no immediately obvious cause of death underwent necropsy. Sudden infant death syndrome was diagnosed in 12 girls and 9 boys. All were ethnic Chinese. The deaths occurred with a fairly even distribution throughout the year except in December,. when more than twice as many infants died. There were 70,519 births during the study period, making the incidence of SIDS 0.3/1,000 live births.

For analysis of the influence of local risk factors, each SIDS victim was matched with 2 control infants, 1 in the hospital and 1 from the community. Usual sleeping position was the only significant difference between patients and controls. Seven percent of the controls habitually slept prone, compared with 44% of the SIDS victims.

The low incidence of SIDS in Hong Kong was confirmed. The incidence of SIDS in Western countries is about 2 to 4 per 1,000 live births, compared with 0.3/1,000 in Hong Kong. The demographic pattern is also different: in Hong Kong there is a slight preponderance among girls, a peak incidence below the age of 2 months, absence of young parents, no obvious high prevalence of low birth weight and premature victims, and no excess previous morbidity. Methods of child care may play a more important role in SIDS than is believed and merit further study.

▶ This paper is a variation on a familiar but potentially useful theme: find a group of infants whose incidence of SIDS is high or low and see what might be different about them or their environment. However, it is not clear that these data are all that unique for "Hong Kong" because a similarly low incidence of SIDS was reported in 1983 from another Asian country, Japan (1). However, it is intriguing that 2 different Oriental cultures would have such dramatically lower SIDS rates than Western cultures have.

That this study was published in 1989 underscores that we do not know the cause or causes of SIDS and must keep open minds as we move ahead into the 1990s. It also serves to remind us that the determinants of SIDS may not all lie with the infant. An emerging theme is that some infants may pass through a period of "vulnerability" during the first 6–8 months of life. Whether a particular infant dies of SIDS may depend heavily on the home environment and how the infant is cared for. In this context, the suggestion that overcrowding, sleeping position, and differences in child care practices are important determinants of the incidence of SIDS is intriguing. A recent British study reported that "family problems," "housing in poor repair," and "inadequate family finance" were associated with an increased risk of SIDS (2). Perhaps overcrowding and the impact of poverty on the family function are dramatically different in Hong Kong than in England. The issue of positioning is particularly intriging in light of the Netherlands Study. Data from Hong Kong is perfectly in keeping with the Dutch hypothesis regarding the dangers of the prone position.

As if studying a condition with probable multiple etiologies was not complicated enough, each of the various causes may consist of complex interactions among multiple factors, thus complicating the design of future studies.—J.L. Carroll, M.D. and G.M. Loughlin, M.D.

*References*

1. Takahashi E, Takano Y: *Incidence of SIDS: The Report of SIDS Study Group.* Japan, Ministry of Health and Welfare, p 37, 1983, quoted in Guntheroth WG: *Crib Death,* ed 2, New York, Futura, p 79, 1989.
2. Nicholl JP, O'Cathain A: Epidemiology of babies dying at different ages from the sudden infant death syndrome. *J Epidemiol Community Health* 43:133–139, 1989.

---

**Intrauterine Growth Retardation and Risk of Sudden Infant Death Syndrome (SIDS)**

Buck GM, Cookfair DL, Michalek AM, Nasca PC, Standfast SJ, Sever LE, Kramer AA (State Univ of New York, Buffalo)

*Am J Epidemiol* 129:874–884, May 1989 5–30

---

A study was conducted to estimate the risk of sudden infant death syndome (SIDS) associated with variables of infant growth, to determine whether symmetric or asymmetric intrauterine growth retardation (IUGR) is associated with an increased risk of SIDS, and to ascertain whether the results varied according to the control group used.

Of a live birth cohort of 132,948 infants in 1974, 148 later died of SIDS. Two control groups were used for comparison: 114 infants who died suddenly of other causes and 355 live infants randomly selected and matched according to maternal age, race, parity, residence, and the infant's birth date. Data from vital certificates, medical records, and autopsy reports were analyzed. Compared with live controls, significantly more SIDS victims had gestations of less than 37 weeks, birth weights less than 2,500 g, and birth lengths of 47 cm or less. Birth length of 47 cm or less was the only significant risk factor determined in a comparison of SIDS victims with other dead infants. The risk of SIDS decreased as length of gestation and birth size increased. Infants born at 42 weeks' gestation or later had the lowest risk of SIDS. When gestational age was controlled for, SIDS victims were found to be lighter and shorter, suggesting that the mechanisms responsible for SIDS begin early in pregnancy.

▶ Mounting evidence suggests that SIDS victims are abnormal before death, but another growing body of evidence indicates that these infants are abnormal before birth. This commendable work is representative of a welcome trend in SIDS research: large, multicenter, well-controlled studies using logistic regression to control for confounding variables. Another recent report examined a cohort of 53,721 infants, of which approximately 200 died of SIDS (1). Yet another report was a study of effects of maternal smoking in a cohort of 305,730 live births, of which 2,720 infants died (2).

As data from these studies roll in, many traditional beliefs about the epidemiology of SIDS are falling by the wayside. Neurologic abnormalities, previously thought to be associated with SIDS, largely drop out when adjusted for birth weight. Adjusting for birth weight and maternal education markedly reduces the negative association with breast-feeding (1). However, 2 factors with staying power are birth weight and size. Other studies, including the National Institute of Child Health and Development Cooperative SIDS Study, have found that even after adjusting for gestational age, birth weight and size remain risk factors for SIDS (1,3). Although the cause of the intrauterine growth retardation is as yet unclear and the ability of these studies to separate specific SIDS risk factors from general risk factors for infant mortality is not fully worked out, these studies represent a major step forward.—J.L. Carroll, M.D.

*References*


1. Kraus JF, Greenland S, Bulterys M: Risk factors for sudden infant death syndrome in the US Collaborative Perinatal Project. Int J Epidemiol 18:113–120, 1989.
2. Malloy MH, Kleinman JC, Land GH, et al: The association of maternal smoking with age and cause of infant death. *Am J Epidemiol* 128:46–55, 1988.
3. van Belle G, Hoffman H, Peterson D: Intrauterine growth retardation and the sudden infant death syndrome, in Harper RM, Hoffman HJ (eds): *Sudden Infant Death Syndrome: Risk Factors and Basic Mechanisms.* New York, PMA Publishing Corp, 203–219, 1988.

**Decreased Lung Surfactant Disaturated Phosphatidylcholine in Sudden Infant Death Syndrome**

Gibson RA, McMurchie EJ (Flinders Med Ctr, Bedford Park; Glenthorne Lab, O'Halloran Hill, Australia)

*Early Hum Dev* 17:145–155, August–September 1988 5–31

The lipid composition of lung surfactant in 40 infants dying of sudden infant death syndrome (SIDS) was determined by analyzing samples taken at autopsy by lung lavage. Samples from 12 infants dying of other causes also were analyzed. Most SIDS deaths occurred at age 4–20 weeks.

There were no major group differences in the proportions of phospholipid classes, especially phosphatidylcholine. The proportion of phosphatidylcholine in disaturated form was, however, significantly reduced in the SIDS group. The proportion in infants at the high-risk age range of 1–26 weeks was significantly less than in the entire control group.

Reduced disaturated phosphatidylcholine lung surfactant could lead to a more fluid surfactant, especially at exhalation, which could influence pulmonary function and contribute to sudden infant deaths. If the chemical abnormality weakens the ability of the surfactant to reduce the surface tension of the alveolar lining layer, the findings are consistent with a form of SIDS resulting from widespread alveolar collapse.

▶ Again, that this study was published in these modern times provides more evidence that we are still groping blindly for clues. Another familiar theme: first find something wrong in some system, and then strongly suggest that it might have something to do in some way with SIDS. It has been known for years that the presence of respiratory tract infection (presumably viral) at the time of death is strongly associated with SIDS.

In another recent study from Australia (1) SIDS victims were reported to have grossly elevated lung IgG, IgM, and (to a lesser extent) IgA in lung lavage fluid. These studies represent a commendable attempt to examine clues to specific pulmonary abnormalities in victims of SIDS. In combination with the finding that the incidence of SIDS is sevenfold greater in infants with bronchopulmonary dysplasia, these results are interesting and suggest specific directions for research. However, extreme caution should be exercised before making the leap from association to causation, particularly because widespread alveolar collapse was not commonly encountered in the postmortem evaluation of SIDS victims.—J.L. Carroll, M.D., and G.M. Loughlin, M.D.

*Reference*

1. Forsyth KD, Weeks SC, Koh L, et al: Lung immunoglobulins in the sudden infant death syndrome.

*Additional Reading*

1. Morley C et al: Lung surfactant and sudden infant death syndrome. *Ann NY Acad Sci* 533:289–295, 1990.

**Risk of Sudden Infant Death Syndrome Among Infants With In Utero Exposure to Cocaine**

Bauchner H, Zuckerman B, McClain M, Frank D, Fried LE, Kayne H (Boston City Hospital; Boston Univ)

*J Pediatr* 113:831–834, November 1988 5–32

The risk of sudden infant death syndrome (SIDS) among infants exposed to cocaine in utero was assessed prospectively with 966 mother-infant pairs. Of 175 women (17.5%) who used cocaine during pregnancy, more were black and poor, and consumed more alcohol than the women who did not use cocaine.

Only 1 infant exposed to cocaine in utero died of SIDS, a risk of 5.6 in 1,000, compared with 4 of the 821 nonexposed infants, a risk of 4.9 to 1,000. The relative risk for SIDS among infants whose mothers used cocaine during pregnancy compared with those whose mothers did not use cocaine was 1.17 (95% confidence interval, 0.13, 10.43).

The risk of SIDS among infants exposed to cocaine in utero is less than previously reported. The increased risk of SIDS among these infants probably reflects other risk factors that are independently associated with SIDS.

▶ This question is extraordinarily difficult to study because of the many confounding behaviors such as maternal smoking, use of other drugs, socioeconomic status, and other factors that may be related to SIDS. It therefore is not surprising that controversy abounds. Previous estimates of SIDS risk in infants exposed to cocaine in utero have been as high as 83 to 151 per 1,000 live births. An obvious point is that this question cannot be approached except with large, carefully controlled studies that effectively deal with the confounding effects of related risk factors for SIDS. This work is an important first step in the right direction. The authors openly discuss the limitations of their work, pointing out that because of the sample size of the cocaine group the confidence interval is wide: between 0.1/1,000 and 31/1,000 live births. However, the upper limit still is much lower than previous estimates.

It is important not to forget that, whether or not cocaine per se is a risk factor, the combination of many other risk factors in infants of drug-abusing mothers appears to place them at high risk for SIDS. In this study the incidence of 1 major risk factor, maternal smoking, was 2.5 times higher in mothers who abused cocaine. A recent study from Sweden (1) reported that cigarette smoking during pregnancy doubled the incidence of SIDS. Therefore, whatever the precise association might turn out to be, this is a group of infants in need of further study and effective intervention.—J.L. Carroll, M.D.

*Reference*

1. Haglund B, Cnattingius S: Cigarette smoking as a risk factor for sudden infant death syndrome: A population-based study. *Am J Public Health* 80:29–32, January 1990.

### Elevated Levels of Hypoxanthine in Vitreous Humor Indicate Prolonged Cerebral Hypoxia in Victims of Sudden Infant Death Syndrome

Rognum TO, Saugstad OD, Øyasæter S, Olaisen B (Natl Hosp, Oslo)
*Pediatrics* 82:615–618, October 1988 5–33

Some researchers believe that sudden infant death syndrome (SIDS) may be caused by a prolonged disease process, such as long-standing hypoxia. Hypoxanthine levels in plasma, CSF and urine are increased during tissue hypoxia. Postmortem assessment of the vitreous humor hypoxanthine concentration may provide some information as to whether death in SIDS victims was preceded by hypoxia.

Hypoxanthine levels in vitreous humor from 32 infants who died of SIDS were compared with those in 8 children who died of trauma, drowning, or hanging and those in 7 infants who died suddenly without long-standing hypoxia. A partial pressure of oxygen electrode method or high-performance liquid chromatography was used to test hypoxanthine levels. The median hypoxanthine level in infants dying of SIDS was 380 μmol/L, compared with 118 μmol/L in children who died violently. The difference was significant. The SIDS victims' hypoxanthine levels were also significantly higher than those of neonates who died without long-standing antemortem hypoxia.

The hypothesis that deaths as a result of SIDS are preceded by hypoxia was supported. Thus, SIDS may not be caused by a sudden event, as some researchers believe and the term suggests.

▶ The "sudden" in SIDS refers to the terminal event, which most likely is quite sudden. The conclusion that "SIDS is probably not a sudden event" is not quite accurate. It is doubtful that in 1990 anyone believes that the majority of SIDS victims are perfectly healthy children who suddenly become abnormal and die.

Hundreds of investigators spanning 3 decades have sought to discover "the underlying cause" of SIDS, usually with the presumption that these infants are not completely normal. Indeed, the validity of various pathologic markers of chronic hypoxia has been a favorite topic of debate for many years.

This is precisely the value of this work. It appears to provide a comparatively simple, objective, and apparently reliable method for detecting whether SIDS victims have been chronically hypoxic before death. Vitreous humor hypoxanthine levels also appear to be independent of age, a finding which, if confirmed, could be extremely useful. For example, Nicholl and O'Cathain (1) have recently analyzed sudden infant death risk factors as a function of age, concluding that there are different causes of SIDS, depending on the age at death. Application of the vitreous humor hypoxanthine test in a large study of SIDS, assessing evidence for chronic premortem hypoxemia as a function of age at death, could yield potentially important insights into the nature of possible etiologies.—J.L. Carroll, M.D.

*Reference*

1. Nicholl JP, O'Cathain A: Epidemiology of babies dying at different ages from the sudden infant death syndrome. *J Epidemiol Community Health* 43:133–139, 1989.

# 6 Basic and Clinical Progress in Lung Cancer

## Introduction

In the absence of significant progress in the treatment of lung cancer as well as many other epithelial malignancies, increasing attention is focused on cancer prevention and control measures to deal with these virulent problems. The National Cancer Institute recently has mandated that a program dedicated to cancer prevention in addition to other, more traditional cancer specialties will be a prerequisite for formal recognition as a federally designated comprehensive cancer center. Lung cancer is the most obvious example of disease for which a shift in emphasis toward primary prevention approaches could be beneficial. Recently, a range of papers in the literature has explored aspects of lung cancer prevention and control issues.

Clinical research in lung cancer continues to focus on identifying favorable subsets that would benefit from refinements of available treatment modalities. These studies frequently involve interdigitating combinations of modalities, which most often is an attempt to enhance control of local relapse of a primary tumor. Our tools for local control include either high-dose radiation therapy or surgery. In multiple clinical studies, the ability of either of these modalities to effect local control has been demonstrated. The challenge is to elucidate the clinical situation in which improved local control can impart a survival advantage. This issue is most clearly demonstrated in the current trials involving neoadjuvant approaches to the treatment of non-small-cell lung cancer. Neoadjuvant approaches involve the use of systemic chemotherapy in anticipation of a definitive local procedure for patients with regionally advanced (usually stage IIIA) disease. The goal is to increase the frequency of complete removal of evident tumor. Further clinical experience with these studies will be discussed.

In the area of basic research in lung cancer, new genetic mechanisms potentially central to pathogenesis have been described. In lung cancer cell lines at least two specific gene deletions termed *tumor suppressor genes* have been reported. In another area, the independent effect of genes reported to be of importance in lung cancer pathogenesis can be studied specifically in vitro. This is accomplished by transfecting particular oncogenes into appropriate nonmalignant human pulmonary cell lines. In this manner the biology of lung-cancer-related oncogenes can be systematically explored. Other related topics in this fast-moving area will be reviewed.

James L. Mulshine, M.D.

## Cancer Prevention and Cancer Control

### General Issues

---

**Vegetable Consumption and Lung Cancer Risk: A Population-Based Case-Control Study in Hawaii**

Le Marchand L, Yoshizawa CN, Kolonel LN, Hankin JH, Goodman MT (Univ of Hawaii, Honolulu)

*J Natl Cancer Inst* 81:1158–1164, Aug 2, 1989 6–1

---

Epidemiologic studies have suggested a negative association between consumption of vegetables and lung cancer, but the exact foods or their constituents that may be protective remain uncertain. A population-based study of diet and lung cancer in the multiethnic Hawaii population between March 1, 1983, and September 30, 1985, included 332 lung cancer patients and 865 controls matched for age and sex. A quantitative dietary history helped in estimating the usual intake of foods rich in vitamins A and C and carotenoids.

Total intake of vitamin A was inversely related to lung cancer risk in both men and women, but was statistically significantly so only for men (Table 1). A clear dose-dependent negative relation was demonstrated between dietary intake of β-carotene and lung cancer risk in men and women. After adjustment for smoking and other co-variates, men in the lowest quartile of intake of β-carotene had an odds ratio of 1.9, compared with those in the highest quartile. The corresponding odds ratio for women was 2.7.

There were no clear associations between cancer risk and vitamin C, folic acid, iron, dietary fiber, or fruits. All vegetables were more strongly inversely associated with cancer risk than was β-carotene. The effect of vegetable consumption held for all cell types (Table 2).

Apart from β-carotene, constituents of vegetables such as lutein, lycopene, and indoles may protect against lung cancer.

▶ Lung cancer eventually develops in only 1 in 10 smokers. Another fraction of smokers succumbs to other cigarette-induced diseases (including heart and respiratory disease), and another subset of patients tolerates cigarette smoking without incurring lethal disease. For this reason, investigators have long searched for factors that may explain this disparity. In this case-control study the consumption of vegetables and β-carotene was inversely associated with cancer risks. This confirms the findings of an earlier case control study done with males in New Jersey (1). Such data form the basis of cancer clinical trials with dietary interventions. In considering such approaches the limitations of small case-control studies need to be considered. Also in trying to understand

TABLE 1.—Odds Ratio* for Lung Cancer by Quartile (Q) of Nutrient Intake† and Sex, Hawaii 1983–1985

| Nutrient intake | Males (230 cases, 597 controls) | | | | | Females (102 cases, 268 controls) | | | | |
|---|---|---|---|---|---|---|---|---|---|---|
| | $Q_4$ (high) | $Q_3$ | $Q_2$ | $Q_1$ (low) | *P* for trend | $Q_4$ (high) | $Q_3$ | $Q_2$ | $Q_1$ (low) | *P* for trend |
| Total vitamin A | 1.0 | 1.3 | 1.9 | 1.8 | .003 | 1.0 | 2.0 | 1.5 | 2.5 | .14 |
| Retinol | 1.0 | 1.0 | 0.9 | 0.9 | .70 | 1.0 | 1.1 | 1.3 | 1.0 | .75 |
| Beta-carotene | 1.0 | 1.5 | 2.4 | 1.9 | .001 | 1.0 | 1.9 | 2.4 | 2.7 | .01 |
| Other carotenoids with vitamin A activity | 1.0 | 1.6 | 2.1 | 2.0 | .003 | 1.0 | 1.9 | 2.3 | 2.9 | .009 |
| Total vitamin C | 1.0 | 1.2 | 2.4 | 2.3 | .001 | 1.0 | 0.6 | 0.7 | 0.7 | .31 |
| Vitamin C from foods | 1.0 | 2.0 | 1.9 | 1.9 | .01 | 1.0 | 0.7 | 1.1 | 1.4 | .42 |
| Vitamin C supplements | 1.0 | 1.7 | 2.8 | 2.5 | .001 | 1.0 | 0.9 | 0.6 | 0.7 | .22 |
| Iron | 1.0 | 1.0 | 1.1 | 1.0 | .79 | 1.0 | 1.2 | 0.7 | 1.4 | .72 |
| Folic acid | 1.0 | 1.7 | 1.2 | 1.8 | .07 | 1.0 | 0.8 | 1.8 | 1.9 | .06 |
| Dietary fiber | 1.0 | 1.3 | 1.5 | 1.5 | .09 | 1.0 | 1.1 | 1.5 | 1.8 | .12 |

*Adjusted for age, ethnicity, smoking status, pack-years of cigarette smoking, and cholesterol intake for male subjects only.

†Interquartile ranges (25th to 75th percentile) for daily nutrient intakes were as follows: total vitamin A—male subjects (M), 6,300–16,100 IU; female subjects (F), 6,400–16,800 IU: retinol—M, 230–780 µg; F, 190–550 µg; B-carotene—M, 1,800–5,000 µg; F, 2,000–5,300 µg; other carotenoids—M, 750–2,100 µg, F, 800–2,300 µg; total vitamin C—M, 110–490 mg, F, 120–490 mg; vitamin C from foods—M, 85–220 mg, F, 90–205 mg; iron—M, 5.5–11.2 mg, F, 4.6–9.1 mg; folic acid—M, 100–250 µg, F, 95–220 µg; and dietary fiber—M, 7–16 g, F, 6.5–14 g.

(Courtesy of Le Marchand L, Yoshizawa CN, Kolonel LN, et al: *J Natl Cancer Inst* 81:1158–1164, Aug 2, 1989.)

TABLE 2.—Odds Ratios* (and 95 Percent Confidence Intervals ) for Lung Cancer by Vegetable Consumption Level and Cell Type Among Male Subjects, Hawaii 1983–1985

| Tertile (T) of intake | Squamous cell carcinoma ($n = 79$†) | Small cell carcinoma ($n = 34$) | Adenocarcinoma ($n = 87$) |
|---|---|---|---|
| $T_3$ (high) | 1.0 | 1.0 | 1.0 |
| $T_2$ | 3.6 (1.8-7.3) | 2.0 (0.7-5.6) | 1.6 (0.9-3.1) |
| $T_1$ (low) | 2.9 (1.4-6.0) | 2.5 (0.9-6.4) | 2.3 (1.2-4.4) |
| | $P = .003$‡ | $P = .09$ | $P = .01$ |

*Adjusted for age, ethnicity, smoking status, pack-years of cigarette smoking, and cholesterol intake.

†Number of cases. All 597 controls were included in each of 3 cell type models.

‡Trend test.

(Courtesy of Le Marchand L, Yoshizawa CN, Kolonel LN, et al: *J Natl Cancer Inst* 81:1158–1164, Aug 2, 1989.)

such effects, no comprehensive mechanistic explanation fits with all the experimental data. In light of its minimal associated toxicity, such research deserves serious ongoing attention (although the toxicity associated with the consumption of cruciferous vegetables is a matter of taste). Elucidation of the basis for the protective effect of specific foods is critically important.—J.L. Mulshine, M.D.

*Reference*

1. Ziegler RG et al: *M J Epidemiol* 123:1080, 1986.

**Lung Cancer Risk, Occupational Exposure, the Debrisoquine Metabolic Phenotype**

Caporaso N, Hayes RB, Dosemeci M, Hoover R, Ayesh R, Hetzel M, Idle J (Natl Cancer Inst, Bethesda, Md; St Mary's Hosp Med School; Whittingon Hosp, London)

*Cancer Res* 49:3675–3679, July 1, 1989 6–2

The ability to metabolize debrisoquine by oxidation has been related to susceptibility to lung cancer. Lung cancer risk was evaluated in smokers with reference to debrisoquine metabolic phenotype and also to occupational exposure to lung carcinogens, specifically, asbestos and polycyclic aromatic hydrocarbons. A total of 245 patients with lung cancer seen in a 1-year period were compared with 234 controls having asthma, bronchitis, or emphysema. All the study subjects were white and of northern European origin and had smoked cigarettes.

Persons who metabolized debrisoquine extensively were at a fourfold increased risk of lung cancer compared with poor metabolizers after age, sex, and pack-years of smoking were controlled. Occupationally exposed persons were excluded from that analysis. Risk was greatest for squamous and small-cell tumors and least for adenocarcinoma. Men ex-

Relative Risk[a] of Lung Cancer in Men by Occupational Exposure to Lung Carcinogens and by Debrisoquine MP Occupational Exposure

| | Debrisoquine MP | | | | | |
|---|---|---|---|---|---|---|
| | PM/IM | | | EM | | |
| | Case | CTL | RR (95% CI) | Case | CTL | RR (95% CI) |
| Asbestos[b] | | | | | | |
| None | 14 | 53 | 1.0 | 97 | 68 | 6.0 (3.0–12.0) |
| Possible | 2 | 12 | 0.6 (0.1–3.0) | 29 | 14 | 8.0 (3.3–19.6) |
| Likely | 1 | 3 | 1.8 (0.2–19.6) | 16 | 3 | 18.4 (4.6–74) |
| PAH[c] | | | | | | |
| None | 12 | 38 | 1.0 | 64 | 53 | 3.9 (1.8–8.4) |
| Possible | 4 | 26 | 0.4 (0.1–1.8) | 68 | 31 | 7.8 (3.5–17.4) |
| Likely | 1 | 4 | 0.7 (0.1–6.7) | 10 | 1 | 35.3 (3.9–317) |

*Abbreviations: MP,* metabolic phenotype; *PM,* poor metabolizer; *IM,* intermediate metabolizer; *EM,* extensive metabolizer; *RR,* relative risk; *CI,* confidence interval; *PAH,* polycyclic aromatic hydrocarbons.

[a]Adjusted for age and smoking (pack-years).

[b]Also adjusted for PAH exposure (unlikely, possible, probable).

[c]Also adjusted for asbestos exposure (unlikely, possible, probable).

(Courtesy of Caporaso N, Hayes, RB, Dosemeci M, et al: *Cancer Res* 49:3675–3679, July 1, 1989.)

posed to occupational carcinogens had a relative risk of 2.8 after age and smoking were controlled (table). The combined risk from extensive metabolism of debrisoquine and likely occupational exposure to asbestos was increased 18-fold.

If these findings are confirmed, debrisoquine phenotyping could provide a useful means of targeting susceptible persons for screening or for lung cancer prevention measures.

▶ Another way to evaluate the risk of lung cancer developing eventually is suggested by profiling the patterns of metabolizing the drug debrisoquine. This is one of several recent reports on this approach. The new field of biochemical epidemiology involves attempt to relate patterns of carcinogen metabolism with cancer risk. As the genes and enzymes responsible for xenobiotic metabolism of carcinogens become known, the usefulness of phenotyping these systems to assess cancer risk may improve (1). Using debrisoquine for metabolic profiling is a model of this type of approach. Further clinical evaluation of the usefulness of debrisoquine phenotyping is ongoing.—J.L. Mulshine, M.D.

*Reference*

1. Harris C: *Ann Intern Med* 105:607, 1986.

**Radon and Lung Cancer**

Samet JM (Univ of New Mexico, Albuquerque)

*J Natl Cancer Inst* 81:745–757, May 22, 1989 6–3

Epidemiologic Studies of Domestic Exposure to Radon and Lung Cancer

| Location (reference) | Study design | Subjects | Exposure measure | Findings |
|---|---|---|---|---|
| Southern Sweden (*78*) | Case-control | 37 cases and 178 controls | Residence type: wood, "mixed," or stone | RR = 1.8 ($P < .05$) for stone and mixed vs. wood |
| Oeland, Sweden (*79*) | Case-control | 23 cases and 202 controls | Residence type and measurements lasting 4 mo | RR = 4.3 [90% confidence interval (CI), 1.7–10.6] for low- vs. high-exposure home type; RR = 2.7 (90% CI, 1.4–18.5) for low- vs. high-exposure home type by measurement |
| Southern Sweden (*80*) | Case-control | 23 cases and 202 controls | Measurement with alpha-sensitive film | RR increased for highest vs. lowest exposure categories; multiplicative interaction with smoking |
| Northern Sweden (*81*) | Case-control | 15 nonsmoker and 15 smoker case-control pairs | Construction characteristics | Estimated mean exposure significantly higher for smoking cases than controls; exposure not different for nonsmokers |
| Sweden (*81*) | Case-control | 11 nonsmoker and 12 smoker case-control pairs | Construction characteristics | Estimated mean exposures comparable for cases and controls regardless of smoking |
| Northern Sweden (*82*) | Case-control | 589 male cases, 582 deceased controls, and 453 living controls | Residence type: wood or nonwood | RR not increased, with or without smoking adjustment; RR increased for those never employed in occupations not associated with lung cancer |
| Stockholm, Sweden (*83*) | Case-control | 292 female cases and 584 controls | Geology and living near ground level | RR = 2.2 (95% CI, 1.2–4.0) for exposed vs. unexposed; exposure-response relationship not found |
| Southern Sweden (*84*) | Case-control | 177 cases and 677 controls | Residence type and geology, all homes; measurements lasting 2 mo, some homes | Exposure associated with increased risk for rural, but not urban, dwellers |
| Maryland, United States (*85*) | Cohort | 298 cases over a 12-yr period | Housing characteristics | No associations of incidence rates with housing characteristics |
| Ontario, Canada (*86*) | Case-control | 27 cases and 49 controls | Reconstructed exposures on the basis of measurements | RR = 2.4 (95% CI, 0.8–7.1) with smoking adjustment for exposed vs. unexposed |

(Courtesy of Samet JM: *J Natl Cancer Inst* 81:745–757, May 22, 1989.)

Radon, an inert gas released during the decay of $^{238}U$, is ubiquitous in both indoor and outdoor air and contaminates many underground mines. Extensive epidemiologic evidence from studies of miners suggests that radon causes lung cancer, even in nonsmokers. Confirmatory animal data are available. Radon also is a potentially important cause of lung cancer in the general population, exposed through contamination of indoor air by radon from soil, water, and building materials.

For underground miners, the risk of lung cancer is increased with the cumulative exposure to radon decay products. The interaction of radon decay products with environmental tobacco smoke conceivably might contribute to lung cancer in both active smokers and nonsmokers passively exposed to smoke. Several case-control studies in the general population have examined lung cancer risk in relation to radon exposure, with mixed results (table).

The highest acceptable level of annual average exposure is 4 pCi/L, which presently serves as a national standard. Whether home testing is effective in controlling radon exposure remains to be determined.

▶ Other than cigarettes, the most significant carcinogen for lung cancer is radon. The Environmental Protection Agency predicts that as many as 20,000 deaths may occur annually as a result of radon exposure. The bulk of this mortality is thought to result from lung cancer. Exposure to radon is carefully monitored in uranium mines. The recent discovery of frequent household exposure to this carcinogen has precipitated a variety of new concerns. This issue was discussed last year in this chapter relative to the question of safe exposure thresholds.

In the comprehensive review of Dr. Samet, the rationale for establishing the highest acceptable level of exposure at 4 pCi/L by the Environmental Protection Agency is discussed. In the absence of definitive epidemiologic data establishing the precise lung cancer risk with radon exposure, risk-estimation procedures have been employed. With an exposure level of approximately 1.5 pCi/L per year the model of the National Council for Radiation Protection and Measurements predicts an incidence of 9,000 lung cancer deaths annually from indoor exposure to radon. Other models based on a different set of assumptions such as the BEIR IV model predict somewhat higher lung cancer rates.—J.L. Mulshine, M.D.

---

**Estimating Rn-Induced Lung Cancer in the United States**
Lubin JH, Boice JD Jr (Natl Cancer Inst, Besthesda, Md)
*Health Physics* 57:417–427, September 1989 6–4

---

There is considerable evidence that prolonged exposure to the α-emitting decay products of radon ($^{222}$Rn, $^{214}$Po, $^{218}$Po) increases the risk of lung cancer in underground miners. Radon is an inert, radioactive gas arising from the decay of $^{226}$Ra and ultimately from $^{238}$U. Levels of radon in the home typically are substantially less than those in mines and below occupational health standards, but exposures at home occur over a lifetime. As a result, cumulative home exposure can approach the level of cumulative occupational exposure.

The risk model developed by the Committee on the Biological Effects of Ionizing Radiations of the National Academy of Sciences predicts that about 14% of lung cancer deaths among residents of single-family homes in the United States, or about 13,300 deaths per year, may be caused by indoor radon exposure. The estimated attributable risks are similar for men and women and in smokers and nonsmokers. Higher baseline risks, however, result in much larger absolute numbers of radon-attributable cancers in men and in smokers. Because of the apparent skewness of the exposure distribution, most of the contribution to the attributable risks is from exposure rates less than 148 becquerels/m$^3$ (4 pCi/L), that is, below the EPA "action level."

Radon definitely is a cause of lung cancer, and it appears that residential exposures do contribute to the present cancer burden. It remains necessary to validate the risk models developed for underground miners in studies of populations exposed to indoor radon.

▶ New data from studies conducted in New Jersey and Connecticut reported by the Centers for Disease Control support the existing guidelines of the Environmental Protection Agency (1). In the first major study of radon exposure and lung cancer that directly measured home radon exposures and obtained detailed smoking histories, the results of comparing the clinical features of 433 lung cancer patients from New Jersey with 402 case controls was consistent with the previously observed outcome with uranium miners. The risk of lung cancer from radon exposure was dose-dependent in that analysis. Radon-exposed persons who smoke more than 15 cigarettes per day had the strongest association with lung cancer risk.

In Connecticut three studies confirmed the findings of the New Jersey study and further strengthened the basis for relating exposure in living areas to ambient radon levels in basements. In that study the ratio between radon concentrations in the basement and those in the living room was consistently 3:2 and highly statistically significant. These studies validate that domestic radon exposure is a significant and potentially preventable health risk. The new data allow for more straightforward public health planning by providing more conclusive data for risk assessment and make concern about secondary exposure to domestic cigarette smoke a stronger issue because so many households already contain biologically significant concentrations of radon. The interaction of radon and secondary cigarette smoke as it relates to the risk of lung cancer will require large samples to quantitate accurately. A back-of-the-envelope calculation based on available data suggests that this issue is of more than theoretic interest.

The issue of radon exposure is getting serious international attention. Excellent epidemiologic data from Sweden largely support the findings of the Environmental Protection Agency. Swedish authorities are similarly formulating appropriate preventive strategies. In the most recent Swedish report (2) the association of radon exposure was strongest with the development of small-cell lung cancer as was observed in certain uranium mining populations. This histologic association with domestic radon exposure must be studied with other populations for confirmation.—J.L. Mulshine, M.D.

*Reference*

1. Ctrs for Disease Control: *J Am Med Assoc* 262:2659, 1989.
2. Svensson C et al: *Cancer Res* 49:1861, 1989.

SMOKING ISSUES

▶ ↓ This year may be a watershed in the public health campaign against tobacco consumption. Legislating smoking restrictions has become politically acceptable. Doctor Louis Sullivan, in assuming the Cabinet position as head of the Department of Health and Human Services, has intensified public pressure on the tobacco industry. A strategic development supporting the general restriction of public tobacco use has been the compelling data outlining the previously unappreciated threat of passive exposure to smoke.—J.L. Mulshine, M.D.

**Trends in Smoking, Cancer Risk, and Cigarette Promotion: Current Priorities for Reducing Tobacco Exposure**
Ernster VL (Univ of California, San Francisco)
*Cancer* 62:1702–1712, Oct 15, 1988 6–5

More than one fourth of the general population continues to smoke, and several thousand American teenagers begin smoking each day. Smoking rates for men and women are much closer than ever before (Fig 6–1). Data from 1981 to 1983 indicate high rates of smoking in young white women (about 40% in the group aged 18 to 24 years). Today the decision to begin smoking rarely is made after reaching adulthood. Both socioeconomic status and educational level are inversely related to smoking.

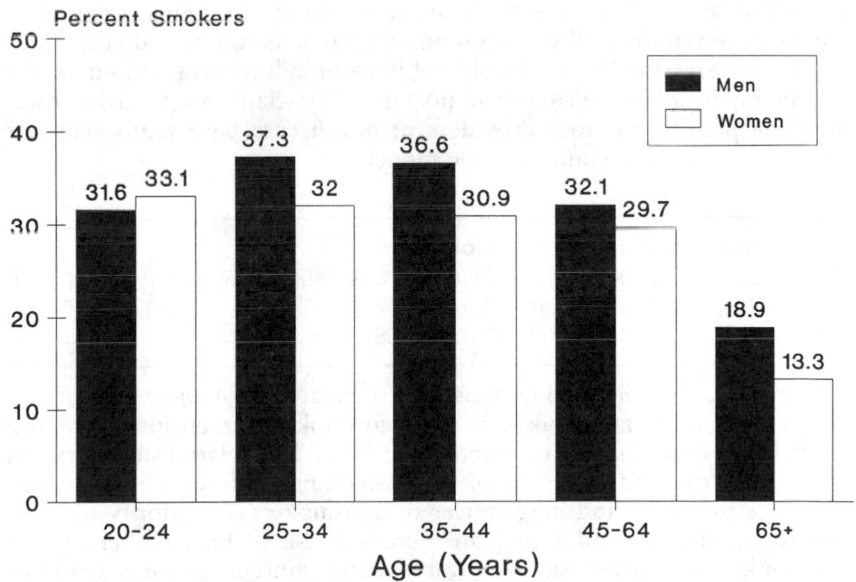


**Fig 6–1.**—Smoking prevalences by age and sex, United States white adults, 1985. (Data from US Dept of Health and Human Services: DHHS pub. no. [PHS] 87-1232. Hyattsville, Md, 1986. Courtesy of Ernster VL: *Cancer* 62:1702–1712, Oct 15, 1988.)

Probability of Death From Smoking-Related Disease Before Specified Age, According to Smoking Status of Man Aged 35 Years

| Disease/Smoking Status | 65 | 75 | 85 |
|---|---|---|---|
| Lung cancer | | | |
| Former smoker | 1.9 | 4.4 | 6.5 |
| Current smoker <25 | 2.5 | 6.3 | 9.3 |
| Current smoker ≥25 | 6.3 | 13.0 | 17.9 |
| Coronary Heart Disease | | | |
| Former smoker | 1.7 | 4.0 | 5.5 |
| Current smoker <25 | 4.6 | 7.4 | 7.7 |
| Current smoker ≥25 | 6.8 | 10.2 | 11.5 |
| All Smoking-Related Diseases | | | |
| Former smoker | 4.2 | 10.9 | 14.8 |
| Current smoker <25 | 8.7 | 16.9 | 21.0 |
| Current smoker ≥25 | 15.6 | 28.3 | 36.4 |

(Courtesy of Ernster VL: *Cancer* 62:1702–1712, Oct 15, 1988.)

An estimated 30% of all cancer deaths in the United States are associated with cigarette smoking, the leading known preventable cause of cancer. Age-adjusted lung cancer rates have risen steadily during this century, first in men and later in women. A man aged 35 years who smokes 25 or more cigarettes a day has a 28% risk of dying before age 75 years because of smoking (table).

Huge amounts of money are spent currently by the tobacco industry on advertising and promoting cigarette smoking. Programs targeted to smoking prevention and cessation among women, youth, and ethnic minorities deserve the highest priority. Limits on advertising and on smoking in public places also are important. Physicians must advise their smoking patients to stop. Providers of health care have many ways of serving as positive community role models.

### Health Effects of Involuntary Smoking

Fielding JE, Phenow KJ (Univ of California, Los Angeles; Johnson and Johnson Health Management, Inc, Santa Monica, Calif)

*N Engl J Med* 319:1452–1460, Dec 1, 1988 6–6

The medical, social, and legal aspects of passive smoking, which occurs when nonsmokers are exposed to tobacco smoke in an enclosed environment, have been subject to extensive debate. The relationship between lung cancer risk and low levels of active smoking reinforce a link between exposure to smoke and lung cancer in nonsmokers. A majority of case-control studies have indicated an increased risk of lung cancer among nonsmokers married to smokers (table). Until more evidence is available it is reasonable to consider tobacco smoke a danger to the health of adult nonsmokers.

Results and Possible Bias From Case-Control Studies of Lung Cancer and Passive Smoking*

| Smoking Exposure | Risk Ratio (Confidence Interval)† | Dose–Response Relation? | Study Conclusion Significant? |
|---|---|---|---|
| Trichopoulos et al.[34] (cigarettes/day) | | Yes | Positive/Yes |
| Ex-smokers | 1.9 (0.9–2.2) | | |
| Smokers | | | |
| 1–20 | 1.9 (0.9–4.1) | | |
| >20 | 2.5 (1.7–3.8) | | |
| Correa et al.[35] (pack-years) | | Yes | Positive/Yes |
| 1–40 | 1.5 (0.6–3.8) | | |
| >40 | 3.1 (1.1–8.5) | | |
| Chan and Fung[36] | | No | Negative/No |
| All smokers | 0.8 (0.5–3.1) | | |
| Koo et al.[37] (hr) | | No | Negative/No |
| <35,000 | 1.3 (0.8–2.4) | | |
| ≥35,000 | 1.0 (0.2–2.7) | | |
| Kabat and Wynder[38] | | No | Negative/No |
| All smokers | 0.9 (0.3–2.1) | | |
| Wu et al.[39] (age — yr) | | No | Positive‡/No |
| 1–20 | 1.4 (0.4–4.9) | | |
| ≥21 | 1.2 (0.4–3.7) | | |
| Garfinkel et al.[40] (cigarettes/day) | | Yes | Positive/Yes |
| <10 | 1.2 (0.8–1.6) | | |
| 10–19 | 1.1 (0.8–1.5) | | |
| ≥20 | 2.1 (1.1–4.5) | | |
| Lee et al.[41] | | No | Negative/No |
| All smokers | 1.1 (0.5–2.4) | | |
| Akiba et al.[42] (cigarettes/day) | | Yes | Positive/Yes |
| 1–19 | 1.3 (0.7–2.3) | | |
| 20–29 | 1.5 (0.8–2.8) | | |
| ≥30 | 2.1 (0.7–2.5) | | |
| Dalager et al.[43] (cigarettes/day)§ | | Yes | Positive/Yes |
| 1–19 | 1.4 (0.4–4.2) | | |
| 20–39 | 1.3 (0.5–3.5) | | |
| ≥40 | 2.7 (0.8–8.5) | | |
| Pershagen et al.[44] (cigarettes/day) | | No | Positive/Yes |
| ≤15 | 1.0 (0.6–1.8) | | |
| >15¶ | 3.2 (1.0–9.5) | | |
| Humble et al.[45] (cigarettes/day) | | No | Positive/No |
| <20 | 2.0 (0.9–4.6) | | |
| ≥20 | 1.6 (0.5–4.9) | | |
| Lam et al.[46] (cigarettes/day) | | Yes | Positive/Yes |
| 1–10 | 2.18 (1.14–4.15) | | |
| 11–20 | 1.85 (1.19–2.87) | | |
| ≥21 | 2.07 (1.07–4.03) | | |

*Updated and adapted from Department of Health, Education, and Welfare: *The Health Consequences of Smoking: A Report of the Surgeon General.* Washington, DC, Government Printing Office, DHEW Publication no. (HMS) 72-7516, 1972; and Department of Health, Education, and Welfare: *Smoking and Health: A Report of the Surgeon General.* Washington, DC, Government Printing Office, DHEW Publication no. (PHS) 79-50066, 1979.

†All risk ratios are relative to a baseline value of 1.0 for nonsmokers.

‡Only a weak positive association was found.

§Includes data from Correa P, Pickle LW, Fontham E, et al: Passive smoking and lung cancer. *Lancet* 2:595–597, 1983.

¶Either 15 cigarettes were smoked per day or 50 g of pipe tobacco was smoked per week.

(Courtesy of Fielding JE, Phenow KJ: *N Engl J Med* 319:1452–1460, Dec 1, 1988.)

Apart from lung cancer, chronic respiratory symptoms have been related to smoke exposure in some, though by no means all, studies. Asthmatic symptoms may be exacerbated by exposure to tobacco smoke. Further epidemiologic studies are needed on the relationship between smoke exposure and specific cardiovascular disorders.

A consistently greater rate of upper and lower respiratory problems has been found among young children of smoking parents. Cross-sectional studies suggest a 30% to 80% excess of chronic respiratory symptoms among children of smokers. Both cross-sectional and longitudinal studies have shown a decline in lung function in children as the number of smokers in the home increases.

---

**The Impact of a Total Ban on Smoking in The Johns Hopkins Children's Center**

Becker DM, Conner HF, Waranch HR, Stillman F, Pennington L, Lees PSJ, Oski F (Johns Hopkins Univ)

*JAMA* 262:799–802, Aug 11, 1989 6–7

---

A 1988 survey of 774 college-affiliated hospitals found that less than 8% are totally free of smoke. In 1986, the Johns Hopkins Children's Hospital administration instituted a ban on smoking in all areas of its hospital and clinics, limiting smoking to designated lounges. Because of noncompliance among both visitors and staff, a total smoking ban was instituted in July 1987.

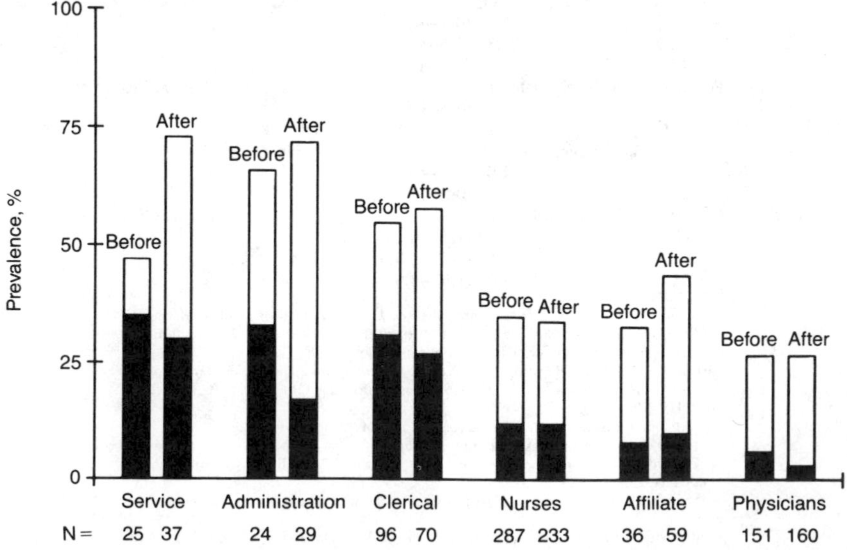


Fig 6–2.—Prevalence of current *(shaded bars)* and former *(open bars)* smokers before and after the smoking ban by occupation. *Service* indicates kitchen and housekeeping employees; and *affiliate*, dietitians, teachers, and social workers. (Courtesy of Becker DM, Conner HF, Waranch HR, et al: *JAMA* 262:799–802, Aug 11, 1989.)

TABLE 1.—Agreement With Smoking Attitude Statements by Smoking Status 6 Months Before and After the Ban on Smoking

| | Current Smokers, % | | Nonsmokers, % | |
|---|---|---|---|---|
| **Statement** | **Before (N=115)** | **After (N=95)** | **Before (N=622)** | **After (N=591)** |
| A hospital should be smoke free | 43 | 66† | 83 | 93† |
| Employees should ask visitors to put out cigarettes | 43 | 47 | 79 | 86‡ |
| Passive smoking exposure is unhealthy | 67 | 88 | 95 | 98 |
| A smoking ban is unfair to smokers | 50 | 82† | 17 | 42† |

*Changes were analyzed using 2 × 2 contingency tables (agree/disagree vs. before and after ban) separately for smokers and nonsmokers. The $\chi^2$ statistic was used to determine significance.

†$P < .01$.

‡$P < .05$.

(Courtesy of Becker DM, Conner HF, Waranch HR, et al: *JAMA* 262:799–802, Aug 11, 1989.)

A 6-month campaign started on January 1, 1987, and involved surveying all employees on their personal smoking habits and their attitude toward a total smoking ban in hospitals. After the total smoking ban had been in effect for 6 months, the employees were surveyed again. Unobtrusive observations of active smoking in visitor lounges and waiting areas were carried out just before and 6 months after the total smoking ban went into effect. Passive diffusion nicotine monitors were placed in the lounge areas for several days before and after the ban went into effect.

A comparison between baseline and follow-up employee survey data showed that 15% of the respondents were smokers 6 months before the ban, but that 13.8% were still smokers 6 months after the total smoking ban. The difference was not statistically significant. The prevalence of current smoking was highest among housekeeping and kitchen personnel (Fig 6–2). However, the percentage of smokers who smoked at work declined from 82% before to 43% after the ban. Before the ban, 43% of the smokers and 83% of the nonsmokers agreed that a hospital should be smoke free. After the ban, 66% of the smokers and 93% of the nonsmokers agreed with that statement (Table 1). Smoking in public areas declined from 53% at 1 month before to no smoking 6 months after the ban. Measuring environmental nicotine vapor concentrations showed a

TABLE 2.—Average Nicotine Vapor Concentrations Before and After the Ban on Smoking

| | Average Nicotine Concentration, μg/m³* | | |
|---|---|---|---|
| **Location** | **1 mo Before Ban** | **6 mo After Ban** | **P†** |
| Elevator lobby lounges | 13.01 | 0.48 | .03 |
| Restrooms | 7.33 | 6.69 | .99 |
| Other (patient rooms, conference rooms, utility rooms, and offices) | 0.43 | 0.17 | .06 |
| Total outpatient clinics | 0.28 | 0.36 | .31 |

*Concentrations less than or equal to 0.24 μg/m³ were below the analytic limit of detection. The midpoint between zero and 0.24 μg/m³ was used to calculate averages.

†Calculated using Student's *t* test (2 failed).

(Courtesy of Becker DM, Conner HF, Waranch HR, et al: *JAMA* 262:799–802, Aug 11, 1989.)

marked decrease in nicotine vapor levels in elevator and lobby lounge areas, confirming a high rate compliance with the total smoking ban (Table 2).

The total smoking ban virtually eliminated public smoking in all areas of the hospital, including visitor lounges and other public areas. Although a total smoking ban did not alter smoking prevalence among employees, it generally was complied with.

▶ Perhaps the most provocative data on the benefit of public smoking restrictions comes from a series of analyses performed around the time of the smoking ban at the Hopkins Children's Center. The ambient nicotine levels in the lobbies around elevators were reduced more than 20-fold, which was statistically significant. The role of nicotine in the debility induced by cigarette consumption recently has been well reviewed. Especially significant is the aspect of nicotine as the world's most widely used psychoactive drug (1). Unintentional exposure of patients to potentially active concentrations of this toxin in a medical environment is not acceptable. The support of this smoking ban at Johns Hopkins by two thirds of smokers and more than nine tenths of nonsmokers indicates a profound reservoir of public support for such measures.—J.L. Mulshine, M.D.

*Reference*

1. Benowitz N: *N Engl J Med* 319:1318, 1988.

**Deaths From Lung Cancer and Ischaemic Heart Disease Due to Passive Smoking in New Zealand**

Kawachi I, Pearce NE, Jackson RT (Wellington School of Medicine, Wellington; Univ of Auckland, New Zealand)

*NZ Med J* 102:337–340, July 12, 1989 6–8

Passive smoking increasingly is being recognized as a public health hazard. Among New Zealanders who have never smoked, an estimated 13% of men and 16% of women are exposed to spousal smoking. The estimated prevalence of exposure to passive smoking in the workplace is 34% for men who have never smoked and 23% for women who have never smoked.

Pooled relative risk estimates of death from lung cancer were 1.3 for both men and women exposed to passive smoking at home, and 2.2 for both men and women exposed at work (table). It was calculated that 30 lung cancer deaths in New Zealand in 1985 were attributable to involuntary smoking.

It also was estimated that another 91 deaths from ischemic heart disease were caused by passive smoking at home and 152 were caused by passive smoking in the workplace. The assumed relative risks were 2.3 for men and 1.9 for women. The estimated total annual number of

Estimates of Relative Risk of Death from Lung Cancer and Ischemic Heart Disease Caused by Passive Smoking

| Disease | Relative risk from exposure at home | | Relative risk from exposure at work | |
|---|---|---|---|---|
| | Men | Women | Men | Women |
| Lung cancer | 1.3 (1.1-1.5) | 1.3 (1.1-1.5) | 2.2 (1.4-3.0) | 2.2 (1.4-3.0) |
| Ischaemic heart disease | 1.3 (1.1-1.6) | 1.2 (1.1-1.4) | 2.3 (1.4-3.4) | 1.9 (1.4-2.5) |

*Note:* 95% confidence interval.
(Courtesy of Kawachi I, Pearce NE, Jackson RT: *NZ Med J* 102:337–340, July 12, 1989.)

deaths from lung cancer and ischemic heart disease caused by passive smoking was 273.

Passive smoking is a major public health problem in New Zealand that warrants taking action. Protection of the health of nonsmokers, especially in the workplace and in enclosed public places, must be a priority.

▶ These preliminary data from New Zealand further broaden the scope of the concern about passive exposure to cigarette smoke. In addition to an additive risk of lung cancer from the combined passive exposure to smoke both at home and in the workplace, the risk of ischemic heart disease secondary to passive smoking is increased demonstrably. In the face of such mounting evidence, retiring Surgeon General Dr. Koop felt compelled to use his last official visit to Congress to discuss the health impact of smoking (1). His final recommendation focused on limiting access of tobacco products to minors. These sentiments were amplified in an editorial by Dr. Stjernsward of the World Health Organization (2), who cites preliminary data from the National Cancer Institute SEER registry indicating that measure to reduce smoking are being reflected in lower rates of lung cancer in younger cohorts. In noting this first glimmer of success with antitobacco measures, he also identifies the pivotal role of the United States in tobacco production and trade. In the face of such negative domestic pressure on smoking, any federal support of tobacco export by this country is troubling.—J.L. Mulshine, M.D.

*References*

1. Koop CE: *JAMA* 262:2892, 1989.
2. Stjernsward J: *J Natl Cancer Inst* 81:1524, 1989.

## Intermediate End Points

▶ ↓ Current diagnostic technology for lung cancer detection still is defined by the use of chest x-ray films as the primary tools for detection. This year witnessed yet another derivative analysis of the NCI-sponsored Early Lung Cancer Project, which again concluded that chest x-ray examination is not effective as an early detection tool (1). This modality routinely detects disease at a very late stage. Chest radiography remains the major available test for detection of lung cancer at a surgically manageable stage and therefore warrants continued selective use in a case finding mode. A reasonable research question is whether other clinically useful markers exist that can indicate the likelihood of lung cancer development before chest x-ray examination can. A number of biologic tools are to be evaluated for such utility.—J.L. Mulshine, M.D.

*Reference*

1. Eddy: *Ann Intern Med* 111:232, 1989.

---

**Correlation of DNA Adduct Levels in Human Lung With Cigarette Smoking**

Phillips DH, Hewer A, Martin CN, Garner RC, King MM (Inst of Cancer Research, London; Univ of York, England)

*Nature* 336:790–792, Dec 22–29, 1988 6–9

---

Lung cancer causes 25% to 40% of all cancer deaths in the United Kingdom, and cigarette smoking is accepted as the major cause. The presence of covalently bound adducts in human DNA provides evidence of exposure to carcinogens, but systematic data on levels of DNA adducts in the human lung are not available. Use of the $^{32}$P-post-labeling technique showed that smokers have higher adduct levels than nonsmokers and that adduct levels are related linearly to cigarette consumption.

Autoradiographs of chromatograms of $^{32}$P-post-labeled digests of

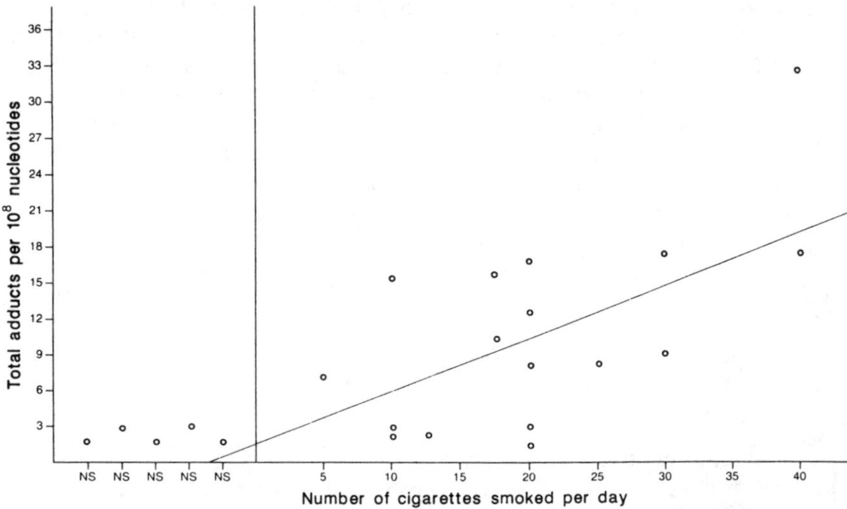


**Fig 6–3.**—Relationship between cigarettes smoked per day and lung DNA adduct levels estimated by $^{32}$P-post-labeling. *NS,* nonsmoker. (Courtesy of Phillips DH, Hewer A, Martin CN, et al: *Nature* 336:790–792, Dec 22–29, 1988.)

DNA from smokers' lungs showed a strong band of radioactive material and a weaker, faster-migrating band, a pattern like that found in lung DNA from mice treated topically with condensate of cigarette smoke. A linear relationship was found between the number of cigarettes smoked each day and DNA adduct levels (Fig 6–3). A linear relationship with lifetime cigarette consumption also was observed.

These observations strongly support epidemiologic findings that the risk of lung cancer increases with the amount of smoking. Cessation of smoking can lower the level of DNA adducts, although this may take months to years. The reduced risk of cancer after stopping smoking may in part reflect a loss of the promutagenic lesions that initiate the process.

► A conceptually attractive marker of the effects of tobacco exposure on a host's genetic material would be the quantitation of DNA adducts. The clinical application of this approach is being evaluated. Technical issues ensuring reproducibility of this analysis are critical. Such limitations can be ameliorated by evaluating more than 1 measure of DNA damage, such as the frequency of sister chromatid exchange (1). This type of analysis still is relatively imprecise, and it implies homogeneity of the genome in regard to cancer risk in the face of carcinogen exposure. As more information about the molecular genetics of cancer become available, it seems evident that specific gene loci are more closely linked to carcinogenesis than others.—J.L. Mulshine, M.D.

*Reference*

1. Liou SH et al: *Cancer Res* 49:4929, 1989.

**Nuclear DNA Content by Cytofluorometry of Stage I Adenocarcinoma of the Lung in Relation to Postoperative Recurrence**

Asamura H, Nakajima T, Mukai K, Shimosato Y (Natl Cancer Ctr Research Inst, Tokyo)

*Chest* 96:312–318, August 1989 6–10

Cytofluorometry was used to measure the nuclear DNA content (NDC) of 46 lung adenocarcinomas, all pathologic stage I lesions. Half the patients had tumor recurrences within 5 years of surgery. Tumors of the 2 groups were of similar size and histologic differentiation. The mean disease-free interval for patients with recurrence was 23 months.

The nuclear DNA content was greater in patients with recurrent disease, as reflected by mean nuclear DNA content, DNA histogram pattern, and occurrence of the aneuploid stem cell line, which was present in 91% of patients with recurrence and 74% of those without.

The nuclear DNA content is a good predictor of outcome in patients with stage I adenocarcinoma of the lung, especially in those with more differentiated and smaller tumors. Even patients with well-differentiated

T1 tumors need close follow-up. Adjuvant therapy should be considered if aneuploid stem cell lines are present.

▶ Another practical tool for evaluating biologic aggressivity for a particular patient's tumor is to measure the nuclear DNA content. As with measuring DNA adducts, technical issues can be confounding as reflected by conflicting reports of clinical correlations with cytofluorometric parameters in the literature. The bulk of the data support a relationship between aneuploidy in a tumor specimen and an aggressive clinical course in patients. The paper of Asamura and co-workers parallels the recently proposed approach to managing early stage breast cancer (1). Using ploidy as a tool to select early-stage patients with a greater risk of recurrence theoretically may define a more appropriate cohort for adjuvant chemotherapy. Formal clinical validation of selecting adjuvant therapy based on this in vitro parameter will be required before this intuitively attractive approach could be endorsed.—J.L. Mulshine, M.D.

*Reference*

1. McGuire WL: *N Engl J Med* 320:525, 1989.

---

**Expression of the Embryonal Neural Cell Adhesion Molecule N-CAM in Lung Carcinoma: Diagnostic Usefulness of Monoclonal Antibody 735 for the Distinction Between Small-Cell Lung Cancer and Non-Small-Cell Lung Cancer**

Kibbelaar RE, Moolenaar CEC, Michalides RJAM, Bitter-Suermann D, Addis BJ, Mooi WJ (The Netherlands Cancer Inst, Amsterdam; Medizinische Hochschule Hannover, Hannover, West Germany; Brompton Hosp, London)

*J Pathol* 159:23–28, September 1989 6–11

---

Many monoclonal antibodies have been raised against small cell lung cancer (SCLC) specimens or cell lines in the search for 1 that distinguishes between SCLC and non-small-cell lung cancer (NSCLC). The antigen of monoclonal antibody 123C3 recently was identified as the neural cell adhesion molecule N-CAM.

Paraffin sections of 19 resected SCLCs, 33 NSCLCs of various types, and 4 bronchial carcinoids were immunostained with monoclonal antibodies 735 and anti-Leu 7, both of which recognize sugar epitopes on N-CAM. With monoclonal antibody 735 all SCLCs were stained focally or diffusely and 1 carcinoid was stained focally. Only 3 of the 33 NSCLCs were faintly and focally positive with monoclonal antibody 735; these 3 tumors showed relatively small tumor cells and small, oval nuclei. Anti-Leu 7 stained all the carcinoids, only 8 SCLCs, sometimes focally, and 8 NSCLCs.

Monoclonal antibody 735 was superior to anti-Leu 7 in distinguishing between SCLC and NSCLC. Because monoclonal antibody 735 stained all SCLC strongly and is applicable on paraffin sections, it provides a needed addition to the immunomarkers used in the diagnostic distinction of SCLC and NSCLC.

▶ The First International Lung Cancer Antibody Workshop established several cluster designations of antibodies based on similar binding specificities to a panel of tissues (1). Cluster 1 defined a number of antibodies that bind to a neuroendocrine antigen, which was later found to be a neural cell adhesion molecule. Kibbelaar and co workers evaluated the diagnostic utility of this antigen. Interest in markers of neuroendocrine differentiation has increased as more reagents to study this phenomenon become available.

Linnoila and co-workers recently described a panel of 3 monoclonal antibodies, including Leu 7 (which is a cluster 1 marker), to immunohistochemically detect tumors with neuroendocrine differentiation (2). This panel was used in a retrospective analysis to evaluate the hypothesis that non-small-cell tumors with neuroendocrine differentiation behave clinically more like small-cell lung cancer. In that preliminary report non-small-cell patients with neuroendocrine features had a better response rate to chemotherapy (3).

A French group recently reported frequent concordance of the occurrence of tumor aneuploidy and neuroendocrine differentiation in non-small-cell tumors (4). The true clinical significance of the presence of neuroendocrine differentiation in a lung cancer is still unknown.

Using a monoclonal antibody not as a histologic discriminant as proposed by Kibbelaar, but as a probe to evaluate more about the underlying biology of a particular cancer may be a more appropriate application of hybridoma technology. Restricting molecular biology analyses to their correlation with light microscopic histology classification ultimately may restrict greatly the utility of these newer tools.—J.L. Mulshine, M.D.

*References*

1. Souhami RL et al: *Lung Cancer* 4:1, 1988.
2. Linnoila RI et al: *Am J Clin Pathol* 90:641, 1988.
3. Graziano SL et al: *J Clin Oncol* 7:1398, 1989.
4. Pujol JL et al: *Cancer Res* 49:2797, 1989.

---

**Considerations in the Development of Lung Cancer Screening Tools**

Mulshine JL, Tockman MS, Smart CR (Natl Cancer Inst, Bethesda, Md; Johns Hopkins Univ, Baltimore)

*J Natl Cancer Inst* 81:900–906, June 21, 1989 6–12

---

Death from lung cancer continues to increase in rate and is the major cancer death among men and women. Predictions suggest that in 1989 lung cancer will be diagnosed in 155,000 new patients, and an estimated 142,000 persons will die of the disease. However, the issues and problems surrounding mass screening programs for lung cancer have not changed.

| Potential Targets in Bronchial Fluids and Sputum for Early Lung Cancer Detection |
| --- |
| Differentiation markers (e.g., glycolipid expression) |
| Specific tumor products (e.g., mucins, matrix proteins, surfactant) |
| DNA ploidy |
| Polyamines |
| Nucleosides |
| Growth factors |
| Oncogenes or oncogene products |
| Cytogenetic changes |
| Specific chromosomal deletions or rearrangements |
| DNA repair enzymes |
| DNA adducts |

(Courtesy of Mulshine JL, Tockman MS, Smart CR: *J Natl Cancer Inst* 81:900–906, June 21, 1989.)

By the time bronchogenic carcinoma becomes symptomatic, it is usually advanced and incurable. Occasionally cancers in symptomatic patients are small, localized, and considered treatable when first diagnosed. A third of the patients with early-stage cancers constitute two thirds of all those who survive for 5 years. Screening for lung cancer therefore involves the search for cancers in asymptomatic persons because it is most likely that they will have disease that can be "cured" by available treatment approaches.

Chest radiography plus sputum cytology can detect presymptomatic early-stage carcinoma, resulting in higher resectability and survival rates for the study groups than for the nonscreened control groups. Ultimately, however, no cancer-related mortality benefit was associated with this combined screening approach. Therefore, until a reduction in morbidity or mortality can be shown, lung cancer screening programs for the general population cannot be supported. For now, screening programs are limited to well-controlled clinical trials among patients in various high-risk groups.

The negative outcome of early-detection trials has prompted investigation of tumor biology. Research is focusing on techniques for developing relevant probes that would reproducibly identify early lung cancer (table). Also, even more support is being given to vigorous smoking prevention efforts that for now remain the only apparent, meaningful, long-term solution to reducing lung cancer mortality.

► The rationale for using biologic parameters as potential tools for the early detection of lung cancer is reviewed in this commentary. In regard to the sputum immunocytology approach to the early detection of lung cancer outlined in this chapter last year (1), further information is available. In that report, 2 monoclonal antibodies were used to stain sputum specimens obtained from an archive that contained serial material from smokers through time, so that the correlation between positive antibody staining and the development of cancer could be established (90% accuracy in predicting lung cancer 2 years before clinical detection). As recently published, one of the antibodies used for that analysis recognizes a blood group-like antigen, difucosylated Lewis X (2). The distribution of related molecules has been mapped in fetal lung, normal lung, and malignant lung tissue (3, 4). Using families of differentiation markers to define the process of retrodifferentiation in carcinogen-exposed bronchial epithelial cells with sputum immunocytology remains a compelling direction for research in identifying early lung cancer. A confirmatory clinical trial of this sputum immunocytology approach is ongoing.—J.L. Mulshine, M.D.

*References*

1. Tockman M et al: *J Clin Oncol* 6:1685, 1988.
2. Kyogashima M et al: *Arch Biochem Biophys* 275:309, 1989.
3. Combs SG et al: *J Histochem Cytochem* 32:982, 1984.
4. Miyake M et al: *Cancer Res* 48:7150, 1988.

## Studies of the Clinical Management of Lung Cancer

### Diagnostic Issues

**Indeterminate Mediastinal Invasion in Bronchogenic Carcinoma: CT Evaluation**

Glazer HS, Kaiser LR, Anderson DJ, Molina PL, Emami B, Roper CL, Sagel SS (Washington Univ)

*Radiology* 173:37–42, October 1989 — 8–13

Gross mediastinal invasion by bronchogenic carcinoma can be diagnosed reliably with CT, but contiguity of tumor to adjacent mediastinal structures is not equivalent to definite invasion and is not necessarily a contraindication to surgical resection. Data were reviewed on 80 patients with bronchogenic carcinoma contiguous to the mediastinum on CT scanning, all of whom underwent thoracotomy. Definite infiltration of mediastinal fat and extension about central vessels or main stem bronchi were not found in these cases. Thirty patients had contrast CT.

In 66 patients (82%) masses classified as indeterminate for mediastinal invasion on CT scans were technically resectable. Eighteen of these masses focally invaded the mediastinum but were considered technically resectable. Invasion did not correlate well with the size of the tumor mass. If, however, there was as much as 3 cm of contact with the mediastinum and less than 90 degrees of contact with the aorta, resectability was likely. Fat between the mass and mediastinal structures also indicated that resectability was likely.

The CT findings helped predict technical resectability in nearly half of these patients classified as indeterminate for mediastinal invasion.

▶ Where CT imaging fits into the preoperative staging of non-small-cell lung cancer is not established. In certain institutions CT imaging of the chest is performed routinely before all lung cancer operations, and at other centers this study is done only occasionally. A critical variable in that regard is an operating surgeon's approach to surgical staging of the mediastinum. Where a mediastinal staging procedure always is performed before a lung resection, the reliance on the CT may be less.

The utility of noninvasive mediastinal staging with CT has grown as the salient radiologic parameters for this procedure have been defined. The group from Washington University touches on one of the thorny issues in interpreting mediastinal CT results. The experience of the diagnostic radiologist or the confidence of the operating surgeon in the radiologist are critical parameters that are difficult to control for in clinical trials.—J.L. Mulshine, M.D.

---

**Cost-Effectiveness of CT Scanning Compared With Mediastinoscopy in the Preoperative Staging of Lung Cancer**

Eddy RJ (Univ of British Columbia, Vancouver)

*J Can Assoc Radiol* 40:189–193, August 1989 6–14

---

Mediastinoscopy long has been the standard means of staging lung cancer before operation, but recently CT scanning has been proposed as an alternative strategy. If enlarged mediastinal nodes are found with CT, directed mediastinoscopy is carried out; otherwise surgery may be done without mediastinoscopy. The expected sequence of events for patients receiving management by these alternative approaches are compared in Figure 6–4. Costs were determined by calculating a fully allocated unit price for all relevant services.

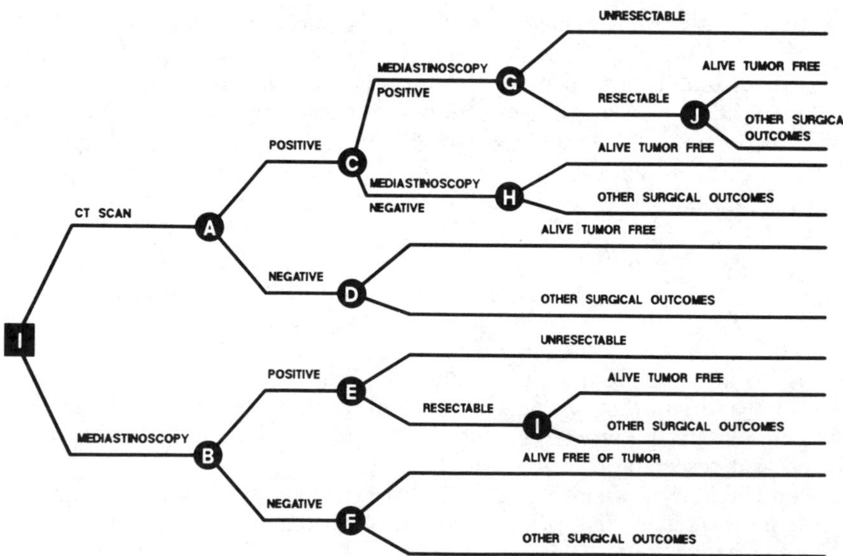


**Fig 6–4.**—Decision tree for alternative staging strategies in lung cancer. Mediastinoscopy includes bronchoscopy. When findings on CT scan are negative, patients undergo bronchoscopy before surgery. (Courtesy of Eddy RJ: *J Can Assoc Radiol* 40:189–193, August 1989.)

Estimated Economic and Complication Outcomes for Different Rates of Positive CT Scans

Economic Outcomes (per 1000 patients)

| % of positive CT Scans | Costs for CT-Directed Biopsy | Costs for mediastinoscopy/ bronchoscopy |
|---|---|---|
| 40 | $ 980,094 | |
| 50 | $1,082,050 | |
| 60 | $1,185,206 | $1,427,570.00 |
| 70 | $1,287,762 | |
| 80 | $1,390,318 | |

Complication Outcomes (per 1000 patients)

| % of positive CT Scans | CT-Directed Biopsy Hospital Days | Mediastinoscopy Hospital Days |
|---|---|---|
| 40 | 151 | |
| 50 | 161 | |
| 60 | 170 | 206 |
| 70 | 180 | |
| 80 | 190 | |
| | Deaths | Deaths |
| All tested patients | 1 | 1 |

(Courtesy of Eddy RJ: *J Can Assoc Radiol* 40:189–193, August 1989.)

Most of the difference in cost between combined mediastinoscopy-bronchoscopy and either bronchoscopy or CT scanning alone was related to high procedure-related costs such as use of the operating and recovery rooms and fees of the surgeon and anesthetist. Complication rates were similar for these 3 approaches, but complications of mediastinoscopy are much more likely to lead to a long hospital stay or to cause death.

At a CT positive rate of 40%, the cost savings of the CT-directed biopsy were as high as 30% (table). When results of 80% of CT scans were positive, however, the cost difference was quite small. The difference in hospital time also became small as the positive rate for CT scans approached 80%.

A strategy of CT-directed biopsy appears to allow substantial cost savings and to lower morbidity and mortality. It should be promoted and preferred over the continued use of mediastinoscopy alone.

▶ The report of Dr. Eddy attempts to standardize for some of the confounding variables, which were previously discussed. The use of CT is defined by a schema as shown in Figure 6–4. Although not fully described, the criteria for positive scan appeared to be restricted to the size of the mediastinal lymph nodes (nodes more than 1 cm in short axis diameter). Based on these parameters it is concluded that CT used as a prescreen for surgical mediastinal exploration has a role and is cost-effective. This study is not definitive, but systematic efforts such as this to define optimal management of common diseases is recommended not only because of the economic factors but also for the possibility of decreasing patient morbidity.—J.L. Mulshine, M.D.

**Pulmonary Microvascular Cytology in the Diagnosis of Lymphangitic Carcinomatosis**

Masson RG, Krikorian J, Lukl P, Evans GL, McGrath J (Framingham Union Hosp, Framingham, Mass; Boston Univ)

*N Engl J Med* 321:71–76, July 13, 1989 6–15

Lymphangitic carcinomatosis is often difficult to diagnose on radiographic information only, as the chest radiograph may mimic other pathologies. Although a lung biopsy study is usually diagnostic of lymphangitic carcinomatosis, it is often too hazardous to attempt in severely ill patients. Bronchoalveolar lavage only occasionally reveals malignant cells. Cytologic assessment of blood drawn from a wedged pulmonary-artery catheter can identify the characteristic microembolic material in amnion-fluid embolism or fat embolism. Whether the technique also could be used to detect cancer cells in patients with lymphangitic carcinomatosis was determined.

Pulmonary microvascular cytology was performed in 48 patients, of whom 8 had lymphangitic carcinomatosis, 17 had cancer without pulmonary metastases, and 23 had no cancer, but had various nonmalignant pulmonary disorders. The sites of primary tumors in the 8 patients with lymphangitic carcinomatosis were the breast in 4, the prostate in 1, the esophagus in 1, and the lung in 2. Lymphangitic carcinomatosis had been confirmed as the primary cause of respiratory distress by subsequent autopsy, lung biopsy, or clinical evaluation in all 8 patients.

Malignant cells were found in 7 of the 8 patients with lymphangitic carcinomatosis. Cytologic findings were normal for 16 of the 17 patients with cancer without pulmonary metastases, and for 22 of the 23 patients with nonmalignant pulmonary disorders (table). Forty-six of the 48 specimens showed only pulmonary megakaryocytes and megakaryocyte nu-

Results of Pulmonary Microvascular Cytology in All 48 Study Patients

| | Status on PMVC | | 95% Confidence Interval for Positive Test |
|---|---|---|---|
| | positive | negative | |
| | *no. of patients* | | |
| Patients with lymphangitic carcinomatosis | 7 | 1 | 47–100 |
| Control patients | | | |
| Cancer other than lymphangitic carcinomatosis | 1* | 16 | 0–30 |
| Nonmalignant pulmonary disorders | 1† | 22 | 0–23 |

*Tumor in hepatic veins.
†Pulmonary infarction.
(Courtesy of Masson RD, Krikorian J, Lukl P, et al: *N Engl J Med* 321:71–76, July 13, 1989.)

clei, confirming that the blood samples came from the pulmonary capillary bed.

When a lung biopsy to confirm a suspected diagnosis of lymphangitic carcinomatosis is refused or considered too hazardous, pulmonary microvascular cytology may be an acceptable alternative diagnostic procedure.

▶ The implication of this study is that patients with obstructed pulmonary lymphatics might also have an element of vascular stasis with regurgitation of malignant cells into the terminal pulmonary vasculature. In developing new diagnostic tests such as pulmonary microvascular cytologic sampling, a clear understanding of the pathophysiology is useful for predicting the theoretic utility of a proposed technique.—J.L. Mulshine, M.D.

## Therapeutic Issues

### Determinants of Perioperative Morbidity and Mortality After Pneumonectomy

Wahi R, McMurtrey MJ, DeCaro LF, Mountain CF, Ali MK, Smith TL, Roth JA (Univ of Texas, Houston)

*Ann Thorac Surg* 48:33–37, 1989 8–16

Data on 197 consecutively seen patients who had pneumonectomy between 1982 and 1987 were reviewed to identify perioperative risk factors. Indications for the procedure were primary lung carcinoma in 161 patients, mesothelioma in 15, and metastatic disease in 15. Operative mortality was 7%.

Mortality was 12% after a right pneumonectomy and only 1% after a

TABLE 1.—Predicted Postoperative Lung Function

| Variable | | No. of Patients | Deaths[a] | *p* Value[b] |
|---|---|---|---|---|
| $FEV_1$ (L) | ≥1.65 | 47 | 0 (0) | <0.05 |
| | <1.65 | 126 | 12 (9) | |
| FVC (L) | ≥2.13 | 78 | 2 (2.5) | <0.05 |
| | <2.13 | 95 | 10 (11) | |
| Percent $FEV_1$ | ≥41% | 122 | 4 (3) | <0.05 |
| | <41% | 51 | 8 (16) | |
| Percent FVC | ≥51% | 83 | 1 (1) | <0.05 |
| | <51% | 90 | 11 (12) | |

*Abbreviations:* $FEV_1$, forced expiratory volume in 1 second; *FVC*, forced vital capacity.

[a]Numbers in parentheses are percentages.

[b]Determined by chi-square analysis.

(Courtesy of Wahi R, McMurtrey MJ, DeCaro LF, et al: *Ann Thorac Surg* 48:33–37, 1989.)

TABLE 2.—Lung Function in Patients Requiring Prolonged Ventilation

| Variable | Ventilation[a] >48 Hours (n = 18) | ≤48 Hours (n = 179) | $p$ Value[b] |
|---|---|---|---|
| Percent predicted normal $FEV_1$ (preoperative) | 69% ± 0.04% | 79% ± 0.01% | <0.05 |
| Predicted (postoperative) $FEV_1$ (L) | 1.26 ± 0.04 | 1.49 ± 0.07 | <0.05 |
| Percent predicted (postoperative) $FEV_1$ | 43% ± 0.02% | 48% ± 0.01% | <0.05 |
| Predicted (postoperative) FVC (L) | 1.93 ± 0.12 | 2.08 ± 0.05 | NS |
| Percent predicted (postoperative) FVC | 45% ± 0.02% | 52% ± 0.01% | <0.05 |

*Abbreviations: $FEV_1$*, forced expiratory volume in 1 second; *FVC*, forced vital capacity; *NS*, not significant.

[a]Data are reported as mean ± standard deviation.

[b]Determined by Student's *t*-test.

(Courtesy of Wahi R, McMurtrey MJ, DeCaro LF, et al: *Ann Thorac Surg* 48:33–37, 1989.)

left pneumonectomy. Chest wall resection, extrapleural pneumonectomy, and diaphragmatic resection all increased operative mortality, as did the need for transfusion of more than 3 units. Mortality was higher among patients with a preoperative forced vital capacity of less than 85% of predicted normal value. No deaths occurred among patients with a predicted postoperative forced expiratory volume in 1 second of 1.65 L or greater (Table 1).

Atrial arrhythmias were the most frequent complication of pneumonectomy. Cardiac failure occurred in 9% of patients. Lower lung function predicted the need for prolonged ventilation (Table 2).

Regional ventilation-perfusion studies and lung function testing can identify patients at increased risk after pneumonectomy. More intensive evaluation and hemodynamic monitoring are appropriate in these cases. The risk of surgery must be balanced against the survival benefit for patients who need extended resection.

▶ The utility of aggressive surgery in patients with more advanced intrathoracic disease must be carefully reconciled to the specific risk profile for each patient. The relevant issues in contemplating a pneumonectomy are outlined in this report. A role for preoperative imaging studies to refine the level of surgical risk to potentially difficult surgical candidates is suggested.—J.L. Mulshine, M.D.

**A Prospective Study of Adjuvant Surgical Resection After Chemotherapy for Limited Small-Cell Lung Cancer: A University of Toronto Lung Oncology Group Study**

Shepherd FA, Ginsberg RJ, Patterson GA, Evans WK, Feld R, Univ of Toronto Lung Oncology Group (Toronto Gen Hosp; Mount Sinai Hosp; Ontario Cancer Inst, Toronto; Univ of Toronto)

*J Thorac Cardiovasc Surg* 97:177–186, February 1989 6–17

Small-cell lung cancer (SCLC) accounts for approximately 25% of all bronchogenic neoplasms, but only about 5% are operated on at detection. Most patients with SCLC have regional lymph node involvement, and many have hematogenous dissemination, rendering them ineligible for potentially curative operations. Although current chemotherapy combinations for SCLC achieve response rates of 80% or more with complete clinical response in approximately 50% of patients with limited-stage disease, most patients relapse early. The primary tumor site or the regional mediastinal lymph nodes are the first site of relapse, which has stimulated efforts at obtaining better local control of the intrathoracic cancer. Adjuvant surgical treatment after remission induction with chemotherapy was studied in 72 patients aged 39–77 years, of whom 21 had clinical stage I; 16, stage II; and 35, stage III disease. All patients underwent combination chemotherapy consisting of either cyclophosphamide, doxorubicin, and vincristine given intravenously every 3 weeks for 5–6 cycles or etoposide and cisplatin given intravenously daily for 3 days every 3–4 weeks for up to 6 cycles. Twenty-seven patients with complete responses and 30 with partial responses were considered eligible for surgery.

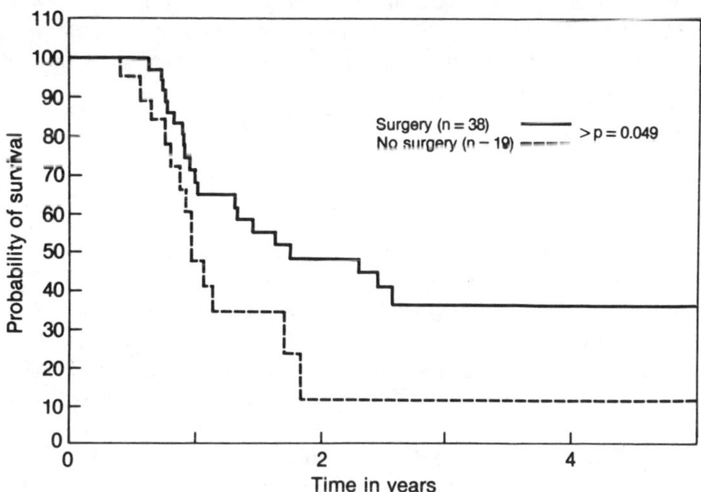


Fig 6–5.—Comparison of survival in 38 patients receiving adjuvant surgical therapy and 19 eligible patients who did not receive adjuvant surgical therapy for SCLC. (Courtesy of Shepherd FA, Ginsberg RJ, Patterson GA, et al: *J Thorac Cardiovasc Surg* 97:177–186, February 1989.)

Of the 57 surgically eligible patients, 38 underwent thoracotomy, of whom 8 required a pneumonectomy and 25, a lobectomy. Five patients did not have resection at thoracotomy. Of the 19 remaining patients eligible for surgery, 10 were randomized to receive radiation only, and 9 refused the operation.

No operative deaths occurred. The 38 operated patients had a median survival time of 91 weeks; the projected 5-year survival rate was 36%. The median survival for operated patients with pathologic stage II tumors was 69 weeks, and for those with stage III tumors, it was 52 weeks. The median survival for operated patients with pathologic stage I tumors had not yet been reached. The median survival for the nonoperated patients was 51 weeks (Fig 6–5). Thus, surgery did not improve survival for patients with stage II or stage III disease. At reporting time, 18 of the 38 surgical patients and 9 of the 34 nonsurgical patients were still alive.

Apparently, surgical therapy can contribute significantly to improve survival for patients with early-stage SCLC who have a complete or partial response to preoperative combination chemotherapy.

▶ Local control issues are very topical in the management of lung cancer. Combined-modality hyperfractionated radiation therapy with chemotherapy has been provisionally reported as promising (1, 2). Now the Toronto thoracic oncology group presents a further option in the process of improving local control of SCLC. The critical issue is minimizing the morbidity or mortality of the local procedure while attempting to achieve effective local control. The Lung Cancer Study Group also is evaluating surgical management of selected small-cell patients. Whether the provocative findings of the Toronto group are confirmed in a randomized multi-institutional trial will be closely watched. If these 2 local control modalities eventually are found to be comparable, quality-of-life issues associated with either approach may be the deciding factor. The problem of distant failure, which is the most common reason for patient relapse even among stage I patients, is not likely to be affected by either of these measures.—J.L. Mulshine, M.D.

*References*

1. Turrisi AT: *Oncology* 2:19, 1988.
2. Johnson BJ et al: *Proc Am Assoc Clin Oncol* 8:228, 1989.

---

**The Importance of Surgical and Multimodality Treatment for Small Cell Bronchial Carcinoma**

Karrer K, Shields TW, Denck H, Hrabar B, Vogt-Moykopf I, Salzer GM (Vienna; Northwestern Univ, Chicago; Ljubljana, Yugoslavia; Heidelberg, West Germany; Innsbruck, Austria)

*J Thorac Cardiovasc Surg* 97:168–176, February 1989 6–18

---

Most medical oncologists still treat all small-cell lung tumors with chemotherapy, alone or combined with radiotherapy, regardless of stage. In

TABLE 1.—Change in Clinical to Final Pathologic Stage Groupings

| Stage advanced ($n$ = 30) | | | Stage unchanged ($n$ = 74) | | | | Stage decreased ($n$ = 8) | | |
|---|---|---|---|---|---|---|---|---|---|
| *No.* | *Clinical TNM* | *Pathologic TNM* | *No.* | *Clinical TNM* | | *Pathologic TNM* | *No.* | *Clinical TNM* | *Pathologic TNM* |
| 19 | I | II | 35 | I | = | I | 1 | II | I |
| 6 | I | IIIa | 16 | II | = | II | 2 | IIIa | I |
| 5 | II | IIIa | 23 | IIIa | = | IIIa | 4 | IIIa | II |
| | | | | | | | 1 | IV | IIIa |
| 30 | | | 74 | | | | 8 | | |

(Courtesy of Karrer K, Shields TW, Denck H, et al: *J Thorac Cardiovasc Surg* 97:168–176, February 1989.)

this cooperative international trial, 112 patients having surgical resection were randomized to receive 1 of 2 intensive chemotherapeutic regimens, a sequential alternating regimen or a standard non-alternating 1, followed by prophylactic cranial irradiation in disease-free patients. Thirty-

TABLE 2.—Median Survival, Initial Resection and Adjuvant Chemotherapy

| | Category | |
|---|---|---|
| | *Dead* * | *Alive* † |
| All patients | 14.9 | 26.6 |
| Pathologic stages | | |
| TNM stage I | 18.9 | 21.6 |
| TNM stage II | 11.1 | 26.5 |
| TNM stage IIIa | 15.8 | 35.9 |
| T3 N0-1 | 22.5 | 47.3 |
| Any T N2 | 15.0 | 25.8 |
| N0 | 19.6 | 26.6 |
| N1 | 11.6 | 26.7 |
| N2 | 15.0 | 25.8 |

*Patients who have died during period of observation.

†Living patients; median survival calculated from date of operation to April 1, 1988.

(Courtesy of Karrer K, Shields TW, Denck H, et al: *J Thorac Cardiovasc Surg* 97:168–176, February 1989.)

eight patients had stage I disease, 39 had stage II disease, and 35 had stage III disease.

Survival differences related to the chemotherapeutic regimen used were not significant. Initial clinical stage was advanced in pathologic staging in 30 cases and was lowered in 8 (Table 1). Survival at 3 years was 61%, 50%, and 41% in stage I, II, and IIIa cases, respectively. The projected 3-year survival for patients having no disease was 65%. Median survival of the 45 patients who have died was 15 months (Table 2).

Pathologic stage I and stage II small-cell lung cancer is effectively treated with resection and intensive chemotherapy. The same approach may be used for stage IIIa cases without N2 involvement. For those with N2 disease the results are uncertain, but at the least, surgical "overtreatment" does not seem to be a disadvantage.

▶ This randomized trial compares the effects of 2 different chemotherapy arms delivered after a thoracic resection to remove the primary tumor. Because of the excellent survival outcome of the patients with limited-stage disease, the authors conclude that initial surgical management of stage I and II small-cell lung cancer patients is appropriate. Unfortunately, the original study was not designed to address this question, so this conclusion is overreaching, but it does suggest the feasibility of this approach. A randomized evaluation of combination chemotherapy coupled with either primary surgery or radiation therapy would need to be done to determine the role of surgery in the initial management of small-cell lung cancer.—J.L. Mulshine, M.D.

**Neoadjuvant Vindesine, Etoposide, and Cisplatin for Locally Advanced Non-Small-Cell Lung Cancer: Final Report of a Phase 2 Study**

Vokes EE, Bitran JD, Hoffman PC, Ferguson MK, Weichselbaum RR, Golomb HM (Univ of Chicago; Michael Reese Hosp and Med Ctr, Chicago)

*Chest* 96:110–113, July 1989 6–19

Patients with locoregionally advanced non-small-cell lung cancer (NSCLC) have a poor outlook. Surgery or radiation therapy have cured patients only occasionally. Two cycles of neoadjuvant chemotherapy with etoposide, vindesine, and cisplatin were evaluated in 27 patients with regionally advanced NSCLC.

Thirteen of the 23 evaluable patients had partial responses to chemotherapy, and 10 had stable disease or progression. The overall response rate was 48%. Seven patients were free of disease after completion of local therapy. Ten patients received further chemotherapy. The overall median survival was 8 months. Progressive disease was documented in 20 patients.

Myelosuppression was the chief form of toxicity. Only 2 patients had serum concentrations of creatinine greater than 2 mg/dL. Five patients had neuropathy, and 1 died of a wasting syndrome. One patient died of intracerebral bleeding while thrombocytopenic.

No clear survival benefit from neoadjuvant chemotherapy was apparent in this study, but further such studies are warranted, preferably with more active drug combinations. The optimal number of cycles and the need for additional adjuvant chemotherapy remain to be determined.

▶ The thoracic oncology group from the University of Chicago played a role in establishing the feasibility of neoadjuvant chemotherapy and surgery approaches to NSCLC. The goal was to cytoreduce the primary tumor with the initial chemotherapy, thus facilitating more frequent complete resection of regionally advanced lung cancer. The chemotherapy that consistently seemed more active in this context was potentially more effective in controlling microdissemination in this fashion.

The single-institution experience of the Chicago group therefore is disappointing because the median survival for all patients was only 8 months. The authors appropriately look to the results of larger cooperative group trials, which are just now maturing, before making a definitive disposition on the utility of neoadjuvant approaches. In addition they suggest that more active chemotherapy is required, as most patients with regionally advanced lung cancer die of distant relapse.

The inadequacy of current lung cancer chemotherapies is underscored by another recent publication of the University of Chicago group. In a report of experience with high-does alkylator therapy given with autologous bone marrow support to patients with NSCLC, the median response duration was 12 weeks, despite a 14% induction mortality (1). Four randomized studies of dose intensity of cisplatin delivery in NSCLC have not shown benefit from higher doses. As a result, although the use of marrow protective cytokines was endorsed as a worthwhile research direction at a recent small-cell treatment workshop, there was a shared concern that these new tools would not make a major difference in treatment outcome in lung cancer patients (2).—J.L. Mulshine, M.D.

*References*

1. Williams SF et al: *Cancer* 63:238, 1989.
2. Carney DN et al: Lung Cancer 5:143, 1989.

---

**A Phase II Study of Oral Etoposide in Elderly Patients With Small-Cell Lung Cancer**

Smit EF, Carney DN, Harford P, Sleijfer DT, Postmus PE (State Univ Hosp, Groningen, The Netherlands; St Luke's Hosp, Dublin)

*Thorax* 44:631–633, 1989 6–20

---

In elderly patients with small-cell lung cancer (SCLC) aggressive combination chemotherapy may cause life-threatening toxicity, particularly myelosuppression. As a result elderly patients often are excluded from clinical phase II trials.

Etoposide, an epipodophyllotoxin derivative that can be given orally, has produced response rates up to 65% when used alone in previously untreated patients. Thirty-five previously untreated, consecutively seen patients with proved SCLC who were aged more than 70 years received cycles of etoposide therapy, which consisted of a total dosage of 800 mg/m$^2$ given over 5 days.

Seventy-one percent of 33 evaluable patients responded, and 6 had complete remission. The median survival was 16 months for patients with limited disease and 9 months for those with extensive disease. One patient remains alive 22 months after the start of treatment. The incidence of bone marrow suppression was low, and no patient was admitted to a hospital because of drug-related toxicity. Gastrointestinal toxicity was easily managed.

Oral etoposide therapy is an effective and well-tolerated approach to elderly patients with SCLC.

▶ In view of the narrow therapeutic index for combination chemotherapy in SCLC, especially in patients with poor performance status or elderly patients, the availability of a less toxic treatment option is attractive.—J.L. Mulshine, M.D.

---

**A Simple Outpatient Treatment With Oral Ifosfamide and Oral Etoposide for Patients With Small-Cell Lung Cancer (SCLC)**

Cerny T, Lind M, Thatcher N, Swindell R, Stout R (Christie Hosp and Holt Radium Inst, Manchester, England)

*Br J Cancer* 60:258–261, August 1989 6–21

---

A 2-drug combination of ifosfamide and etoposide, given intravenously, has given results comparable to those achieved with 3- and 4-drug regimens in patients with small-cell lung cancer (SCLC). In the present study the 2-drug combination was given orally to 65 patients with SCLC who were aged 65 years or older or were medically unfit for intensive chemotherapy. Patients with metastases to the CNS or an elevated serum level of creatinine were excluded. Two grams of ifosfamide was given on days 1 to 3, and 100 mg of etoposide was given daily for 8 consecutive days.

The 60 evaluable patients had an overall response rate of 90% and a complete remission rate of 32%. Symptomatic relief occurred rapidly. Median survival was 11 months for all patients and 13 months for those with a complete response to treatment. Toxicity generally was mild, but 1 patient died of septicemia in the first course of treatment. Mild reversible toxicity of the CNS, chiefly somnolence, occurred in 25% of courses and was severe in 5%.

This simple and well-tolerated outpatient-based treatment regimen for SCLC is as effective as more toxic and costly treatments. The low risk of severe toxicity may promote the acceptance of palliative chemotherapy in patients with SCLC.

▶ This paper reflects another approach to lessening the morbidity of chemotherapy for SCLC. The support for this approach must await validation in a randomized clinical trial. The quality-of-life data are critical in correctly comparing conservative treatment with the more standard approach. A disparity between objective end points of clinical trials and patient perceptions of subjective benefit occasionally occur (1).—J.L. Mulshine, M.D.

*Reference*

1. Bleehen N et al: *Respir Med* 83:51, 1989.

---

**Clinical Pharmacology of Gallium Chloride After Oral Administration in Lung Cancer Patients**

Collery P, Millart H, Lamiable D, Vistelle R, Rinjard P, Tran G, Gourdier B, Cossart C, Bouana JC, Pechery C, Etienne JC, Choisy H, De Montreynaud JMD (Centre Hospitalier Universitaire, Reims; Coopération Pharmaceutique Française, Melun, France)

*Anticancer Res* 9:353–356, March–April 1989 6–22

---

Gallium, like platinum, is a metal ion used in cancer treatment, and oral administration may avoid the renal toxicity that complicates parenteral use. Pharmacokinetic parameters were examined in 18 patients with lung cancer after an oral dose of 800 mg/day of gallium chloride for 15 days. Serum levels of gallium were monitored in 45 patients who received doses of 100 to 1,400 mg/day of gallium chloride.

Large individual variations in pharmacokinetic parameters were noted after administration of a single oral dose of gallium chloride. Steady-state serum concentrations did not correlate with pharmacokinetc values in individual patients. Serum levels rose with doses up to 400 mg daily but not with further dose increases up to 1,400 mg. Tissue assays in 2 patients showed gallium concentrations in metastases that exceeded 10 μg/g. Concentrations in primary tumor were 3.6 μg/g.

Treatment with oral gallium chloride can be used in conjunction with other cytotoxic agents because of the lack of renal and hematologic toxicity. The optimal daily dose in lung cancer patients appears to be 400 mg.

▶ Gallium is a metal ion that has been studied extensively because of its effect on iron metabolism (1). Clinical evaluation of gallium chloride in phase I trials as outlined above or gallium nitrate in phase II trials for eventual use in the treatment of lung cancer patients has been started recently. This ion is known to inhibit transferrin-dependent growth in small number of lung cancer cell lines (2). Gallium may have only a limited effect on advanced lung cancer, but its mechanism of action suggests another application. Transferrin or closely related molecules appear to have a significant role as lung cancer autocrine factors. These factors may play a fundamental role during the promotion phase of lung carcinogenesis. Gallium independent of its evaluation as a traditional antineoplastic also might be evaluated for its utility as an antagonist of tumor promotion. With the limited effectiveness of the drugs currently available for lung cancer therapy, new rationally derived approaches warrant serious consideration.—J.L. Mulshine, M.D.

*References*

1. Weiner R: *Nucl Med Biol* 17:141, 1990.
2. Vostrejs M et al: *J Clin Invest* 82:331, 1988.

## Studies of Lung Cancer Biology

### Growth Factors

▶ ↓ Growth factors play a central role in lung carcinogenesis, understanding that biology can lead to both diagnostic and therapeutic applications.—J.L. Mulshine, M.D.

---

**Immunoreactive Gastrin-Releasing Peptide as a Specific Tumor Marker in Patients With Small-Cell Lung Carcinoma**

Maruno K, Yamaguchi K, Abe K, Suzuki M, Saijo N, Mishima Y, Yanaihara N, Shimosato Y (Natl Cancer Ctr, Tokyo; Tokyo Med and Dental Univ; Univ of Shizuoka School of Pharmaceutical Sciences, Shizuoka, Japan)
*Cancer Res* 49:629–632, Feb 1, 1989 6–23

---

Gastrin-releasing peptide (GRP) is a bombesin-like peptide that is commonly produced by small-cell lung cancer (SCLC), which suggests that the plasma GRP could be a useful tumor marker. A highly sensitive radioimmunoassay for GRP involves immune-affinity chromatography for plasma extraction. Plasma immunoreactive GRP was measured in 17 untreated patients with SCLC and 21 with other forms of lung cancer.

All controls and patients without SCLC had plasma GRP levels below 4 pg/mL, whereas 13 of 17 untreated patients with SCLC had elevated values ranging from 4.6 to 58 pg/mL. More than two thirds of patients with limited disease had high GRP values. In most patients GRP became undetectable with treatment. In 1 patient with a response, a rise in plasma GRP preceded the appearance of a new bone metastasis.

There is evidence that GRP can function as an autocrine growth factor for SCLC and that it may be a reliable tumor marker for patients with that neoplasm.

▶ Gastrin-releasing peptide was the first described and most extensively studied of the lung cancer autocrine growth factors (1). Maruno and co-workers suggest that quantitation of the amount of this neuropeptide in the plasma of small-cell patients could be a useful clinical management tool. Because of its rapid serum degradation, previous approaches to GRP quantitation were problematic. An alternative approach is to measure the more stable co-translationally produced C-flanking peptide (2). Detecting GRP immunohistochemically is also technically difficult. Recently, an in situ hybridization technique was reported to detect the more biologically stable prohormone form of this peptide (3). New molecular techniques can provide opportunities to study biologic problems with greater precision, potentially revealing attractive targets for effective therapy.—J.L. Mulshine, M.D.

*References*

1. Cuttitta F et al: *Nature* 316:823, 1985.
2. Holsted JJ et al: *J Clin Oncol* 7:1831, 1989.
3. Hamid QA et al: *Cancer* 63:266, 1989.

---

**Inhibition of Growth of Human Lung Adenocarcinoma Cell Lines by Anti-Transforming Growth Factor-α Monoclonal Antibody**

Imanishi KI, Yamaguchi K, Kuranami M, Kyo E, Hozumi T, Abe K (Natl Cancer Ctr Research Inst, Tokyo; Wakunaga Pharmaceutical Co, Hiroshima)

*J Natl Cancer Inst* 81:220–223, Feb 1, 1989 6–24

---

Previous study showed that human transforming growth factor-α (hTGF-α) stimulates the in vitro growth of 2 human lung adenocarcinoma cell lines, A-549 and PC-9. An anti-hTGF-α monoclonal antibody now has been used to determine whether hTGF-α acts as an autocrine growth factor in these cell lines. A radioreceptor assay for hTGF-α was used to study the effects of monoclonal antibody on growth of the human carcinoma cell lines and on colony formation by NRK-49F cells.

Exogenous addition or the anti-hTGF-α monoclonal antibody in vitro inhibited growth of both the human lung adenocarcinoma cell lines. This inhibition was specifically reversed in other experiments by exposing the lung cancer cells to higher concentrations of hTGF-α. In addition, the antibody blocked the stimulatory effect of hTGF-α on colony formation with NRK-49F cells.

These findings suggest that hTGF-α can act as an autocrine growth factor in human lung adenocarcinomas.

▶ Transforming growth factor-α or the closely related molecule, epidermal growth factor, joins gastrin-releasing peptide, insulin-like growth factor I, and transferrin as the 4 potential autocrine growth factors for lung cancer. In this report a monoclonal antibody is used to block growth factor effect in vitro. A clinical trial using a comparable antibody is under way at Memorial Sloan Kettering (1). The clinical benefit of antagonizing growth factor effects in advanced lung cancer remains to be established. Complex interrelationships between the various growth factors are possible (2). As discussed with the clinical evaluation of gallium as a therapeutic intervention agent, growth factor antagonists have the theoretic potential for greatest patient benefit if employed as antitumor promotion agents.—J.L. Mulshine, M.D.

*References*

1. Divgi CR et al: *Proc Am Soc Clin Oncol* 8:183, 1989.
2. Mulshine JL et al: *Basic and Clinical Concepts of Lung Cancer.* 1989, p 107.

---

**Pro-Opiomelanocortin Gene Expression and Peptide Secretion in Human Small-Cell Lung Cancer Cell Lines**

White A, Stewart MF, Farrell WE, Crosby SR, Lavendar PM, Twentyman PR, Rees LH, Clark AJL (Univ of Manchester; St Bartholomew's Hosp, London; MRC Clinical Oncology and Radiotherapeutics Unit, Cambridge, England)
*J Mol Endocrinol* 3:65–70, July 1989 6–25

---

Adrenocorticotropic hormone (ACTH) is synthesized as part of a precursor, pro-opiomelanocortin (POMC), which is cleaved to yield an intermediate ACTH-containing peptide (pro-ACTH). Expression of the RNA coding for POMC was demonstrated in 5 human small-cell lung cancer (SCLC) cell lines. A 2-site immunoradiometric assay for precursors is based on monoclonal antibodies to ACTH and γ-melanocyte–stimulating hormone.

Northern and slot-blot hybridization analysis of RNA and the use of bovine POMC complementary DNA as a probe showed processed POMC RNA from SCLC cells to be about 1,350 nucleotides long, larger than that found in the normal human pituitary gland. Measurement of ACTH precursors secreted by the cells confirmed expression of the POMC gene. Levels of POMC in medium accumulated throughout the growth of the cells, but POMC RNA was expressed at a relatively constant level.

The abnormalities detected in processing POMC peptide and in the size of POMC messenger RNA in SCLC cells are consistent with the occurrence of ectopic ACTH syndrome.

▶ This report establishes that SCLC cell lines are a relevant model for studying the genetic regulation of peptide production.—J.L. Mulshine, M.D.

### Small-Cell Lung Cancer Cell Lines Secrete Predominantly ACTH Precursor Peptides not ACTH

Stewart MF, Crosby SR, Gibson S, Twentyman PR, White A (Univ of Manchester; MRC Clinical Oncology and Radiotherapeutics Unit, Cambridge, England)
*Br J Cancer* 56:20–24, 1989 6–26

Although the ectopic adrenocorticotropic hormone (ACTH) syndrome occurs in only 2% to 3% of patients with small-cell lung cancer (SCLC), up to 30% of patients have increased plasma levels of immunoreactive ACTH. The precursors of ACTH (Fig 6–6) do not circulate in healthy persons, but may do so in patients with pathologic conditions, including ectopic ACTH syndrome. Eighteen human SCLC cell lines were examined for the production of ACTH and its precursor peptides pro-opiomelanocortin (POMC) and pro-ACTH by using a 2-site immunoradiometric assay based on monoclonal antibodies.

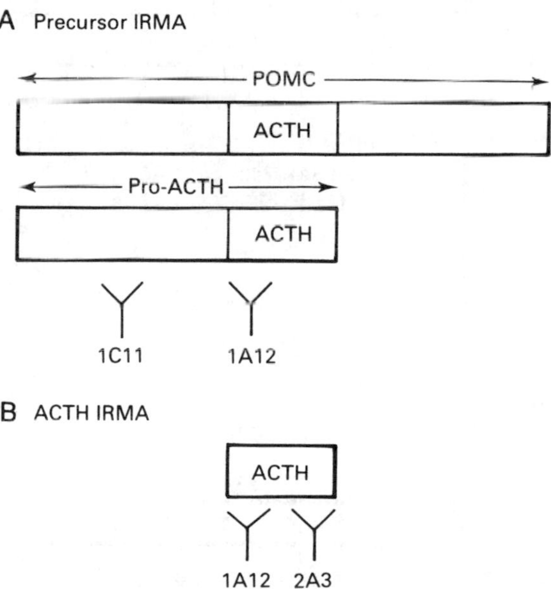


**Fig 6–6.**—Binding sites of monoclonal antibodies (MAbs) used in immunoradiometric assay (IRMA)s for ACTH-related peptides. In precursor IRMA (**A**) $^{125}$I-MAb-1A12 recognizes ACTH 10–18 and solid phase-linked MAb-1C11 recognizes gamma-melanocyte stimulating hormone sequence. In ACTH IRMA (**B**) $^{125}$I-MAb-1A12 recognizes ACTH 10–18 and solid phase-linked MAb-2A3 recognizes ACTH 23–39. (Courtesy of Stewart MF, Crosby SR, Gibson S, et al: *Br J Cancer* 56:20–24, 1989.)

Ten of the 18 cell lines (56%) secreted significant amounts of ACTH precursors. The low levels of ACTH immunoreactivity found in 7 cell lines could be explained by the known cross-reactivity of precursors in the ACTH immunoradiometric assay (Fig 6–7). Cell pellet extracts contained low or undetectable levels of ACTH precursors and ACTH, indicating that these peptides are not stored intracellularly. During the growth of SCLC cells in vitro ACTH precursors accumulated in the culture medium.

Significant levels of ACTH precursors were secreted by more than half

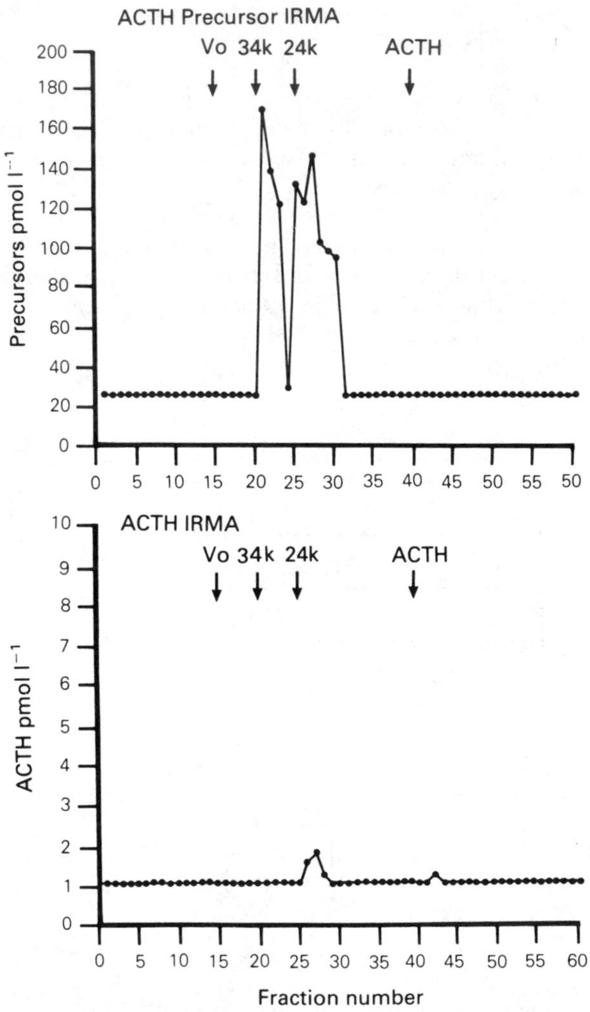


**Fig 6–7.**—Sephadex G-75 chromatography of COR L103 culture medium. The 34K, 24K, and ACTH markers correspond to elution positions of POMC, pro-ACTH, and ACTH 1–39 from human pituitary adenoma cell culture medium. (Courtesy of Stewart MF, Crosby SR, Gibson S, et al: *Br J Cancer* 56:20–24, 1989.)

of the SCLC cell lines examined in this study. Although POMC is processed to pro-ACTH, little if any ACTH 1–39 is synthesized or secreted by these tumor cells.

▶ Further work with the small-cell model suggests an answer to a long perplexing clinical problem. As suggested by the paper, investigators have previously measured high levels of what appeared to be ACTH in the sera of small-cell patients. Clinical stigmata of glucocorticoid excess would develop in relatively few of these patients. The suggestion from this paper is that, although abundant prohormone of ACTH is made, very little if any pro-ACTH is processed to the final biologically active form. This is somewhat perplexing because the same processing enzyme that potentially would cleave pro-ACTH from its precursor, POMC, should also cleave ACTH from its precursor, pro ACTH. The biology of gene expression especially as it relates to peptide processing is an area of intense basic research. Processing abnormalities have similarly been reported for lung cancer patients with the maturation of the peptide gastrin (1). Elucidation of the relevant mechanisms for these events has the potential for explaining more of the current gaps in our understanding of lung cancer biology.—J.L. Mulshine, M.D.

*Reference*

1. Rehfeld JF et al: *Cancer Res* 49:2840, 1989.

**Presence of Thrombosis-Inducing Activity in Plasma From Patients With Lung Cancer**

Maruyama M, Yagawa K, Hayashi S, Kinjo M, Nakanishi M, Ogata K, Iwami T, Ishinose Y, Hara N, Ohta M, Shigematsu N (Kyushu Univ; Sanshin-Kai Hara Hosp; Natl Kyushu Cancer Ctr, Fukuoka, Japan)

*Am Rev Respir Dis* 140:778–781, September 1989 6–27

Abnormalities in coagulation parameters are frequent in patients with malignant disease. Thrombosis-inducing activity (TIA) has been detected in the peripheral blood of patients with advanced lung cancer. Thirty-two men and 10 women aged 61 to 72 years with lung cancer, mostly in an advanced stage, were studied. Twelve patients with pulmonary sarcoidosis, 6 with tuberculosis, 6 with bronchial asthma, 5 with chronic bronchitis, and 3 with benign lung tumors served as controls.

Mice and guinea pigs given plasma intravenously from some of the cancer patients became immobile and died within 30 minutes, with multiple thromboses in the lungs. When heparin was given intravenously 5 minutes before the injection of plasma, thrombosis did not occur and the animals survived. Thirteen of the 42 lung cancer patients had TIA in plasma. Only 2 of 32 patients with chronic lung diseases and 2 of 31 healthy persons had TIA in plasma. The cancer patients with TIA in plasma had elevated levels of fibrinogen and increased levels of fibrin degradation products. The TIA was heat labile and sensitive to phospholipase C, and it bound to concanavalin-A Sepharose.

Massive release of TIA into the circulation may trigger disseminated intravascular coagulation. Thrombosis-inducing activity also appears in plasma from some patients with acute bacterial infection of the respiratory tract.

▶ This is another report that challenges our understanding of tumor biology. If cancer cells represent frozen states of differentiation, what was the adaptive function of a lung cell that produces significant quantities of a thrombogenic substance? Functionally, this report suggests that the clinical reflex of treating with heparin the occasional lung cancer patient whose presenting course is characterized by frequent thrombotic events has an in vitro rationale.—J.L. Mulshine, M.D.

---

**Antiproliferative and Differentiative Effect of Granulocyte-Macrophage Colony-Stimulating Factor on a Variant Human Small-Cell Lung Cancer Cell Line**

Yamashita Y, Nara N, Aoki N (Tokyo Med and Dental Univ)

*Cancer Res* 49:5334–5338, Oct 1, 1989 6–28

---

The presence of monocyte-specific surface antigens on some cell lines of small-cell lung carcinomas (SCLCs) suggests an origin related to cells of myeloid derivation, such as macrophages or their precursors. In the present study the effects of hematopoietic growth factors including granulocyte-macrophage colony-stimulating factor (GM-CSF) were examined on a variant clone adopted during passage of an SCLC cell line, GKT3-1.3.

This clone exhibits distinct morphological features and stains positively with nonspecific esterase. The surface-specific markers OKM5, HLA-DR, Mol, and My7 are increased. Proliferation occurs rapidly, as with immature cells.

The clone had specific binding capacity for GM-CSF; the number of binding sites was comparable to that in myelomonocytes or monocytic cell lines. Cell proliferation was inhibited by GM-CSF in clonogenic assay and suspension culture. The percentage of cells with surface marker Mol was increased after addition of GM-CSF. The antiproliferative effect of GM-CSF reflected a block at $G_0$ or $G_1$; it was abolished by anti–GM-CSF antibody.

These variant cells may represent a clone within the tumor population that becomes dominant when passaged in vitro and exhibits monocyte-like features. Eventually SCLC may be treated with differentiation-inducing colony-stimulating factors in conjunction with chemotherapy.

▶ The speculation in this paper regarding the joint origin of SCLC and myeloid cells represents an overinterpretation of the significance of the relatively promiscuous expression of certain putative tissue-specific markers. Much more important in this paper is the finding of lack of growth stimulation associated with growing SCLC in the presence of GM-CSF in vitro. In the initial phase of GM-CSF development, there was a theoretic concern that the cytokine might have a generalized mitogen effect of tumor cell proliferation. Fortunately, no stimulatory effect of tumor growth has been reported either in vitro or in vivo.—J.L. Mulshine, M.D.

## Issues With Molecular Genetics

### MDR1 Gene Expression in Lung Cancer

Lai S-L, Goldstein LJ, Gottesman MM, Pastan I, Tsai C-M, Johnson BE, Mulshine JL, Ihde DC, Kayser K, Gazdar AF (Natl Cancer Inst, Bethesda, Md)
*J Natl Cancer Inst* 81:1144–1150, Aug 2, 1989 6–29

The MDR1 (PGY1) gene often is overexpressed in multidrug-resistant cell lines. Expression of this gene appears to suffice to produce the full multidrug-resistance phenotype. In this study RNA slot blot analysis was used to investigate expression of the MDR1 gene in 24 lung cancers, 10 nontumorous lung tissue samples, and 67 tumor cell lines of varying histologic type.

Nearly all the tumors, nontumorous lung tissues, and cell lines expressed low levels of MDR1 RNA. Relatively higher levels were found in a subgroup of non-small-cell lung cancers that expressed neuroendocrine markers. There was no evidence of amplification or rearrangements of the MDR1 gene. The level of expression of MDR1 gene in cell lines failed to correlate with in vitro chemosensitivity of the cells (Fig 6–8), status of previous treatment, or clinical response to therapy.

Clinical multidrug resistance of many lung cancers cannot be explained exclusively by expression of the MDR1 gene. Other possible mechanisms of resistance include changes in the cellular glutathione system and altered function of DNA topoisomerase II.

▶ The surprising finding from this paper is the low or absent expression of MDR1 RNA in two thirds of the 67 lung cancer cell lines that were analyzed. Furthermore, the subset of non-small-cell patients with the greatest in vitro chemosensitivity paradoxically had the highest levels of expression of MDR1. These data strongly suggest that the profound clinical resistance seen initially with non-small-cell lung cancer and ultimately with small-cell lung cancer is not related to P-glycoprotein-dependent drug efflux pumps. This negative information will lead to different approaches to overcoming drug resistance in lung cancer potentially involving other putative drug resistance mechanisms.—J.L. Mulshine, M.D.

### Differential Expression of the c-*erbB*-2 Gene in Human Small-Cell and Non-Small-Cell Lung Cancer

Schneider PM, Hung M-C, Chiocca SM, Manning J, Zhao X, Fang K, Roth JA (Univ of Texas, MD Anderson Cancer Ctr, Houston)
*Cancer Res* 49:4968–4971, Sept 15, 1989 6–30

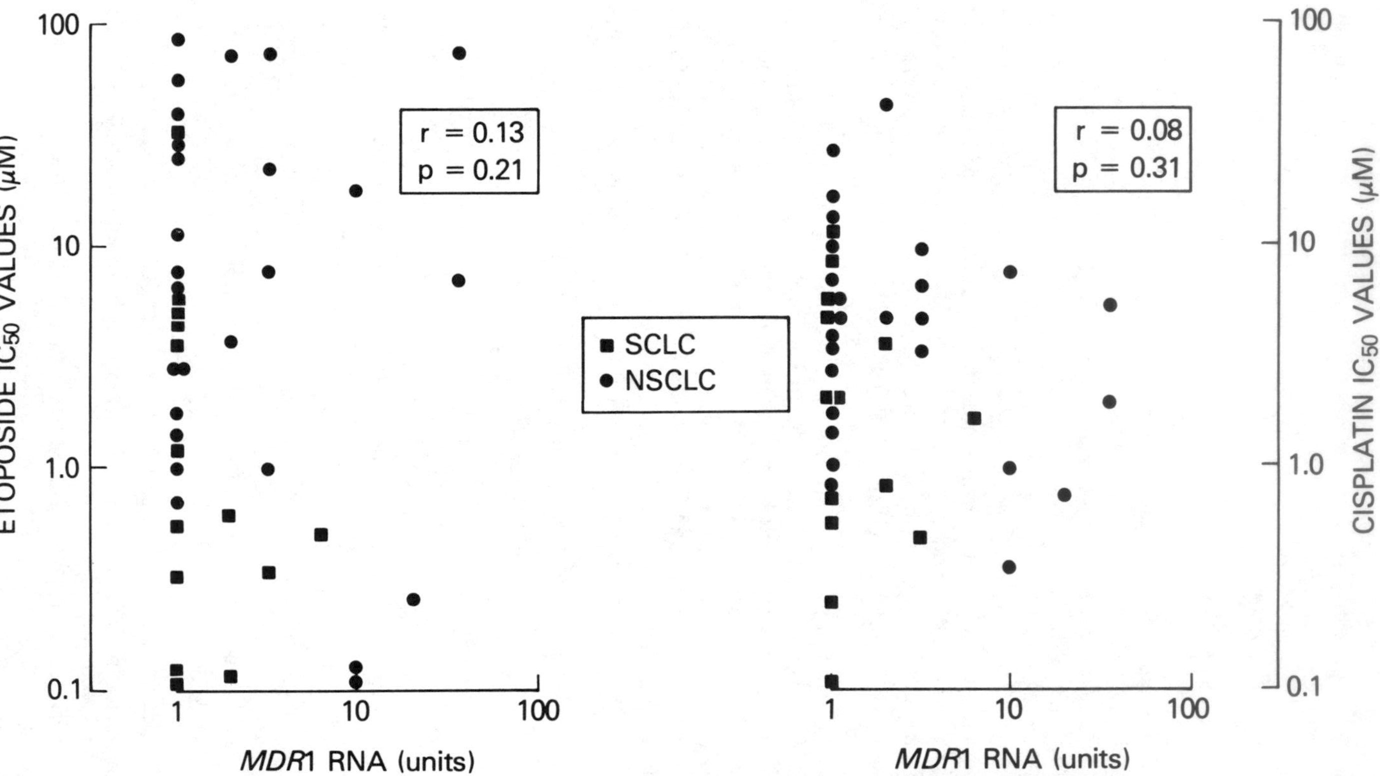


**Fig 6–8.**—Lack of correlation between MDR1 RNA expression and in vitro chemosensitivity to etoposide and cisplatin. Comparison of MDR1 RNA levels to sensitivity to other drugs tested (doxorubicin, carmustine, and melphalan) also demonstrated lack of correlation. For purposes of clarity, carcinoids and NSCLC-NE subtypes are included among NSCLC tumors. (Courtesy of Lai S-L, Goldstein LJ, Gottesman MM, et al: *J Natl Cancer Inst* 81:1144–1150, Aug 2, 1989.)

The c-*erbB*-2 gene, which produces a protein that has extensive sequence homology to EGFR, is amplified in some human tumors. In human breast cancer amplification of this gene reportedly correlates with the spread of disease and relapse and survival. Abnormalities were sought in the c-*erbB*-2 gene in 60 patients who had non-small-cell lung cancer (NSCLC). In addition, 11 human lung cancer cell lines, 4 derived from SCLC and 7 from NSCLC, were examined for altered c-*erbB*-2 gene expression.

Southern blot analysis of paired tumor and normal lung samples showed that amplification of the c-*erbB*-2 gene is rare in NSCLC, occurring in only 2 of 60 cases. It is not restricted to adenocarcinomas. One patient had an *Eco*RI restriction fragment length polymorphism for the c-*erbB*-2 locus. All NSCLC lines had high levels of expression of c-*erbB*-2 messenger RNA, whereas all SCLC lines had minimal or no expression. Adenocarcinomas expressed the most c-*erbB*-2 messenger RNA.

Expression of c-*erbB*-2 differs between SCLC and NSCLC. Levels of expression are consistently high in lung adenocarcinomas, and it is possible that expression of c-*erbB*-2 is important in the pathogenesis of human lung adenocarcinoma.

▶ The gene c-*erbB*-2 produces a protein product in various human tumors. This protein product has extensive homology to the epidermal growth factor receptor and is suspected to play a role, especially, in breast carcinogenesis. Again this analysis is largely negative, suggesting at most that c-*erbB*-2 expression may play a central role in the development of some adenocarcinomas of the lung. Continued study in this area is required before a satisfying explanation of the role of oncogenes in lung carcinogenesis is evident.—J.L. Mulshine, M.D.

---

**Tumorigenicity of Human Mesothelial Cell Line Transfected With EJ-ras Oncogene**

Reddel RR, Malan-Shibley L, Gerwin BI, Metcalf RA, Harris CC (Natl Cancer Inst, Bethesda, Md)

*J Natl Cancer Inst* 81:945–948, June 21, 1989 6–31

---

To determine whether human mesothelial cells are capable of undergoing neoplastic change in vitro and to observe their interaction with the activated c-Ha-ras (HRAS1) oncogene EJ-ras, which has a role in the development of many human tumors, the activated oncogene was transfected into a nontumorigenic cell line, MeT-5A.

This line was established from normal human mesothelial cells after transfection with a plasmid containing simian virus 40 early-region genes. The transfected plasmid contained the EJ-ras gene and the neomycin-resistance gene. A population resistant to the neomycin analogue G418 was selected.

Cells from the transfected cell line formed rapidly growing subcutaneous tumors in athymic nude mice, but no tumors formed from untransfected MeT-5A cells or cells transfected with the vector DNA and selected for G418 resistance. The tumors formed by EJ-ras–transfected cells were established in vitro and cells from these tumor cell lines had altered morphology and the same isoenzyme phenotype as the parent cells. They expressed the mutant EJ-ras p21 protein.

Cells from human mesothelium can undergo transformation to a fully malignant phenotype in vitro. Presently the relevance of ras oncogenes to the formation of naturally occurring mesotheliomas is under study.

▶ The use of oncogene-transfected "normal tissue" cell lines provides an opportunity to identify specific gene-dependent functions. The EJ-ras–transfected mesothelial cells develop the new property of tumorigenic growth in nude mice. In addition they manifest a variety of other in vitro properties of more aggressive growth. In a similar study from the same group, a v-Ha-ras construct was transfected into a human bronchial epithelial cell line (1) and again more aggressive in vitro and in vivo behavior was observed in the oncogene transfected line. These studies provide a model for identifying the biology associated with the expression or overexpression of a particular oncogene. Further research in this area ultimately will explore the feasibility of nullifying malignant oncogene effects through the use of anti-sense oncogene constructs. Whether this elegant technology will filter into clinical practice will be watched closely.—J.L. Mulshine, M.D.

*Reference*

1. Bofil RD et al: *J Natl Cancer Inst* 81:587, 1989.

---

**p53: A Frequent Target for Genetic Abnormalities in Lung Cancer**

Takahashi T, Nau MM, Chiba I, Birrer MJ, Rosenberg RK, Vinocour M, Levitt M, Pass H, Gazdar AF, Minna JD (Natl Cancer Inst; Uniformed Services Univ of the Health Sciences, Bethesda, Md; Univ of Pittsburgh)
*Science* 246:491–494, Oct 27, 1989 6–32

---

Specific chromosomal deletions are described in various human tumors, suggesting a pathogenetic role for antioncogenes ("tumor suppressor" genes). Allelic loss characterizes chromosomal regions that harbor recessive oncogenes. In lung cancer there often is a loss of heterozygosity on 17p, and the p53 gene located on 17p13 appears to have many features of an antioncogene. Allelic loss for chromosome regions 3p and 17p is found in both small-cell lung cancer (SCLC) and non-SCLC.

The genetic abnormalities of p53 include homozygous deletions and abnormally sized messenger RNAs in addition to a range of point or small mutations which map to the p53 open reading frame and change amino acid sequencing in a region that is highly conserved between mouse and man. Very low or absent expression of p53 messenger RNA was found in lung cancer cell lines compared with normal lung cell lines.

Studies of 30 lung cancer cell lines indicate that the p53 gene is affected in all types of lung cancer. There is substantial evidence that normal p53 may function as an antioncogene. In many SCLC and non-SCLC cell lines alterations of the *Rb* gene on 13q and p53 genes on 17p13 coexist with 1 or more deletions in chromosome region 3p. An obviously important question is whether correction of these lesions reverses the malignant phenotype.

▶ After the molecular characterization of the retinoblastoma gene, Minna and co-workers used the appropriate probes to study that gene expression in lung cancer (1). In about 20% of small-cell lung tumor and cell lines, structural abnormalities of the retinoblastoma gene were found. Likewise in the paper of Dr. Takahashi and co-workers structural abnormalities of the p53 gene frequently are found in all forms of lung cancer. In both these papers, the gene in question is believed to be constitutively involved in the regulation of the genome to suppress the development of a cancer. With the gene mutation comes an abrogation of that repressor function permitting the development of a lung cancer. The concept of tumor repressor genes currently is being evaluated to explain the pathogenesis of a range of human malignancies. Its relevance to human lung cancer both in terms of pathogenesis and in permitting the development of innovative therapies are being studied intensively.—J.L. Mulshine, M.D.

*Reference*

1. Harbour JW et al: *Science* 241:353, 1988.

# 7 Respiratory Structure and Function

## Introduction

This chapter is divided into three sections: Pulmonary Function, Sleep Disordered Breathing, and Miscellaneous Studies.

Pulmonary function testing is the theme that ties together the first series of articles. Abstract 7–1 discusses the statistical phenomenon of regression to the mean and how this process can lead to faulty decision making based on "clinical experience." How to select the best spirogram continues to be a topic of controversy despite the American Thoracic Society Standards. This topic is treated in one of the summarized articles, which suggests that the size of the forced expiratory volume in 1 second is more dependent on the size of the forced vital capacity than the maximal expiratory effort.

Two articles treat the association of impairment of pulmonary function with subsequent mortality. Both standard spirometry and simple peak flowmeter testing seem to give us valuable information about study populations. Because of the association of tobacco cigarette smoking with coronary heart disease as well as impaired lung function, many patients with obstructive airway disease are candidates for coronary artery bypass surgery. The magnitude of fall in spirometry after coronary artery bypass surgery is shown in one study, which suggests that the type of procedure influences the amount of subsequent derangement.

Last year I discussed the relationship between heart-lung transplantation and the development of bronchial hyperresponsiveness. This year, a study of bone-marrow transplant patients also finds an increase in bronchial hyperresponsiveness in 20% of them. Ozone is an increasing problem: too much in the lower atmosphere and too little in the upper. Exposure to ozone on one day apparently can influence responses the following day, particularly in those who exercise in the polluted air.

Our understanding of the mechanisms, pathophysiology, and treatment of sleep-disordered breathing continues to increase. Studies summarized in this volume show that patients with the most severe desaturations during sleep apnea have the most depressed hypoxic ventilatory drive. The bony facial structure of patients with sleep apnea is different from that of normals, showing foreshortening of the maxilla in the anteroposterior axis. One study of healthy persons who snore suggests that the primary mechanism for the depression of alveolar ventilation with sleep is an increase in airway resistance. Two studies show that a single night of sleep deprivation can lead to poor performance on spirometry the following day, as well as the previously reported reduction in hypercapnic responsiveness.

The parodoxical increase in sodium excretion at night in patients with obstructive sleep apnea syndrome may result from the secretion of atrial natriuretic hormone at night caused by distention of the heart.

Although treatment for sleep apnea syndrome with continuous positive airway pressure (CPAP) or tracheostomy is effective in preventing apneic episodes, the benefits and complications of these treatments remain speculative. One dramatic, though unrandomized, study shows that tracheotomy virtually eliminates 5-year mortality among patients with severe sleep apnea. One study shows that continuous positive airway pressure does improve neuropsychological impairments in sleep apnea patients, but another shows that oxygen treatment of snorers does not do the same.

The hope for a pharmacologic treatment for sleep apnea is spurred on by the demonstration that large doses of salicylate preferentially stimulate the upper airway dilating muscles. Finally, two case series show that effective sleep apnea treatments—tracheostomy and CPAP—both can have complications that at times can be life-threatening.

In the section Miscellaneous Studies, two articles are discussions of interaction of respiration with other organ systems, specifically the heart and the gastrointestinal tract. An increasing consensus about the mechanics that influence the respiratory wave of blood pressure is apparent in one of the key recent articles in this area. The common association of asthma exacerbations with esophageal reflux is relevant to the study of the effects of negative pressure ventilation on lower esophageal sphincter tone. An intriguing study of the ventilatory pattern "fingerprint" or "ventilatory personality" suggests that all of us possess an intrinsic respiratory rhythm and pattern which persists over years. Finally, two articles address how the diaphragm is activated. Activation of the diaphragm motor units apparently occurs in a carefully scripted sequential pattern that maximizes endurance and prevents fatigue. In the case of special stereotyped respiratory maneuvers such as sneezing or gasping, however, the respiratory muscles may be supramaximally contracted beyond maximal voluntary stimulation.

**Robert A. Wise, M.D.**

## Pulmonary Function

**Relationship of Lung Function Loss to Level of Initial Function: Correcting for Measurement Error Using the Reliability Coefficient**

Irwig L, Groeneveld H, Becklake M (Univ of Pretoria; Univ of Witwatersrand, Johannesburg, South Africa)

*J Epidemiol Community Health* 42:383–389, December 1988 7–1

Determining whether a change in level of a certain variable over time is related to its initial measurement is useful in epidemiology. The estimate of such an association is biased if the initial random measurement is in error. Various ways of reaching unbiased estimates of regression coefficients were applied to determine whether lung function loss in 433 men aged 18–23 years was associated with the initial level of function.

Use of the reliability coefficient to correct the regression coefficient for random error of measurement was the best method for both conceptual and practical reasons. This method shows the proportion of the variance that can be attributed to true variability, and the correlation between repeated determinations of the underlying level is a simple way of estimating this. In the men studied, no relation was suggested between initial level and changes in forced vital capacity, forced expiratory volume in 1 second, and forced expiratory flow in the middle of expiration.

Estimating the random error of measurement is necessary in epidemiologic research. For this purpose, the reliability coefficient is preferable to the coefficient of variation.

▶ This article in its original form is rather hard reading for all but the most statistically oriented. The subject, though, is one well worth considering, as it affects not only the statistical interpretation of data, but also the way physicians make day-to-day decisions. The phenomenon treated here is *regression to the mean.* Briefly stated, given a set of data that has random variability, second observations will tend to be closer to the mean of all values than the initial observation. Thus, initially high values will tend to be lower on a second measurement, and initially low values will tend to be higher on a second measurement. In measuring the effect of baseline lung function on subsequent change in lung function, one would find that those with high initial values would tend to have greater declines in lung function than those with lower values purely as a consequence of random variability. The scientific literature is filled with examples of misinterpretation of this phenomenon. For example, one study presented at a recent national meeting found that patients with low levels of arterial oxygen tended to have improvement after bronchoscopy, whereas those with high levels tended to have drops after bronchoscopy. A reasonable pathophysiologic explanation for these results could be crafted, but that this was just an artifact of regression to the mean is also likely.

In a related, fascinating article, Tversky and Kahneman describe how such a phenomenon can influence decision making (1). In an experimental study, flying instructors were asked to judge whether praise or censure were more effective in improving the performance of student pilots learning to land airplanes. The quality of the mock landings was random, but the instructors concluded that censure was more effective. Whenever a bad landing was followed by censure, the next landing was likely to be improved, but when a good landing was followed by praise, the next landing was likely to be worse. Such an effect undoubtedly influences our evaluation of clinical experience. A placebo treatment rendered to a patient with a very low blood pressure, for example, will tend to show a rise in blood pressure on subsequent readings if the values are randomly variable. Because physicians tend to confront patients at the nadirs of their health, nearly any nonharmful treatment will appear to be effective to both patient and physician as a consequence of regression to the mean. On a second visit, poor health is likely to improve, and good health is likely to worsen. Only physicians who confront patients at the peak of their health will be confronted regularly with declining patient health.—R.A. Wise, M.D.

*Reference*

1. Tversky A, Kahneman D: Judgement under uncertainty: Heuristics and biases. *Science* 185:1124–1131, 1974.

**Effect of Effort Versus Volume on Forced Expiratory Flow Measurement**
Park SS (Albert Einstein College of Medicine, Bronx, NY)
*Am Rev Respir Dis* 138:1002–1005, October 1988 7–2

The American Thoracic Society (ATS) recommends reporting the best of 3 values of forced expiratory volume in 1 second ($FEV_1$), but recent experience indicates that $FEV_1$ consistently declines with increasing effort in normal research subjects. A similar inverse effort dependence of $FEV_1$ was apparent in routine lung function testing. How $FEV_1$ and forced expiratory flow at 25% to 75% ($FEV_{25-75}$) are affected by using effort-based criteria (the highest peak expiratory flow rate) was compared with volume-based criteria (the largest forced vital capacity (FVC) and the largest sum of FVC and $FEV_1$).

Data from 10 healthy persons and 12 patients with chronic obstructive lung disease were analyzed. The volume-based criteria, including ATS criteria, led to the selection of identical maneuvers and identical test results (table). This confirms the importance of volume as a determinant of forced expiratory flow. Selection based on the highest peak expiratory flow rate resulted in a decline in mean $FEV_1$ and an even more significant decrease in FVC. Individual values for $FEV_1$ often declined on effort only when the accompanying FVC also was lower. The $FEV_{25-75}$ was more obviously affected by the negative result of effort, independently of accompanying FVC.

Mean FVC, $FEV_1$, and $FEF_{25-75}$ From Maneuvers Selected Based on ATS Criteria (I), Largest FVC (II), and Highest PEFR (III)

| | I (*mean*) | II (*mean*) | III (*mean*) | Difference* (*mean* ± *SE*) | p Values† |
|---|---|---|---|---|---|
| **Normal subjects, n = 10** | | | | | |
| FVC, L | 2.983 | 2.983 | 2.938 | 0.045 ± 0.015 | < 0.01 |
| $FEV_1$, L | 2.460 | 2.460 | 2.424 | 0.036 ± 0.019 | < 0.05 |
| $FEF_{25-75}$, L/s | 2.692 | 2.692 | 2.645 | 0.047 ± 0.051 | > 0.05 |
| **COPD patients, n = 12** | | | | | |
| FVC, L | 1.804 | 1.804 | 1.786 | 0.018 ± 0.007 | < 0.01 |
| $FEV_1$, L | 1.053 | 1.053 | 1.031 | 0.022 ± 0.01 | < 0.05 |
| $FEF_{25-75}$, L/s | 0.698 | 0.698 | 0.684 | 0.014 ± 0.009 | > 0.05 |

*Differences between II and III.
†*P* values were obtained based on paired *t*-test, 1-tailed analysis.
(Courtesy of Park SS: *Am Rev Respir Dis* 138:1002–1005, October 1988.)

Volume is an important determinant of the net effect of effort on $FEV_1$. Fully inflated lungs appear to favorably shift the balance so that $FEV_1$ is little affected by effort. Volume-based ATS selection criteria are valid, but this does not apply to $FEV_{25-75}$, which is significantly influenced by the negative effect of effort.

► The ATS standards for spirometry suggest that the largest $FEV_1$ and FVC be selected as the test values even if derived from different maneuvers (1). Evidence, however, suggests that maximal effort, defined by maximal expiratory pleural pressure, is associated with smaller $FEV_1$ values as a consequence of "negative effort dependence." Krowka and colleagues have proposed, therefore, that spirometric indices should be taken from the efforts that are the greatest rather than those with the largest volumes. Because measurement of esophageal pressure is obviously not practical, they propose using the tracing with the maximal peak flow, which they have shown is indicative of maximal expiratory effort (2). The study abstracted above applied 3 criteria for determining the best maneuver. The authors found that the ATS criteria gave results the same as those for the maneuver with the largest FVC. The maneuver with the highest peak flow produced slightly smaller values, which were statistically different but not of much clinical importance for a single test.

Why is this an important issue? Reproducibility is one of the most important characteristics of good spirometry. In the 20% or so of persons with significant negative effort dependence, the pulmonary function technician can be exceedingly frustrated trying to have a person reproduce within 5% a submaximal but larger $FEV_1$. The harder the person tries, the smaller the $FEV_1$ becomes. Thus the test results could be considered of suboptimal quality when they did reflect maximal effort. I suspect that this phenomenon is sometimes responsible for what we erroneously call spirometry-induced bronchospasm where successive efforts show declining $FEV_1$. Because the differences are small, usually less than 0.2 L, it is not likely that this would interfere with clinical decision making or diagnosis. It can, however, be an important consideration in following sequential spirometry in treated patients for whom directional changes of this magnitude can influence therapeutic decisions.

What should the laboratory director do? Unless the ATS changes its standards, it is still reasonable for the laboratory to report spirograms with the largest $FEV_1$ and FVC among those of satisfactory quality. Care should be taken, though, to reject as unsatisfactory those studies that do not have reproducible peak flow rates even if the $FEV_1$ exceeds that of better quality studies.—R.A. Wise, M.D.

*References*

1. American Thoracic Society: Standardization of spirometry: 1987 update. *Am Rev Respir Dis* 136:1285–1298, 1987.
2. Krowka MJ, Enright PL, Rodarte JR, et al: Effect of effort on measurement of forced expiratory volume in one second. *Am Rev Respir Dis* 136:829–833, 1987.

**Pulmonary Function as a Predictor of Coronary Heart Disease**

Marcus EB, Curb JD, MacLean CJ, Reed DM, Yano K (Kuakini Med Ctr, Honolulu; Natl Inst on Aging, Bethesda, Md; Natl Heart, Lung, and Blood Inst, NIH, Honolulu)

*Am J Epidemiol* 129:97–104, January 1989 7–3

There is much disagreement over the possible association between pulmonary function and CHD. Although some investigators have shown an independent effect of pulmonary function on the incidence of CHD, others have found no association between the presence of pulmonary dysfunction or chronic lung disease and evidence of CHD. Cigarette smoking may cause both conditions, rather than pulmonary impairment causing CHD. Pulmonary function may be an independent predictor of CHD.

Among a cohort of Japanese-American men who were participants in a prospective epidemiologic study of CHD and stroke, pulmonary function testing was carried out in 5,924 men aged 45 to 68 years. All participants had been free of CHD at baseline and had been monitored for 15 to 18 years for the development of nonfatal MI and fatal CHD.

After adjusting for age, the percent predicted forced expiratory volume in 1 second (%$PFEV_1$) was significantly inversely related to the incidence of CHD in the total cohort. However, when the data were rearranged by smoking status, %$PFEV_1$ was a predictor of CHD only among past and current smokers, but not among men who had never smoked cigarettes. This measurement was thus a significant, but not an independent predictor of subsequent CHD.

The inverse relationship between pulmonary function and CHD was found to be a result of their mutual association with smoking. The suggested association between pulmonary function and CHD can therefore be explained by cigarette smoking that causes both pulmonary impairment and CHD.

▶ The association between poor pulmonary function and mortality from nonrespiratory causes has been documented in several studies. One of the possible explanations for this is the common pathogenetic mechanism of tobacco smoke exposure. In some studies such as the Glostrup population study (1) and the Framingham population study (2), controlling for cigarette smoking did not account for the entire association between lung function and mortality. This study of Japanese men shows that the presence of CHD is correlated with the degree of abnormality of lung function only in those who smoke, not in nonsmokers. Thus, one interpretation of these data is that the lung function abnormalities are not the consequence of impaired cardiac function, but serve only as a sentinel organ to measure the amount or toxicity of inhaled tobacco smoke. It is interesting that this effect seems to be more impressive in those who have quit smoking than in those who continue to smoke. The age-adjusted relative mortality is 4.5 times greater in those former smokers who are in the lowest 20% of the population than in those who are in the highest 20% of the population. Thus, spirometry still should be considered an important adjunct to assessment of risk for coronary disease as well as for lung disease.—R.A. Wise, M.D.

*References*


1. Schroll M: Smoking habits in the Glostrup population of men and women, born in 1914; Implications for health, evaluated from ten-year mortality, incidence of cardiovascular manifestations, and pulmonary function 1964–1974. *Acta Med Scand* 208:245–256, 1980.
2. Ashley F, Kannel WB, Sorlie RD, et al: Pulmonary function: Relation to aging, cigarette habit, and mortality. *Ann Intern Med* 82:739–745, 1975.


**Peak Expiratory Flow Rate in an Elderly Population**

Cook NR, Evans DA, Scherr PA, Speizer FE, Vedal S, Branch LG, Huntley JC, Hennekens CH, Taylor JO (Brigham and Women's Hosp, Boston: Harvard Med School; Univ of British Columbia, Vancouver; Boston Univ; Natl Inst on Aging, Bethesda, Md)

*Am J Epidemiol* 130:66–78, July 1989 7–4

The peak expiratory flow rate (PEFR) commonly is used to monitor patients with asthma and other lung diseases. Although it is relatively insensitive compared with other measures derived from spirometric testing, PEFR has the advantage of being easily measured with a mini-Wright peak flowmeter, an inexpensive, portable instrument. Examined were the distribution of PEFR among persons aged 65 and older and the relationship between PEFR and other variables, including cardiovascular measures, socioeconomic status, measures of physical function, and performance on simple tests of cognitive function.

The study population consisted of 3,812 persons aged 65 to 105 years, with a median age of 72. All participants were living in East Boston, a geographically defined urban working-class community of approximately 32,000 residents. Participants were visited in their homes by specially trained interviewers. In addition, 3 measurements of PEFR were obtained with the mini-Wright meters during the home visit.

The PEFR was significantly related to age, sex, smoking, and years smoked. After the data had been adjusted for these factors, low PEFR was associated with chronic respiratory symptoms and with certain cardiovascular variables, including history of stroke, angina, and high pulse rate. No significant association was found between PEFR and a history of MI or systolic and diastolic blood pressures. The PEFR was positively related to education and income, measures of functional ability and physical activity, self-assessment of health, and simple measures of cognitive function.

The data from this survey suggest that low PEFR is correlated with respiratory symptoms and is strongly related to certain indices of poor health. Low PEFR may well predict subsequent mortality.

▶ Although the mini-Wright peak flowmeter is a relatively variable instrument with less precision than the more standard spirometers, it is an inexpensive and highly portable instrument (1–3). Such an instrument is tractable for use in this large population study of 85% of the over-65 population of East Boston. Like the more precise spirometric indices such as $FEV_1$, peak flow rates are shown to be good surrogate measures of general health status for population studies. At some variance with this study, Hogans and Keller found that peak flow rates were among the poorest spirometric indices of respiratory disease (4). The explanation for this may be that the peak flow measurement, which is a particularly effort-dependent test, represents a global measure of cognition and vigor as well as lung function.—R.A. Wise, M.D.

*References*


1. Perks WH, Tams IP, Thompson DA, et al: An evaluation of the mini-Wright peak flow meter. *Thorax* 4:79–81, 1979.
2. Burns KL: An evaluation of two inexpensive instruments for assessing airway flow. *Ann Allergy* 43:246–249, 1979.
3. Fisher J, Shaw A: Calibration of some Wright peak flow meters. *Br J Anaesth* 52:461–464, 1980.
4. Higgins MW, Keller JR: Seven measures of ventilatory lung function. *Am Rev Respir Dis* 108:258–272, 1973.


---

**Lung Function After Coronary Artery Surgery Using the Internal Mammary Artery and the Saphenous Vein**

Jenkins SC, Soutar SA, Forsyth A, Keates JRW, Moxham J (King's College Hospital, London)

*Thorax* 44:209–211, March 1989 7–5

---

The internal mammary artery now is used in preference to the saphenous vein graft for coronary artery surgery, even though the former is associated with an increased incidence of pleurotomy. Effects of the 2 grafts on lung function tests and blood gas tensions were compared in a study of 110 men undergoing uncomplicated coronary artery surgery. Seventy-seven patients had internal mammary artery grafts; 72 of them also received saphenous vein grafts; 33 patients had saphenous vein grafts only. Preoperatively, lung function in the 2 groups was similar; the patients had a forced expiratory volume in 1 second of more than 50% predicted and a forced expiratory ratio of more than 60%.

Lung volumes in both groups were reduced after surgery, particularly in those receiving internal mammary arteries (Fig 7–1). Vital capacity, total capacity, and inspiratory capacity were more severely reduced when internal mammary artery grafting was done. This technique is technically more demanding. Respiratory abnormalities after coronary artery surgery involving the internal mammary artery may result from the high incidence of pleurotomy, additional trauma to the chest wall, and placing of the pleural drain. The greater impairment of lung function resulting from this technique should be taken into account for postoperative management.

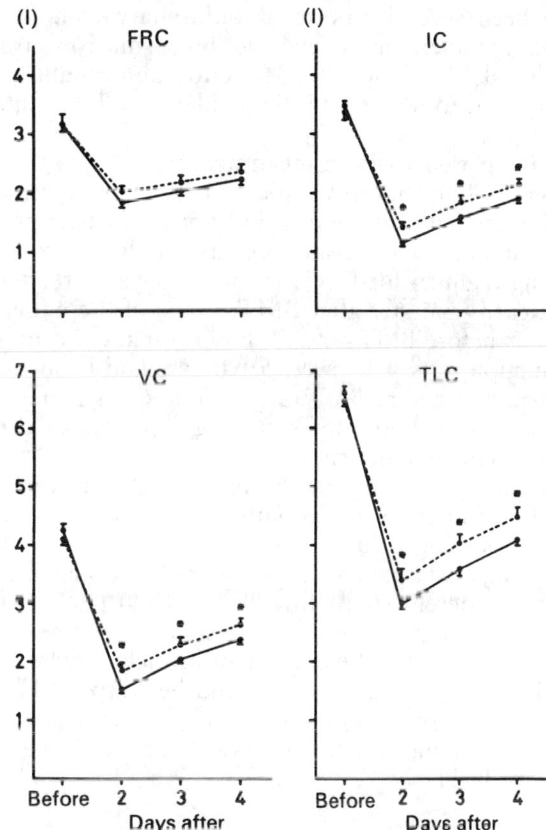


Fig 7–1.—Lung volumes (means with SEM) before and after operation in group 1 (internal mammary artery graft: *black dots with solid line*) and group 2 (no internal mammary artery graft: *black dots with broken line*). *$P < .05$. (Courtesy of Jenkins SC, Soutar SA, Forsyth A, et al: *Thorax* 44:209–211, March 1989.)

▶ This study reminds us that mammary artery implants place greater stress on lung function than saphenous vein bypass grafts. The dramatic finding, though, is the severe degree of lung impairment after surgery. The vital capacity and total lung capacity fall to less than half their initial preoperative values, which may result in part from reflex inhibition of the diaphragm postoperatively as well as the effect of pain and the direct effect of anesthesia on lung compliance. One realizes, however, the importance of identifying and aggressively treating underlying lung disease in patients who are to undergo coronary artery bypass surgery.—R.A. Wise, M.D.

---

**Lung Function in Allogeneic Bone Marrow Transplantation Recipients**

Rodríguez-Roisin R, Roca J, Grañena A, Agustí AGN, Marín P, Rozman C (Universitat de Barcelona, Spain)

*Eur Respir J* 2:359–365, April 1989 7–6

---

There have been several reports of pulmonary complications in patients who have undergone allogeneic bone marrow transplantation (BMT). Subclinical and clinical lung function abnormalities in BMT patients were observed to investigate the incidence of lung function impairment after BMT.

A group of 25 patients with a mean age of 24 years had transplantation of allogeneic bone marrow donated by first-degree relatives. Of these, 17 had acute leukemia and 8 had severe aplastic anemia. All patients underwent pulmonary evaluation at baseline before initiation of the conditioning regimen for BMT, every 30 days thereafter for the first trimester, and each trimester after BMT. None of the patients had respiratory symptoms before BMT, and all had normal chest radiographs and pulmonary function tests. However, 5 patients had bronchial hyperreactivity to metacholine before BMT. Aplastic anemia patients had significantly lower hemoglobin-adjusted diffusing capacity for carbon monoxide (DLCO) than leukemia patients.

After BMT, acute or chronic biopsy-proven graft-vs.-host disease (GVHD) developed in 20 of the 25 patients. Mild to moderate reductions in DLCO and static lung volumes were noted throughout the post-BMT follow-up. The leukemia patients had lower DLCO than the aplastic anemia patients. At different stages of follow-up, 10 patients had transient respiratory clinical complications, but most were mild to moderate in severity. In addition, the overall incidence of bronchial hyperreactivity doubled after BMT. No association was found between GVHD and the observed ventilatory abnormalities. The data presented here are part of a comprehensive screening program to assess the incidence of pulmonary dysfunction after BMT.

▶ Bone marrow transplantation is one of the major advances of modern medicine. It is a curative procedure in 50% to 60% of patients with nonlymphocytic leukemia or chronic myelogenous leukemia in the early stages.

Despite sometimes dramatic cures, experience is sufficient to indicate significant late complications of BMT, which include increased risk for secondary malignancies as well as disabling lung disease. During the first 3 months after BMT, nonbacterial interstitial pneumonia occurs in about one third of patients and is associated with greater than 50% mortality (1). After the initial 3 months, pulmonary complications include progressive, nonspecific interstitial pneumonitis and chronic obstructive lung disease secondary to bronchiolitis obliterans (2, 3). Pulmonary function tests may show either decreased carbon monoxide diffusing capacity or airflow limitation (4, 5).

In the study summarized above, 5 of the 20 patients had bronchial hyperreactivity to methacholine. Similar changes have been found in patients with heart-lung transplantation (6). Because these patients also tend to have bronchiolitis obliterans, this increase in bronchial hyperreactivity may reflect asymptomatic inflammation of the small airways or changes in airway geometry as a reusIt of that inflammation. This may be the result of an occult viral infection in these immunosuppressed subjects, but it appears to be associated with the development of chronic GVHD.—R.A. Wise, M.D.

*References*


1. Meyers JD, Flournoy N, Thomas ED: Non-bacterial pneumonia after allogenic marrow transplantation: A review of ten years experience. *Rev Infect Dis* 4:1119, 1982.
2. Wingard JR, Santos GW, Saral R: Late onset interstitial pneumonia following allogeneic bone marrow transplantation. *Transplantation* 39:21–23, 1985.
3. Sullivan KM, Deeg HJ, Sanders JE, et al: Late complications after marrow transplantation. *Sem Hematol* 21:53–63, 1984.
4. Clark JG, Schwartz DA, Flournoy N, et al: Risk factors for airflow obstruction in recipients of bone marrow transplantation. *Ann Intern Med* 107:648–656, 1987.
5. Prince DS, Wingard JR, Saral R, et al: Longitudinal changes in pulmonary function following bone marrow transplantation. *Chest* 96:301–306, 1989.
6. Glanville AR, Burke CM, Theodore J, et al: Bronchial hyper-responsiveness after cardiopulmonary transplantation. *Clin Sci* 73:299–303, 1987.


## 0.35 ppm $O_3$ Exposure Induces Hyperresponsiveness on 24-h Reexposure to 0.20 ppm $O_3$

Brookes KA, Adams WC, Schelegle ES (Univ of California, Davis)

*J Appl Physiol* 66:2756–2762, June 1989 7–7

Exercise in the presence of ozone ($O_3$) can produce significant respiratory discomfort and pulmonary dysfunction. High ambient levels of $O_3$ may persist for several consecutive days in areas of severe photochemical smog. The effects of 2 levels of $O_3$ exposure were studied in 15 aerobically trained men aged 19–34 years who completed 7 exposures of 1 hour each of continuous exercise. Work rates that produced a mean

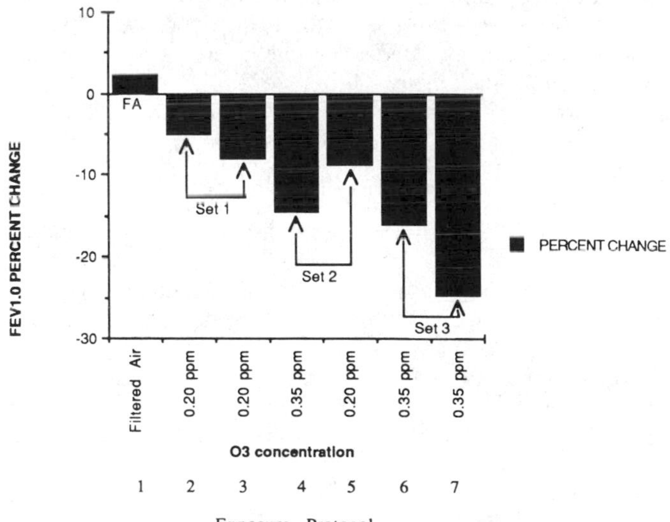


Fig 7–2.—Group mean percent of change in $FEV_1$ on exposure and reexposure at 2 different concentrations of $O_3$. (Courtesy of Brookes KA, Adams WC, Schelegle ES: *J Appl Physiol* 66:2756–2762, June 1989.)

minute ventilation of 60 L/minute were used with levels of $O_3$ exposure of 0.20 and 0.35 ppm.

Initial exposure to either level of $O_3$ had significant effects on lung function and patterns of exercise ventilation. Reexposure to 0.35 ppm of $O_3$ 24 hours after an initial 0.35-ppm exposure led to significant hyperresponsiveness for forced vital capacity and forced expiratory volume in 1 second ($FEV_1$) (Fig 7–2). Those exposed to 0.20 ppm after initial exposure to 0.35 ppm had enhanced responses for $FEV_1$ and tidal volume, but not forced vital capacity. No significantly enhanced responses were seen on reexposure to 0.20 ppm after initial exposure to the same concentration.

Reexposure to a high ambient level of $O_3$ can induce hyperresponsiveness: Hyperresponsiveness, however, may occur only at an $O_3$ dose threshold, somewhat higher than that at which significant effects are observed after initial exposure.

▶ Abundant evidence indicates that intense exposures to $O_3$ comparable to those that occur transiently or locally during a photochemical air pollution alert (0.32 to 0.42 ppm) can reduce lung function and induce respiratory symptoms in healthy persons. Increases in methacholine reactivity develop in some subjects, which is associated with neutrophilic infiltration into the airways, and is thought to be partly mediated by arachnidonic acid metabolites (1). Furthermore, exposure to similar high concentrations on subsequent days causes an increased responsiveness to $O_3$. With repeated exposure, however, there is a progressive adaptation to the exposure, which lasts for several days to a week (2, 3). This adaptation is thought to be caused by the induction of protective antioxidants, but recent animal studies show that this effect can be blocked by colchicine and occurs before the development of increased levels of antioxidant enzymes (4). Smokers with chronic bronchitis show less harmful effects of ozone than healthy persons, suggesting that cigarette smoking may induce a level of adaptation to oxidant injury (5).

There appears to be a threshold dose of $O_3$ that leads to subsequent increases in reactivity. When the first exposure during exercise was 0.35 ppm, a second-day exposure caused increased reductions in lung function on subsequent days. This was not the case when the initial level was 0.20 ppm. The mechanism for this effect is not known, but it is an important finding with respect to determination of public policy for setting permissible exposure levels of ozone. The authors also emphasize that recommendations for maximal permissible levels of ozone should take into account not only the intensity of exposure, but also the duration and the level of ventilation during the exposure.

In the last year, evidence has accumulated that exposure to low levels of ozone (.02 to .12 ppm) by exercising adults and children are associated with symptoms as well as decrements in lung function (6–8).—R.A. Wise, M.D.

*References*

1. Seltzer J, Bigby BG, Stulbarg M, et al: $O_3$-induced change in bronchial reactivity to methacholine and airway inflammation in humans. *J Appl Physiol* 60:1321–1326, 1986.

2. Cal TJ, Sauder LR, Kerr HD, et al: Duration of pulmonary function adaptation to ozone in humans. *Am Ind Hyg Assoc J* 43:832–837, 1982.
3. Schonfeld BR, Adams WC, Schelegle ES: Duration of enhanced responsiveness upon re-exposure to ozone. *Arch Environ Health* 44:229–236, 1989.
4. Nambu Z, Yokoyama E: Antioxidant system and ozone tolerance. *Environ Res* 32:111–117, October 1983.
5. Cal TJ, Milman JH, Sauder LR, et al: Pulmonary function adaptation to ozone in subjects with chronic bronchitis. *Environ Res* 34:55–63, 1984.
6. Folinsbee LJ, McDonnell WF, Horstman DH: Pulmonary function and symptom responses after 6.6-hour exposure to 0.12 ppm ozone with moderate exercise. *JAPCA* 38:28–35, 1988.
7. Spektor DM, Lippmann M, Thurston GD, et al: Effects of ambient ozone on respiratory function in healthy adults exercising outdoors. *Am Rev Respir Dis* 138:821–828, 1988.
8. Spektor DM, Lippmann M, Lioy PJ, et al: Effects of ambient ozone on respiratory function in active, normal children. *Am Rev Respir Dis* 137:313–320, 1988.


## Sleep Disordered Breathing

### Abnormal Breathing During Sleep and Chemical Control of Breathing During Wakefulness in Patients With Sleep Apnea Syndrome

Kunitomo F, Kimura H, Tatsumi K, Okita S, Tojima H, Kuriyama T, Honda Y (Chiba Univ, Chiba, Japan)

*Am Rev Respir Dis* 139:164–169, January 1989 7–8

Patients with obesity hypoventilation syndrome have greater oxygen desaturation during sleep than patients with eucapnic sleep apnea syndrome (SAS), although the role of ventilatory control in relation to sleep apnea is not well understood. To clarify the relationship between ventila-

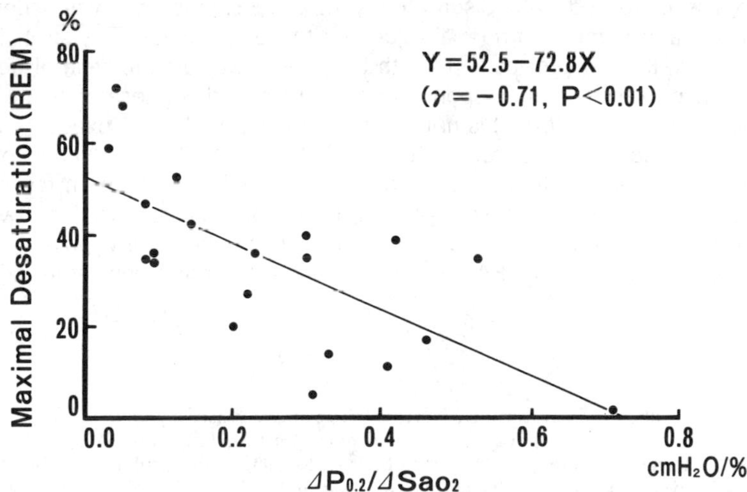


Fig 7–3.—Relationship of hypoxic occlusion pressure response to maximal desaturation during rapid eye movement sleep. (Courtesy of Kunitomo F, Kimura H, Tatsumi K, et al: *Am Rev Respir Dis* 139:164–169, January 1989.)

tory drives and apnea and oxygen desaturation during sleep, 21 patients with SAS were studied while awake and during disordered breathing periods while asleep.

The patients had a mean age of 43 years. Eighteen had more than 130% of ideal body weight. Apnea was defined as cessation of flow at the nose and mouth for at least 10 seconds. Hypopnea occurred when a decrease of 50% or more in airflow was associated with a fall in arterial oxygen saturation of 4% or more.

The awake hypoxic ventilatory drive correlated inversely with the degree of maximal oxygen desaturation during sleep as well as the ratio of duration. Awake hypercapnic ventilatory drive, however, did not show this correlation. The negative correlation was most evident during rapid eye movement sleep (Fig 7–3). Two possible explanations exist for the correlations between awake ventilatory drive to hypoxia and sleep desaturation parameters. The hypoxic ventilatory drive may be blunted during awake conditions by recurrent desaturation during sleep. It is also possible that the magnitude of desaturation during sleep in SAS may be largely determined by hypoxic ventilatory drive.

▶ The relationship between sleep apnea and obesity hypoventilation syndrome is still not clear. Although many patients with obesity hypoventilation syndrome (OHS) have obstructive apneas, clearly not all of them do. Although OHS patients have some reduction in hypercapnic ventilatory response, they have a greater attenuation of hypoxic ventilatory response (1, 2). As a group, patients with obstructive SAS have normal hypoxic and hypercapnic ventilatory responses (2).

Previous studies have not found that the number of disordered breathing events is correlated with disordered ventilatory chemosensitivity. There is, however, a wide range of normal values for these responses. This study found that, within the group of patients with SAS, there was a correlation of depression of hypoxic ventilatory response with the magnitude of desaturation. Which is cause and which is effect is not known. Certainly, prolonged exposure to hypoxia at altitude is associated with a diminution of the hypoxic ventilatory response (3). Alternatively, the duration of apneas and the maximum fall in oxygen tension may be the consequence of depressed hypoxic response. It would be of interest to know whether attenuation of the nocturnal hypoxemia with supplemental oxygen or CPAP would increase the hypoxic ventilatory drive.—R.A. Wise, M.D.

*References*

1. Zwillich CW, Sutton FD, Pierson DJ, et al: Decreased hypoxic ventilatory drive in the obesity hypoventilation syndrome. *Am J Med* 59:343–348, 1974.
2. Garay SM, Rapoport D, Sorkin B, et al: Regulation of ventilation in the obstructive sleep apnea syndrome. *Am Rev Respir Dis* 124:451–457, 1981.
3. Weil JV, Byrne-Quinn E, Sodal IE, et al: Acquired attenuation of chemoreceptor function in chronically hypoxic man at high altitude. *J Clin Invest* 50:186–195, 1971.

**Craniofacial Characteristics in Patients With Obstructive Sleep Apneas Syndrome**

Bacon WH, Krieger J, Turlot J-C, Stierle JL (Université Louis Pasteur; Hôpital Civil, Strasbourg, France)

*Cleft Palate J* 25:374–378, October 1988 7–9

In obstructive sleep apnea syndrome (OSAS), bucconasal airflow ceases several hundred times during the night. The precise means of upper airway occlusion remain uncertain. The possible role of predisposing skeletal craniofacial conditions was examined in a cephalometric study of 32 adults with OSAS and 40 controls with ideal dentofacial characteristics. All patients had more than 10 apneas per hour.

There were no group differences in maxillary or mandibular prognathism. The sagittal dimension of the cranial base was significantly reduced in patients with OSAS, as were the bony pharyngeal opening and the length of the maxilla. Increased lower face height also was noted. Discriminant function analysis succeeded in correctly classifying 80% of the population. The analysis included the sagittal dimension of the anterior cranial fossa, a sagittal measure of the median upper face, and lower face height.

Patients with OSAS consistently have posterior facial compression with narrowing of the pharyngeal airway and vertical hyperdevelopment, as well as a shortened cranial base. The latter feature would seem to be a major influence on the others.

▶ It has been shown previously that sleep apnea patients have decreased cross-sectional areas of the upper airway (1). Because this is a disease of obesity, the assumption that this is the consequence of fat deposition in the upper airway is natural. This is not the case, however, because radiographic images of the upper airway have shown that the excess tissue is nonadipose soft tissue (2, 3). This study extends other studies of craniofacial anthropometry in patients with OSAS to show that there are, indeed, bone structure abnormalities (4). Although micrognathia can lead to OSAS (5, 6), the mandible is not short in most subjects. Rather, the face is elongated and compressed in the anteroposterior direction. A shortened anteroposterior dimension of the maxilla is the major discriminator of patients with OSAS compared with controls. This may be, in part, the reason that some experienced sleep clinicians believe a characteristic facies accompanies OSAS.—R.A. Wise, M.D.

*References*

1. Rivlin J, Hoffstein V, Kalbfleisch J, et al: Upper airway morphology in patients with idiopathic obstructive sleep apnea. *Am Rev Respir Dis* 129:355–359, 1984.
2. Haponik EF, Smith PL, Bohlman ME, et al: Computerized tomography in obstructive sleep apnea. *Am Rev Respir Dis* 127:221–226, 1983.
3. Surratt PM, Dee P, Atkinson RL, et al: Fluoroscopic and computed tomographic features of the pharyngeal airway in obstructive sleep apnea. *Am Rev Respir Dis* 127:484–492, 1983.

4. Riley R, Guilleminault C, Herran J, et al: Cephalometric analyses and flow-volume loops in obstructive sleep apnea patients. *Sleep* 6:303–311, 1983.
5. Conway WA, Bower GC, Barnes ME: Hypersomnolence and intermittent upper airway obstruction: Occurrence caused by micrognathia. *JAMA* 237:2740–2742, 1977.
6. Coccagna G, Di Donato G, Verucchi P, et al: Hypersomnia with periodic apneas in acquired micrognathia (a bird-like face syndrome). *Arch Neurol* 33:769–776, 1976.

---

**Effect of Airway Impedance on $CO_2$ Retention and Respiratory Muscle Activity During NREM Sleep**

Skatrud JB, Dempsey JA, Badr S, Begle RL (Univ of Wisconsin, Madison)
*J Appl Physiol* 65:1676–1685, October 1988 7–10

---

The end-tidal or arterial carbon dioxide pressure ($PaCO_2$) consistently increases from quiet wakefulness to non-rapid eye movement (NREM) sleep in normal persons. A sleep-induced increase in upper airway resistance could explain both $CO_2$ retention and the high inspiratory muscle EMG observed during NREM sleep. The role of high airway impedance was examined in healthy nonsmoking persons. Airway impedance was decreased during sleep by breathing a low-density gas mixture of helium and oxygen.

Total pulmonary resistance increased from the waking state to NREM sleep. The $PaCO_2$ consistently increased, as did the inspiratory muscle EMG activity. Steady-state breathing of the helium-oxygen mixture decreased peak total pulmonary resistance by 38% and the $PaCO_2$ by 2 torr. Both the inspiratory and expiratory muscle EMG activity decreased, the latter by more than half.

A sleep-related increase in upper airway resistance without immediate load compensation is an important factor in $CO_2$ retention, which in turn can augment inspiratory and expiratory muscle activity to greater than waking levels during NREM sleep. More complete unloading might prevent even more of the $CO_2$ retention and respiratory muscle activation.

▶ The facile explanation for the well-documented increase in $PaCO_2$ that occurs during sleep is a depression of the ventilatory sensitivity to $CO_2$. This study shows that the portion of ventilatory drive manifest by an increase in the EMG activity of the upper airway dilator muscles actually is increased during NREM sleep. These authors hypothesize that the primary event that disrupts ventilatory control during sleep is an increase in airway resistance. This leads to compensatory increases in upper airway dilator muscle activity, which is not fully effective and therefore allows an increase in arterial $PaCO_2$. What is not clear, though, is what leads to the increase in airway resistance with sleep if the dilator muscles are supranormally activated. Perhaps synergy or coordination of the upper dilator airway muscles is ineffective during sleep so that activation of these muscles must be greater to maintain a patent airway.

An important aspect not emphasized in the summary is that all but 2 of the 17 subjects were snorers. This may not reflect a pathologic condition, but whether nonsnoring subjects show a similar increase in airway resistance during sleep remains to be determined.—R.A. Wise, M.D.

---

**Sleep Quality and Pulmonary Function in the Healthy Elderly**

Phillips B, Berry D, Schmitt F, Patel R, Cook Y (Univ of Kentucky, Lexington)

*Chest* 95:60–64, January 1989 7–11

---

Previous studies have shown that loss of sleep causes deterioration of pulmonary function and ventilatory responsiveness in healthy human beings and in patients with moderate chronic obstructive pulmonary disease (COPD). It is also well known that gross sleep disturbances worsen parameters of a routine pulmonary function test (PFT). Variations in sleep quality may affect PFT parameters in healthy persons aged more than 60 years.

A group of 48 healthy elderly volunteers, 21 women and 27 men aged 60 to 87 years (mean age, 69.6 years) were studied. All spent a single night of polysomnographic testing in a clinical sleep laboratory, and all underwent routine spirometric evaluation the next day.

Several correlations between indices of sleep quality and daytime spirometric measurements were significant (Fig 7–4). The correlations between sleep quality and pulmonary function were stronger for poor sleepers than for the group as a whole. The correlations between sleep quality and PFT parameters in those with sleep efficiency less than 70% were striking.

These findings suggest that sleep disturbances may well be related to poor performance on spirometric testing performed the next day. Therefore, baseline pulmonary function parameters should be determined for well-rested persons. Another implication from the findings is

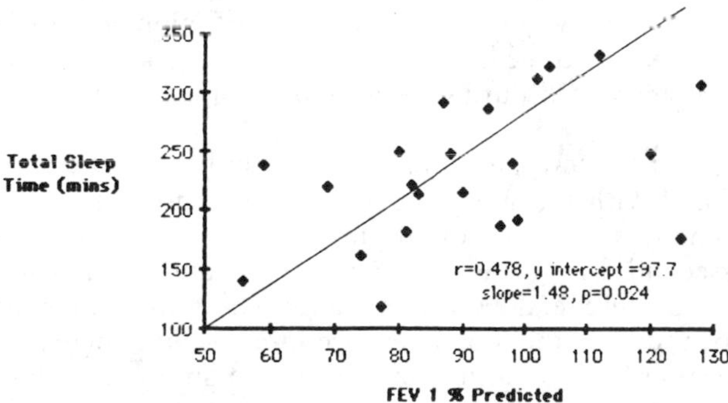


Fig 7–4.—Scattergram of correlation between $FEV_1$ (percent of predicted) and total sleep time. This zero order correlation does not control for age, sex, or height. (Courtesy of Phillips B, Berry D, Schmitt F, et al: *Chest* 95:60–64, January 1989.)

that sleep quality may be an important variable affecting the response to treatment of COPD.

▶ Patients with advanced lung disease have nocturnal hypoxemia and sleep fragmentation, which may contribute to daytime functional impairment. Also, a healthy person with a single night of sleep deprivation has small but consistent decreases in forced vital capacity (FVC) and maximal voluntary ventilation, as well as hypoxic and hypercapnic ventilatory responses (1, 2). Patients with COPD also show small consistent decrements in $FEV_1$ and FVC after losing a single night of sleep (3). Whether sleep deprivation contributes to the spiraling decompensation in exacerbations of chronic obstructive lung disease is not known, but could well be the case. This study now raises the possibility that sleep patterns may be an important influence on the variance of lung function in an elderly population sample. Thus, sleep quality may be one of the pathogenetic links between general health status and lung function.—R.A. Wise, M.D.

*References*

1. Cooper KR, Phillips BA: Effect of short-term sleep loss on breathing. *J Appl Physiol* 53:855–858, 1982.
2. White DP, Douglas NJ, Pickett CK, et al: Sleep deprivation and the control of ventilation. *Am Rev Respir Dis* 128:984–986, 1983.
3. Phillips BA, Cooper KR, Burke TV: The effect of sleep loss on breathing in chronic obstructive pulmonary disease. *Chest* 91:29–32, 1987.

**Supine Position and Sleep Loss Each Reduce Prolonged Maximal Voluntary Ventilation**

Keeling WF, Martin BJ (Indiana Univ, Bloomington)
*Respiration* 54:119–126, October 1988 7–12

The effects of supine posture and sleep deprivation on prolonged maximal voluntary ventilation (MVV) were studied with a group of healthy persons to gauge the impact of these conditions on patients with chronic lung disease. Sixteen volunteers, 11 men and 5 women with a mean age of 25 years, were studied. Lung volume changes and ventilatory responses were measured during periods of supination and sleep deprivation.

Regardless of the test duration, significantly lower maximal ventilation was associated with the supine position. A second series of experiments measured changes in lung volume in different postures. Supination reduced 12-second MVV and end-expiratory lung volume during quiet breathing. Absolute end-expiratory lung volumes supine and upright were identical during the MVV because lung volume increased to greater than the resting level by a greater amount in supination than in an upright position.

Both short- and long-term MVV were decreased by sleep loss, whereas fatigue and confusion were increased on subjective rating scales. Minute-by-minute mean MVV was significantly lower after sleep deprivation (Fig

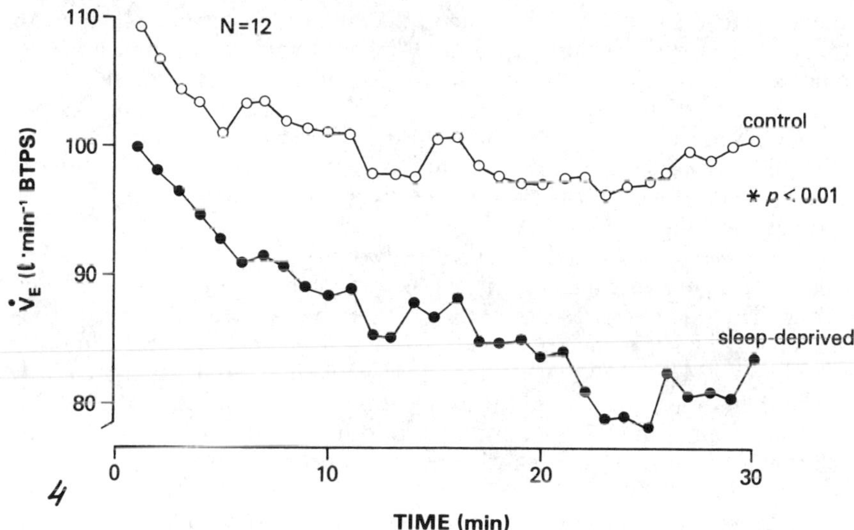


Fig 7–5.—Effect of sleep deprivation on minute-by-minute mean MVV ($\dot{V}_E$) during an isocapnic 30-minute test. Throughout, $\dot{V}_E$ was significantly lower after sleep deprivation (*asterisk*, $P < .01$); *open circles*, control; *shaded circles*, sleep-deprived; no. = 12. (Courtesy of Keeling WF, Martin BJ: *Respiration* 54:119–126, October 1988.)

7–5). Supine posture lowers maximal ventilatory output although relative endurance is unchanged. The decrease in maximal ventilatory output in supination may result from an increase in pulmonary blood volume and pulmonary arterial pressure or from gravitational effects, which cause the abdominal contents to force the diaphragm cephalad.

Supination may relieve dyspnea in some patients with chronic obstructive lung disease and exacerbate it in others. However, supination and sleep deprivation together decrease MVV by approximately 20%, diminishing the ability of patients to voluntarily ventilate at high levels.

► If sleep deprivation leads to a reduction in maximal voluntary ventilation (MVV) by impairment of endurance, then it would be expected to cause a greater decrement in the 10-minute MVV than in the 12-second MVV. This is not the case, so some other mechanism must be involved.—R.A. Wise, M.D.

---

**Long-Term Outcome for Obstructive Sleep Apnea Syndrome Patients: Mortality**

Partinen M, Jamieson A, Guilleminault C (Stanford Univ)

*Chest* 94:1200–1204, December 1988 7–13

---

As the mortality and morbidity of obstructive sleep apnea syndrome (OSAS) remain unknown, a 5-year follow-up study of 198 patients was done to determine death rates from OSAS and to compare outcomes after treatment by tracheostomy or weight loss. The study included 190 men (median age, 52 years) and 8 women (median age, 57 years). The median apnea index for the group was 54.8. Arterial hypertension had been diagnosed in 112 (56.6%) patients, and coronary artery disease, in 33 (16.7%); 127 patients conservatively treated with weight loss, and 71 patients with more severe disease underwent surgery (tracheostomy).

There were 14 deaths during the first 5-year follow-up period; all were men who had received conservative treatment, for a mortality of 11.0 per 100 patients. Eight of the 14 deaths were classified as "vascular." Thus patients who were treated conservatively had a much higher mortality risk and a higher vascular mortality risk at 5 years than those treated surgically. This increase was present even though the surgically treated patients had a higher mean apnea index (69 vs. 43) and a higher mean body mass index (34 vs. 31 kg/m$^2$) than conservatively treated patients.

These findings suggest rigorous treatment for patients with OSAS. Options other than tracheostomy include maxillofacial surgery, uvulopalatopharyngoplasty, and nasal continuous positive airway pressure.

▶ In the 1989 YEAR BOOK OF PULMONARY DISEASE, we reviewed the literature on the mortality related to OSAS. Of the 3 studies available at the time, one showed a greater death rate, one showed no difference, and one showed a reduced death rate compared with sleep laboratory controls (1–3). This study differs from those previously cited because it does not compare sleep apnea patients with non-sleep apnea patients. Instead, it compares tracheotomized patients with "conservatively" treated (i.e., untreated) patients. All the cardiovascular deaths occurred in the untreated patients. The study was not randomized nor prospective, but it certainly provides a strong rationale for the aggressive diagnosis and treatment of OSAS. Because of the high prevalence of obstructive sleep apnea and the great expense for diagnosis and treatment, a clinical trial of treatment for sleep apnea should be of the highest priority for pulmonary research.

To put this into perspective, it is useful to compare the potential benefits of treatment of sleep apnea with the potential benefits of the much publicized and debated recommendations of the National Cholesterol Educational Program. About one third of the population suffers from hypercholesterolemia; about 15% of the male population suffers from obstructive sleep apnea. The Lipid Research Clinics Coronary Prevention Trial showed that cholestyramine drug treatment reduced MI from 9.8% to 8.1% over 7 years. There was no difference, however, in all-cause mortality. The Helsinki Heart Study showed that gemfibrozil treatment reduced MIs from 4.1% to 2.7% over 5 years. In comparison, the study presented above shows a reduction in cardiovascular mortality from 6.3% to 0 over 5 years. But, before we replace shopping center cholesterol screenings with polysomnograms and trade in our oat bran for CPAP masks, we ought to do the proper large-scale epidemiologic and clinical studies.—R.A. Wise, M.D.

*References*

1. Bliwise DL, Bliwise NG, Partinen M, et al: Sleep apnea and mortality in an aged cohort. *Am J Public Health* 78:544–547, 1988.

2. He J, Kryger MH, Zorick FJ, et al: Mortality and apnea index in obstructive sleep apnea: Experience in 385 male patients. *Chest* 94:9–14, 1988.
3. Gonzalez-Rothi RJ, Foresman GE, Block AJ: Do patients with sleep apnea die in their sleep? *Chest* 94:531–538, 1988.


**Urinary Excretion of Guanosine 3′:5′-Cyclic Monophosphate During Sleep in Obstructive Sleep Apnoea Patients With and Without Nasal Continuous Positive Airway Pressure Treatment**

Krieger J, Schmidt M, Sforza E, Lehr L, Imbs J-L, Coumaros G, Kurtz D (CHRU, Strasbourg, France)

*Clin Sci* 76:31–37, January 1989 7–14

Patients with obstructive sleep apnea (OSA) excrete more urinary water and salt during sleep. Application of nasal continuous positive airway pressure reverses most of the symptoms and normalizes urinary salt and water excretion during sleep. Whether increased release of atrial natriuretic factor during sleep could account for the diuresis and natriuresis associated with OSA was examined in 21 patients. Nighttime urine collections were assayed for a variety of chemicals and hormones for 2 nights, 1 in which they received continuous positive airway pressure and 1 during which they were untreated; the results were compared.

Patients had higher urinary sodium and chloride outputs on untreated nights than on treated nights. No differences were found in morning plasma active renin content or in urinary aldosterone excretion during sleep. Urinary excretion of epinephrine, norepinephrine, free dopamine, or total dopamine were similar for treated and untreated nights. Urinary excretion of cyclic guanosine monophosphate (GMP) was higher during untreated nights than during treated nights, but no correlations were found between sodium excretion and cyclic GMP excretion on either night.

Increased outputs of cyclic GMP were found in untreated, but not in treated, patients with OSA. This is consistent with the hypothesis that increased atrial natriuretic factor release in OSA patients accounts for increased urinary water and salt output. Ineffective inspiratory efforts increase thoracic pressures in untreated OSA patients, and increased pressure results in atrial distention and greater release of atrial natriuretic factor.

▶ In last year's YEAR BOOK, we reviewed the effects of sleep apnea on renal function. This study provides a possible explanation for the previously noted association of sleep apnea syndrome with increased urinary excretion of sodium and chloride during the night, which is reversed with CPAP treatment (1, 2). The elevation of urinary cyclic GMP is consistent with the hypothesis that atrial natriuretic hormone (ANF) is the cause of the sodium excretion. Distention of the right and left heart because of markedly negative intrathoracic pressures or hypoxic pulmonary hypertension could lead to secretion of ANF.

The past year has seen several good reviews of the pharmacology and physiology of ANF (3–5). Two recent studies have suggested that ANF can protect against the development of pulmonary edema, possibly through its vasodilating properties.(6, 7)—R.A. Wise, M.D.

*References*

1. Warley ARM, Stradling JR: Abnormal diurnal variations in salt and water excretion in patients with obstructive sleep apnoea. *Clin Sci* 74:183–185, 1988.
2. Krieger J, Imbs JL, Schmidt M, et al: Effects of nasal continuous positive airway pressure: Renal function in patients with obstructive sleep apnea. *Arch Intern Med* 148:1337–1340, 1988.
3. Buckalew VM Jr, Paschal-McCormick C: Natriuretic hormone: Current status. *Am J Nephrol* 9:329–342, 1989.
4. Needleman P, Blaine EH, Greenwald JE, et al: The biochemical pharmacology of atrial peptides. *Annu Rev Pharmacol Toxicol* 29:23–54, 1989.
5. Goetz KL: Physiology and pathophysiology of atrial peptides. *Am J Physiol* 254:E1–15, 1988.
6. Imamura T, Ohnuma N, Iwasa F, et al: Protective effect of alpha-human atrial natriuretic polypeptide (alpha-hANP) on chemical-induced pulmonary edema. *Life Sci* 42:403–414, 1988.
7. Inomata N, Ohnuma N, Furuya M, et al: Alpha-human atrial natriuretic peptide (alpha-hANP) prevents pulmonary edema induced by arachidonic acid treatment in isolated perfused lung from guinea pig. *Jpn J Pharmacol* 44:211–214, 1987.

---

## Neuropsychologic Symptoms in Obstructive Sleep Apnea Improve After Treatment With Nasal Continuous Positive Airway Pressure

Derderian SS, Bridenbaugh RH, Rajagopal KR (Walter Reed Army Med Ctr, Washington, DC; Uniformed Services Univ of the Health Sciences, Bethesda, Md)

*Chest* 94:1023–1027, November 1988 7–15

---

Patients with obstructive sleep apnea may have psychological symptoms including anxiety, irritability, depression, and sleepiness. Various therapeutic interventions for this syndrome often ameliorate many of its symptoms. To assess changes associated with the restoration of normal sleep patterns, the Profile of Mood States questionnaire was administered to patients with obstructive sleep apnea before and after treatment with nasal continuous positive airway pressure (NCPAP).

Seven adult men given NCPAP were compared with 7 untreated men who had similar scores on the sleep apnea index. Administration of NCPAP reduced the mean apnea index score from 40.7 to 0 and improved other sleep parameters including oxyhemoglobin saturation. Depression and fatigue also were improved significantly in patients given NCPAP. The mean score for total mood disturbance decreased from −1.7 before treatment to −7.6 during treatment. This change in total mood disturbance was significantly different from scores of the control group.

Patients with obstructive sleep apnea given NCPAP report feeling better and having a general improvement in mood. The sleep fragmentation and abnormalities of respiration associated with episodes of obstructive sleep apnea may be responsible for the psychological changes characteristic of this syndrome. Nasal continuous positive airway pressure significantly relieves at least some of these disturbances.

▶ In last year's YEAR BOOK OF PULMONARY DISEASE, we reviewed the conflictive evidence about whether sleep apnea syndrome is an important cause of death. Besides death, there may be an enormous, albeit subtle, social and economic cost of sleep apnea as a consequence of its effect on human performance. Traumatic death and occupational injury are more common among the obese, and automobile accidents are more common among persons with sleep apnea. With a volunteer population of asymptomatic snoring men, Berry has shown impressive evidence that nocturnal oxygen denaturation was associated with lower levels of performance on the WAIS performance IQ and tests of verbal fluency and memory (1, 2). Analysis of the associated sleep data suggested that the abnormal cognitive function was a consequence of the hypoxia rather than the disruption of sleep.

That conclusion is supported by a more recent study, which compared neuropsychological function in sleep apnea patients with somnolent patients having other disorders. The sleep apnea group performed worse on perceptual and organizational tasks than the other patients. Among the sleep apnea group, the level of hypoxemia was correlated with the degree of impairment (3)

Another study of 39 persons showed abnormal speech fluency or phonation in patients with sleep apnea, although it is not clear whether this reflects abnormal upper airway geometry or neurophysiologic defects (4). Kales and colleagues reported that 76% of a population of patients with severe sleep apnea had evidence of cognitive impairment consisting of defects in thinking, perception, memory, communication, and inability to learn. There was also a high incidence of psychosocial disruption involving family, social, and work interactions (5). Reynolds found that 40% of 25 consecutive patients with sleep apnea syndrome had evidence of depression or alcoholism, which was associated in part with the degree of sleep disruption (6). In a prospective study of 139 elderly persons, the same group found that sleep-disordered breathing occurred in 11.4% of depressed subjects and 16.7% of subjects with mixed cognitive impairment and depression compared with 5% of healthy elderly controls.

Therefore, the hypothesis that a considerable amount of neuropsychiatric disease can be attributable to sleep-disordered breathing bears consideration. The subjects in the study abstracted above had rather severe apnea, averaging about 40 events per hour. The degree of impairment and reversal of symptoms with CPAP were quite dramatic and could be demonstrated clearly with only 7 patients. It would be of great importance to know whether "asymptomatic" people with less severe apnea also would benefit in subtle ways from the diagnosis and treatment of sleep apnea.

A note of caution: this study did not have a randomized control population, nor was a placebo form of CPAP given. Nonetheless, this study does support the association of sleep apnea with mood disorders. The induction of neuropsychologic dysfunction with the induction of sleep apnea would be needed to solidify the causal relationship.—R.A. Wise, M.D.

*References*

1. Berry DTR, Webb WB, Block AJ, et al: Nocturnal hypoxia and neuropsychological variables. *J Clin Exp Neuropsychol* 3:229–238, 1986.
2. Block AJ, Berry WW: Nocturnal hypoxemia and neuropsychological deficits in men who snore. *Eur J Respir Dis* 69(Suppl 146):405–408, 1986.
3. Greenberg GD, Watson RK, Deptula D: Neuropsychological dysfunction in sleep apnea. *Sleep* 10:254–262, 1987.
4. Monoson PK, Fox AW: Preliminary observation of speech disorder in obstructive and mixed sleep apnea. *Chest* 92:670–675, 1987.
5. Kales A, Caldwell AB, Cadieux RJ, et al: Severe obstructive sleep apnea: II. Associated psychopathology and psychosocial consequences. *J Chronic Dis* 38:427–434, 1985.
6. Reynolds CF, Kupfer DJ, McEachran AB, et al: Depressive psychopathology in male sleep apneics. *J Clin Psychiatry* 45:287–290, 1984.

**Nocturnal Oxygen Therapy Does Not Improve Snorers' Intelligence**

Block AJ, Hellard DW, Switzer DA (Univ of Florida; VA Med Ctr, Gainesville)

*Chest* 95:274–278, February 1989 7–16

Asymptomatic men who snore heavily may have neuropsychological dysfunction that is related significantly to sleep apnea and nocturnal oxygen desaturation. Seventeen asymptomatic men who snore heavily were given inhaled oxygen to determine whether treatment of nocturnal oxygen desaturation improves neuropsychological function.

Oxygen concentrators, modified to produce more than 96% oxygen or air at 2 L/min, were installed in the homes of patients for use each night. Inspirate was administered via nasal cannula. Air was given for 1 month, and oxygen was given for 1 month in random order. Neuropsychological testing was done before and after each month.

On a screening night, oxygen did not improve obstructive sleep apnea but did improve oxygenation. After 1 month of oxygen treatment no significant benefit was observed on multiple measures of neuropsychological function.

These findings suggest that oxygen therapy at 2 L/min by nasal cannula does not improve neuropsychological functioning in men who are heavy snorers. These findings therefore do not support the previously reported association between neuropsychological dysfunction and nocturnal oxygen desaturation.

▶ Snorers have impaired neuropsychological functioning, as noted above, which is correlated with the degree of nocturnal hypoxemia (1). Because hypoxemic patients with obstructive lung disease also have impaired neuropsychological functioning, which is reversible with 1 month of oxygen treatment, it seems reasonable to attempt to apply nocturnal oxygen to snorers (2). In this series of persons chosen on the basis of snoring alone, 1 month of oxygen treatment produced no improvement in neuropsychological functioning. Several explanations for this are plausible. First, nocturnal hypoxemia is not the cause of neuropsychological dysfunction. Second, the dysfunction is caused by hypoxemia, but is not reversible. Third, this group of subjects may not have had significant dysfunction in the first place. Fourth, 1 month of treatment may not have been adequate to reverse it.

Whatever the explanation for the negative results, those who finance health care spending should be pleased. Our society could ill afford giving snorers long-term oxygen. Snoring is common. One survey found that 52% of wives and 15% of husbands were bothered by their spouses' snoring (3).—R A Wise, M.D.

*References*


1. Berry DTR, Webb WB, Block AJ, et al: Nocturnal hypoxia and neuropsychological variables. *J Clin Exp Neuropsychol* 8:229–238, 1986.
2. Krop HD, Block AJ, Cohen E: Neuropsychological effects of continuous oxygen therapy in chronic obstructive pulmonary disease. *Chest* 64:317–322, 1973.
3. Norton PG, Dunn EV, Haight JS: Snoring in adults: Some epidemiologic aspects. *Can Med Assoc J* 128:674–675, 1983.


## Effect of Salicylate on Upper Airway Dilating Muscles in Anesthetized Dogs

Oliven A, Odeh M, Gavriely N (Haifa City Med Ctr; Technion, Haifa, Israel)
*Am Rev Respir Dis* 139:170–175, January 1989 7–17

Large doses of salicylate administered to human beings or animals have been shown to stimulate respiration. The augmenting effect of salicylate on phrenic activity also has been documented previously. However, whether salicylate also stimulates activity in the dilatory muscles of the upper airway is not known. Salicylate was used to stimulate the electrical activity of 3 upper airway muscles in spontaneously breathing, healthy, anesthetized dogs.

The 3 upper airway muscles were the alae nasi, the genioglossus, and the posterior cricoarytenoid. The dogs were intubated to obtain tidal volume measurements. Blood gases were measured via a cannulated femoral artery. Muscle activity was measured by electromyography (EMG) after inserting electrodes into each of the 3 muscles. An electrode also was inserted into the diaphragm. The EMGs of these 3 muscles were compared with the EMGs of the diaphragm before, and at 15-minute intervals after, intravenous administration of salicylate.

Salicylate induced gradual increases in ventilation and in the electrical activity of all 3 upper airway muscles. However, salicylate increased the electrical activity of the genioglossus more than that of the diaphragm. Increases in electrical activity of the upper airway muscle were associated with a significant decrease in upper airway resistance to airflow.

In addition to the stimulatory effect on diaphragm activity and ventilation, salicylate also augmented electrical activity of the upper airway muscles and decreased upper airway resistance. Although salicylate in doses large enough to improve ventilation may not be acceptable as a major clinical treatment modality, that salicylate stimulates ventilation and possibly improves upper airway patency merits further investigation.

▶ Thc reader should not entertain the notion that aspirin is a cure for sleep apnea. The dose of aspirin used in this study is equivalent to an adult dose of 50 aspirin tablets! The significant finding is that the upper respiratory muscles can be stimulated preferentially to the other inspiratory muscles. This leaves open the possibility that specific drugs could be effective in treating sleep apnea. Other drugs shown to stimulate the upper airway dilator muscles include the toxins strychnine (1), which prevents postsynaptic inhibition, and nicotine (2, 3), which stimulates presynaptic ganglia. Drugs that more directly stimulate respiration have been disappointing, however. Theophylline (4), almitrine (5), and progesterone (6) are respiratory stimulants that have not been effective in significantly reducing the number of sleep apneic events.—R.A. Wise, M.D.

*References*


1. Remmers JE, Anch AM, De Groot WJ, et al: Oropharyngeal muscle tone in obstructive sleep apnea before and after strychnine. *Sleep* 3:447–453, 1980.
2. Strohl KP, Gottfried SB, Van de Graaff W, et al: Effects of sodium cyanide and nicotine on upper airway resistance to anesthetized dogs. *Respir Physiol* 63:161–175, 1986.
3. Gothe B, Strohl KP, Lewis S, et al: Nicotine: A different approach to treatment of obstructive sleep apnea. *Chest* 87:11–17, 1985.
4. Guilleminault C, Hayes B: Naloxone, theophylline, bromocriptine, and obstructive sleep apnea: Negative results. *Bull Eur Physiopathol Respir* 19:632–634, 1983.
5. Krieger J, Mangin P, Kurtz D: Effects of almitrine in the treatment of sleep apnea syndromes. *Bull Eur Physiopathol Respir* 19:630, 1983.
6. Orr WC, Imes NK, Martin RJ: Progesterone therapy in obese patients with sleep apnea. *Arch Intern Med* 139:109–111, 1979.


---

## Sleep Apnea: Morbidity and Mortality of Surgical Treatment

Harmon JD, Morgan W, Chaudhary B (Med College of Georgia, Augusta)
*Sough Med J* 82:161–164, February 1989 7–18

---

Surgical intervention has become an increasingly common treatment for sleep apnea, but few data about short- and long-term surgical complications are available. Data on a consecutive series of adults operated on at a single institution during 1981–1987 were evaluated.

A total of 132 patients aged 19–70 years underwent 196 procedures. There were 34 complications (26%). Complications related to uvulopalatopharyngoplasty in 126 patients included oropharyngeal hemorrhage (6%) and rhinolalia (2%). No persistent nasopharyngeal reflux occurred. Septoplasty was performed in 26 patients without complication. In 41 patients who had tracheostomy, complications included peristomal infection (15%), intolerance to the Shiley tracheostomy tube (7%), and tracheomalacia (5%). Because none of the 5 patients in whom the Montgomery tube was used could tolerate it, its use was discontinued. Complications not directly related to a specific operative procedure occurred in 10 (8%) patients. In the first 3 postoperative months, 2 patients died, 1 presumably of pulmonary embolism, the other of cerebral infarction after external carotid artery embolization to stop bleeding after transsphenoidal hypophysectomy and uvulopalatopharyngoplasty.

Despite possible complications of surgical treatment for sleep apnea, morbidity and mortality are lower in patients treated by methods other than tracheostomy.

▶ Although tracheostomy is an effective treatment for the obstructive component of sleep apnea syndrome, there are definite and occasionally serious complications such as local hemorrhage and tracheomalacia, each of which occurred in 5% of the patients in this series. Uvulopalatopharyngoplasty (UPP) had fewer complications overall, but 6% did have pharyngeal hemorrhage. The effectiveness of UPP depends to some degree on selection of patients and the skill of the surgeon in resecting the redundant tissue. Almost always effective in quieting the loud snorer, UPP improves sleep apnea in only about half of the treated subjects (1, 2). Of importance, 70% of patients report some improvement in sleepiness, but only half of these actually have objective improvement in sleep latency (3). In children with tonsillar hypertrophy who have polysomnographically proven obstructive sleep apnea, the response to tonsillectomy usually is dramatic (4).

Therefore, a prudent approach to the treatment of symptomatic sleep apnea follows: first, except in life-threatening disease, try conservative measures such as weight loss and elimination of alcohol and sedatives. If symptoms persist, which is usual, nocturnal continuous positive airway pressure should be implemented. Uvulopalatopharyngoplasty should be reserved for those cases in which snoring is the major source of discomfort (often for the wife) and tracheostomy is not necessary or acceptable. In unusual cases, life-threatening arrhythmias or cor pulmonale are present; tracheostomy may be implemented as an initial approach to treatment. In the future, drug treatments may become available, as may techniques, electrical or mechanical, to open the upper airway dilator muscles.—R.A. Wise, M.D.

*References*


1. Conway W, Fujita S, Zorick F, et al: Uvulopalatopharyngoplasty: One-year follow-up. *Chest* 88:385–387, 1985.
2. Fujita S, Conway WA, Zorick FJ, et al: Evaluation of the effectiveness of uvulopalatopharyngoplasty. *Laryngoscope* 95:70–74, 1985.
3. Zorick F, Roehrs T, Conway W, et al: Effects of uvulopalatopharyngoplasty on the daytime sleepiness associated with sleep apnea syndrome. *Bull Eur Physiopathol Respir* 19:600–603, 1983.
4. Potsic WP: Sleep apnea in children. *Otolaryngol Clin North Am* 22:537–544, 1989.

**Compliance and Side Effects in Sleep Apnea Patients Treated With Nasal Continuous Positive Airway Pressure**

Nino-Murcia G, McCann CC, Bliwise DL, Guilleminault C, Dement WC (Stanford Univ)

*West J Med* 150:165–169, February 1989 7–19

Nasal continuous positive airway pressure (CPAP) is recognized as an effective treatment for sleep apnea; however, the long-term effects of this intervention are unknown. The intermediate-term efficacy and side effects of nasal CPAP were investigated in 139 adults who were followed systematically for 2–25 months. These patients were more obese and had a higher rate of episodes of apnea and hypopnea than patients with sleep apnea who did not agree to use CPAP.

The effectiveness of CPAP was confirmed by polysomnographic data. Pneumothorax did not occur in any patient. Compliance rates ranged from 65% to 83%, depending on the population considered. There was no relation between discontinuance of CPAP and demographic factors such as sex, age, or living with someone; however, discontinuation was related to education, with lesser educated patients better able to tolerate the equipment. The most common side effects were sore eyes and dry nose and throat, but only the latter was associated with the amount of pressure. A relationship between obesity and higher pressures was noted. The presence of side effects was not dependent on the duration of CPAP use.

These intermediate-term results suggest that CPAP is suitable for most of the patients with sleep apnea studied. The long-term consequences are still unknown.

▶ Nasal CPAP is an effective treatment for sleep apnea syndrome (1–3). When this treatment first was used, the main concern was that pneumothorax would develop as a consequence of the high pressures applied during sleep. This has not turned out to be a common complication as shown by this report. Of importance, though, is the frequency of noncompliance, which is about 1 in 4 patients. Most of those who discontinued the device complained of nasal symptoms. Although this is usually in the form of minor nasal dryness, 1 case report in the last year describes life-threatening epistaxis from CPAP (4). A second report of a serious complication of CPAP is about pneumocephalus with development of seizures and a cerebrospinal fluid rhinorrhea (5). Therefore, although CPAP is generally effective and benign, it should not be implemented without careful consideration of the potential risks and benefits. The level of nasal CPAP should be adjusted to the lowest level consistent with obliteration of the apneas. Frequently, this requires several subsequent nights of monitoring in the sleep laboratory, which adds to the expense of implementing this treatment. Recently, Millman has described a promising method for home-monitoring of nasal CPAP to allow adjustment of the mask pressure without additional nights in the sleep laboratory (6).—R.A. Wise, M.D.

*References*


1. Sullivan CE, Issa GF, Berthon-Jones M, et al: Reversal of obstructive sleep apnea by continuous positive airway pressure applied through the nares. *Lancet* 1:862–865, 1981.
2. Sanders MH, Moore SE, Eveslage J: CPAP via nasal-mask: A treatment for occlusive sleep apnea. *Chest* 83:144–145, 1983.
3. Lamphere J, Roehrs T, Wittig R, et al: Recovery of alertness after CPAP in apnea. *Chest* 96:1364–1367, 1989.
4. Strumpf DA, Harrop P, Dobbin J, et al: Massive epistaxis from nasal CPAP therapy. *Chest* 95:1141, 1989.
5. Jarjour NN, Wilson P: Pneumocephalus associated with nasal continuous positive airway pressure in a patient with sleep apnea syndrome. *Chest* 96:1425–1426, 1989.
6. Millman RP, Kipp GJ, Beadles SC, et al: A home monitoring system for nasal CPAP. *Chest* 93:730–733, 1988.


## Miscellaneous Studies

### Effects of Changes in Left Ventricular Loading and Pleural Pressure on Mitral Flow

Robotham JL, Stuart RS, Borkon AM, Doherty K, Baumgartner W (Johns Hopkins Hosp, Baltimore)

*J Appl Physiol* 65:1662–1675, October 1988 7–20

The cause of the inspiratory fall in left ventricular (LV) stroke volume during decreasing pleural pressure remains uncertain. Attempts to separate the effects of preload and afterload were made by measuring mitral and aortic flows simultaneously. If a change in preload only causes the respiratory variation in LV stroke volume, altered LV inflow in diastole always should precede changes in integrated ascending aortic flow in systole. If, however, afterload change is the cause, altered LV output should precede change in LV inflow.

Left ventricular preload and afterload were acutely altered in open-chest dogs, and the LV inflow signal was validated in a closed-chest preparation by esophageal echography and angiography. In addition, the effects of an acute fall in intrathoracic pressure at constant lung volume (the Mueller maneuver) were examined. In closed-chest dogs, LV inflow during a fall in pleural pressure with the Mueller maneuver reached its inspiratory minimum and expiratory maximum before LV outflow in 80% of instances. If rapid change in pleural pressure occurred during systole, LV outflow could vary independently of the preceding inflow.

Both diastolic and systolic events can contribute to the inspiratory fall in LV stroke volume while producing opposite changes in LV volumes. This could explain many of the confusing studies wherein either steady-state ventilatory conditions or changes in multiple beats over an entire respiratory cycle are analyzed.

► This important study clarifies a confusing and controversial topic: the mechanism by which LV stroke volume falls with inspiration. Two major mechanisms have been proposed, and each has been validated by strong experimental and observational evidence. The first mechanism is *ventricular interdependence*. Inspiration causes filling of the right ventricle and distention of the lungs surrounding the left ventricle. Because these forces restrain the filling of the left heart, subsequent ejections have diminished stroke volumes. The second mechanism is *negative pleural pressure afterload*. With this effect, the negative pleural pressure during inspiratory maneuvers prevents the ejection of blood from the left heart by increasing the systolic gradient for blood flow. This effect is similar to a sudden increase in aortic pressure and therefore has been compared to an afterload. Both of these mechanisms have been shown to reduce LV stroke volume, and much controversy has been engendered about which mechanism predominates. This paper provides a unifying hypothesis. When inspiration is initiated during systole, the afterload mechanism predominates. When inspiration is initiated during diastole, the ventricular interdependence mechanism is predominant.

It is likely that the magnitude of the effect depends not only on the phase of the cardiac cycle when inspiration is initiated, but also on the functional status of the left heart. If the heart has poor functional capacity, then it will be more sensitive to afterload, whereas if it has good functional capacity, then it is more sensitive to changes in preload as a consequence of ventricular interdependence.—R.A. Wise, M.D.

**Induction of Lower Esophageal Sphincter (LES) Dysfunction During Use of the Negative Pressure Body Ventilator**

Marino WD, Jain NK, Pitchumoni CS (Our Lady of Mercy Med Ctr, Bronx, New York)

*Am J Gastroenterol* 83:1376–1380, December 1988 7–21

The iron lung and the cuirass respirator, which are negative pressure body ventilators, have been used with increasing frequency in patients with chronic respiratory failure. In patients using such ventilators, regurgitation of gastric contents often has been noted. This regurgitation is believed to be caused by either insufflation of the stomach with resulting generation of a propulsive head of gastric pressure or the induction of lower esophageal sphincter (LES) dysfunction. The mechanism and frequency of occurrence of gastroesophageal reflux during the use of the body ventilator were determined in 16 normal volunteers. Pressure measurements were recorded in the esophagus, stomach, and at the LES before, during, and after a period of negative-pressure mechanical ventilatory assistance in an Emerson tank respirator.

In 8 of the 16 volunteers the LES-to-stomach pressure gradient was abolished or actually reversed. In 2 of the remaining 8 volunteers, it was substantially reduced. In 8, esophageal pH was measured simultaneously. As assessed by the level of decrease in esophageal pH, the occurrence of reflux correlated significantly with the change in LES pressure.

No evidence for gastric insufflation as a mechanism of reflux was found. In 7 of the 16 volunteers heartburn developed during mechanical ventilation. Four of those subjects had complete loss of LES function, and 3 had reduction but not elimination of lower esophageal sphincter pressure $P_{LES}$. The incidence of dyspepsia and the magnitude of esophageal pH change correlated with the magnitude of the change in $P_{LES}$.

An important factor in the development of gastroesophageal reflux during use of the body ventilator seems to be the induction of dysfunction of the lower esophageal sphincter. Consistent use of the upright sitting position during use of the cuirass body ventilator and the use of medication such as metoclopramide, which increases $P_{LES}$, may minimize such reflux. Because LES dysfunction occurred in most volunteers, LES function in patients with respiratory failure during use of body ventilators now is being investigated.

▶ The authors of this paper do not speculate on what the mechanism might be for the decrease in measured lower esophageal sphincter tone and esophageal reflux, which occurs with a negative pressure ventilator. Two potential mechanisms seem worthy of consideration. First, evidence suggests that lung inflation in animals leads to reflex decreases in lower esophageal sphincter tone. Second, contraction of the diaphragm with inspiration may serve as a valving mechanism, which increases the pressure gradient across the lower esophagus. The authors properly remind us that mechanical ventilation, which has been advocated for "rest" therapy of advanced COPD, may add to the risk of aspiration. This is compounded by the detrimental effect of other common drugs such as nitrates, aminophylline, and calcium channel blockers on lower esophageal sphincter tone.

A recent epidemiologic study from Denmark underscores the importance of the relationship between obstructive lung disease and esophageal reflux. Anderson and Jensen found that 44.5% of a group of patients with COPD had manometric or endoscopic evidence of esophageal disease, compared with 30% of a general population (1). In children with unexplained pulmonary symptoms the prevalence of esophageal reflux may be even higher. A Belgian study of children referred for unexplained chronic respiratory symptoms were found to have an astonishing 63% prevalence of esophageal reflux. The respiratory symptoms improved or disappeared with treatment of the reflux in most of the children who demonstrated abnormally low esophageal pH (2).—R.A. Wise, M.D.

*References*

1. Andersen LI, Jensen G: Prevalence of benign oesophageal disease in the Danish population with special reference to pulmonary disease. *J Intern Med* 225:393–402, 1989.
2. Malfroot A, Vandenplas Y, Verlinden M, et al: Gastroesophageal reflux and unexplained chronic respiratory disease in infants and children. *Pediatr Pulmonol* 3:208–213, 1987.

**Individuality of Breathing Patterns in Adults Assessed Over Time**

Benchetrit G, Shea SA, Dinh TP, Bodocco S, Baconnier P, Guz A (Faculté de Médecine; Laboratoire d'Informatique et de Mathématique Appliquées, Grenoble, France; Westminster Med School, London)

*Respir Physiol* 75:199–209, February 1989 7–22

Individuals have diverse patterns of breathing at rest, which are reproducible for a given person. To determine whether this individual pattern is maintained over long periods, 16 healthy persons of both sexes aged 18–55 years were studied twice at an interval of 4–5 years.

Breath-by-breath analysis of airflow, as measured by pneumotachometer, served to quantify the breathing pattern in terms of individual respiratory variables that included inspiratory and expiratory times, total breath duration, and tidal volume. The shape of the airflow profile was quantified by harmonic analysis. All of the variables were significantly more similar within than between individuals. This consistency was evident when viewing average airflow profiles over time (Fig 7–6). Similar breathing patterns prevailed despite changes in body weight, smoking habit, and the occurrence of mild respiratory disorders.

The consistency of breathing patterns for individuals over time probably reflects an inherent property of the respiratory system. Possible explanations include a central respiratory generator, the innervation of the respiratory musculature, the precise anatomy of the ventilatory apparatus, or cortical influences on breathing.

▶ DeJours coined the term *personalite ventilatoire* to refer to the characteristic shape and rhythm of individual ventilatory patterns (1). This study involved an elegant technique of reducing typical tidal breathing patterns into 4 vectors, which retained 95% of the information about the shape of the breath. Of the 16 patients studied up to 5 years apart, only 1 had any appreciable change in "breathing personality."

It may be, then, that the inherent rhythms and orderly progression of respiratory muscle activation is an intrinsic property of the CNS set at an early stage of development. One wonders whether this contributes to the manifestation of diseases in later life.—R.A. Wise, M.D.

*Reference*

1. DeJours P, Bechtel-Labrousse, Monzein P, et al: Etude de la diversite des regimes ventilatoires chez l'homme. *J Physiol* (Paris) 53:320–321.

**Expiratory Neural Activities in Gasping**

St John WM, Zhou D, Fregosi RF (Dartmouth Med School, Hanover, NH)

*J Appl Physiol* 66:223–231, January 1989 7–23

Expiratory-related neural activities in eupnea and gasping are not well understood. To examine these neural activities, 30 adult decerebrate and

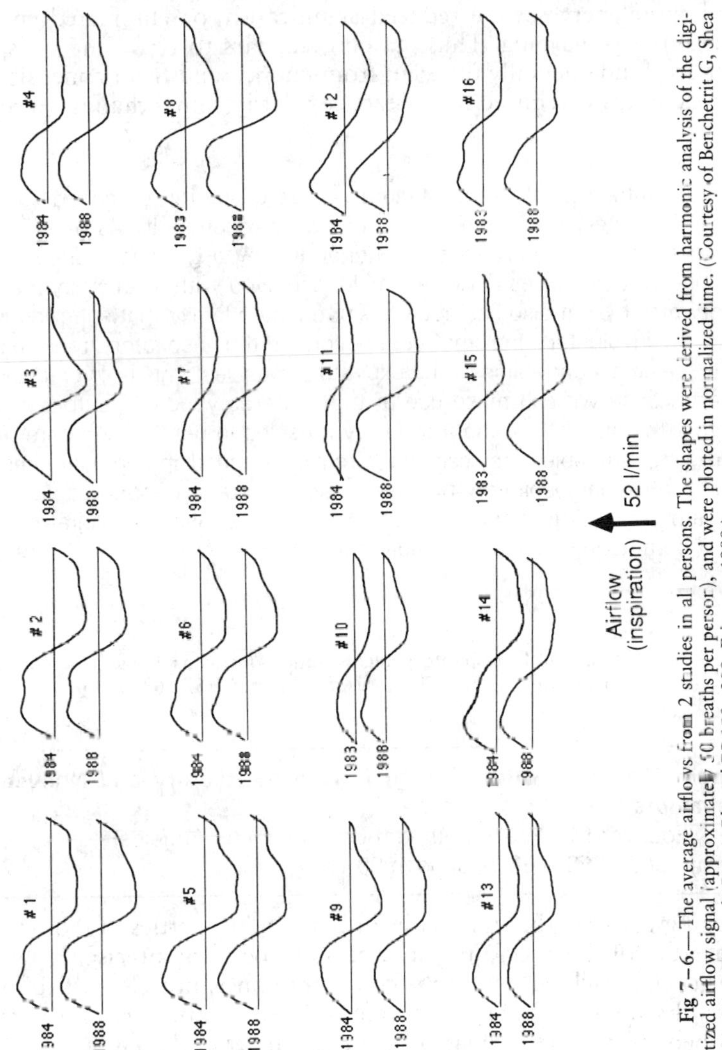


**Fig 7–6.**—The average airflows from 2 studies in all persons. The shapes were derived from harmonic analysis of the digitized airflow signal (approximately 50 breaths per person), and were plotted in normalized time. (Courtesy of Benchetrit G, Shea SA, Dinh TP, et al: *Respir Physiol* 75:199–209, February 1989.)

vagotomized cats were used. Recordings were made of the activities of the phrenic nerve, recurrent laryngeal nerve and its branches, intercostal nerves and their branches, and the abdominal nerve. Neural inspiration was defined by phrenic discharge.

Initial recordings of neural activites were obtained during eupnea. Four procedures were used to alter the ventilatory pattern from eupnea to gasping. Brain stems in 9 cats were frozen at the pontomedullary junction. Asphyxia was used in 5 animals; anoxia, in 5; and ischemic "transection" of the brain stem, in 11.

The principal finding was that phasic expiratory activities of both cranial and spinal nerves were reduced significantly or eliminated entirely with the onset of gasping. Thus, gasping appears to represent a respiratory pattern fundamentally different from eupnea and from apneusis. Expiratory action was reduced to a greater extent in spinal than in laryngeal nerves.

▶ Maximal contraction of the diaphragm can be elicited in untrained subjects by having them perform a sniff maneuver. More recently, it has been shown that the maximal inspiratory pressure generated by a gasping maneuver can develop pressures in excess of what can be achieved with a voluntary maximal inspiratory effort (1). It also has been observed anecdotally that sneezing is initiated by an involuntary maximal contraction of the inspiratory muscles followed by maximal contraction of the expiratory muscles. This is of practical importance because we can make use of these stereotyped respiratory maneuvers to test the strength of the respiratory muscles in persons who are otherwise unwilling or unable. They can sniff a maximal transdiaphragmatic pressure and gasp a maximal inspiratory pressure. Perhaps some pepper (capsaicin for the mediator-minded) to induce sneezing to generate maximal expiratory pressures will be a useful pulmonary function test.—R.A. Wise, M.D.

*Reference*

1. Macefield G, Nail B: Inspiratory augmentation during asphyxic hyperpnoea and gasping: Proprioceptive influences. *Respir Physiol* 64:57–68, 1986.

---

**Diaphragm Motor Unit Recruitment During Ventilatory and Nonventilatory Behaviors**

Sieck GC, Fournier M (Univ of Southern California, Los Angeles)
*J Appl Physiol* 66:2539–2545, June 1989 7–24

---

Matching between the contractile and fatigue properties of motor units and the order of their recruitment appears to be fairly precise. However, whether such matching occurs in the diaphragm is not clear. The forces generated by the cat diaphragm during different ventilatory and nonventilatory behaviors were estimated by measuring transdiaphragmatic pressure (Pdi). Phrenic nerve stimulation was performed, and chemical drive was increased by inhalation of a hypoxic, hypercapnic gas mixture.

The Pdi generated during eupnea was only about 12% of the maximal Pdi generated by bilateral phrenic nerve stimulation. On breathing a mixture of 10% oxygen and 5% carbon dioxide, the Pdi increased to about 28% of maximum (Fig 7–7). On total airway occlusion the Pdi increased to nearly half of maximum. Only during the gag reflex and sneezing was maximal Pdi reached.

It is likely that abdominal muscles are activated during certain nonventilatory behaviors of the diaphragm, which may contribute to the measured Pdi response by producing a lengthening contraction of the diaphragm. Orderly recruitment of diaphragmatic motor units with the step-

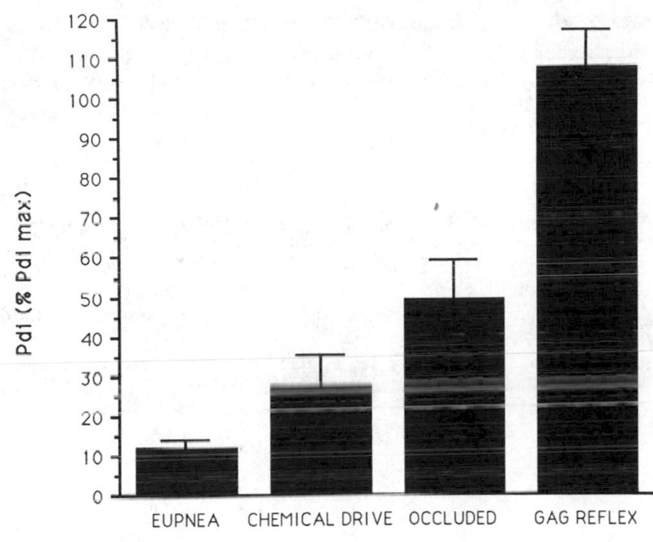


Fig 7–7.—Relative transdiaphragmatic pressures (% $Pdi_{max}$, mean + SD) generated during different ventilatory and nonventilatory behaviors of the diaphragm. (Courtesy of Sieck GC, Fournier M: *J Appl Physiol* 66:2539–2545, June 1989.)

wise addition of unit tetanic tensions may not occur in vivo, but there is evidence supporting a general recruitment order of motor unit types in most motor behaviors. The nervous system may alternate the recruitment of motor units during sustained diaphragmatic contractions, allowing time for rest and recovery from fatigue.

▶ Activation of peripheral skeletal muscle with increasing neural stimulation occurs in an organized and beneficial fashion (1). With low levels of activation, the first motor units to be activated contain small motoneurons that have high membrane resistance and innervate slow twitch motor units. These fibers tend to produce lower tensions, but are resistant to fatigue. As the degree of excitation increases or is prolonged, larger motoneurons are recruited that have lower membrane resistance and innervate fast twitch motor units. These fibers produce higher tensions, but are more prone to fatigue with repeated activation (2, 3).

The first motor units to be activated are those relatively resistant to fatigue, and the last to be recruited are those that are easily fatigued. Thus, with low levels of neural stimulation, the diaphragm is resistant to fatigue and can contract indefinitely. If there is an increase in activation, much greater force can be achieved, but this cannot be sustained without development of fatigue of the fast twitch motor units. External electrical stimulation of the phrenic nerves can contract the diaphragm, which is about twice what can be achieved with maximal voluntary contraction. Presumably, this reserve capacity of muscles is advantageous in protecting the muscle from overstimulation and prolonged fatigue. Of interest, though, brief nonventilatory respiratory actions such as gagging and sneezing can maximally or supramaximally stimulate the diaphragm of the cat. The survival value of this mechanism must be to provide maximal lung volume for subsequent expiratory efforts that protect the airway.—R.A. Wise, M.D.

*References*


1. Zajac FE, Faden JS: Relationship among recruitment order, axonal conduction velocity, and muscle unit properties of type-identified motor units in cat plantaris muscle. *J Neurophysiol* 53:1303–1322, 1985.
2. Dick TEF, Kong J, Berger AJ: Correlation of recruitment order with axonal conduction velocity for supraspinally driven diaphragmatic motor units. *J Neurophysiol* 57:245–259, 1987.
3. Jodkowski JS, Viana F, Dick TE, et al: Electrical properties of phrenic motoneurons in the cat: Correlation with inspiratory drive. *J Neurophysiol* 58:105–124, 1987.

# 8 Occupational and Environmental Lung Disorders

## Introduction

Five areas in occupational and environmental lung disorders captured most of the excitement during the past year: (1) mechanisms of occupational alveolitis; (2) mechanisms of occupational fibrosis; (3) new insights into lung cancer; (4) pulmonary effects of air pollution; and (5) respiratory protective devices.

### Mechanisms of Occupational Alveolitis

Perhaps the most provocative paper was the one by Goodglick and co-workers (Abstract 8–1), who demonstrated that the familiar asbestos–lipid peroxidation effect on macrophage cell membrane was not likely to be the cause of cell death. Control of membrane peroxidation by vitamin E, for example, did not prevent cytotoxicity. Instead, it was hypothesized that repair of oxidant DNA damage (single-strand breaks) may lead to cellular NAD+ depletion and subsequent macrophage toxicity. Proof of their hypothesis lay in showing that inhibition of DNA repair prevented cytotoxicity, even in the presence of membrane peroxidation. Further, their model of asbestos DNA damage, repair, and cytotoxicity might better account for the development of asbestos-related neoplasia.

Garcia and associates (Abstract 8–2) address the mechanisms by which asbestos exerts its fibrogenic effect. Although the asbestos-activated macrophage produces $LTB_4$, "the most potent chemotactic agent generated by arachidonic acid metabolism," there is no difference in BAL-$LTB_4$ levels between asbestos workers with asbestosis and those without it. Instead, the emerging recognition of the role of eosinophil recruitment in the pathogenesis of interstitial fibrosis may provide new insight into the effector cell for fibrogenesis. This report of Garcia may be complementary to the paper by Dubois and colleagues (Abstract 8–3). Dubois studied the autoregulatory effects of $LTB_4$ on macrophage production of tumor necrosis factor after asbestos and silica stimulation. Tumor necrosis factor may have a direct effect on fibroblasts or may act indirectly through eosinophil and leukocyte activation. In contrast, Schwartz and co-workers (Abstract 8–4) in their negative study found no evidence for the expression of fibroblast-stimulating cytokines by peripheral blood monocytes from asbestosis patients. It is possible that cytokine production requires direct activation of macrophages and mono-cytes by asbestos fibers such as that which occurs in the lung. Peripheral blood monocytes may not have been activated directly.

This concept of locally activated pulmonary effector cells is demonstrated with CD4+ T lymphocytes by Saltini and colleagues (Abstract 8–5), who found that chronic beryllium alveolitis results from a specific delayed-typed hypersensitivity response, rather than a nonspecific metal mitogen (e.g., nickel, lithium, zirconium). The authors conclude that chronic beryllium disease is identical to sarcoid, with the essential difference being that, for chronic beryllium disease, the antigen is known.

### Mechanisms of Occupational Fibrosis

Bégin and associates (Abstract 8–6) used their sheep model of nodular silicosis to demonstrate that the increase in the production and release of alveolar phospholipids was suppressed by inhalation of aluminum lactate. Alveolar phospholipids are of interest because these molecules may reduce dust toxicity, but may also be chemotactic for macrophages and other inflammatory effector cells. Ramos and co-workers (Abstract 8–7) show that, in response to silica inhalation, the development of fibrosis depends not only on macrophage activation, cytokine release, and collagen synthesis, but also on the rate of collage degradation. Instead of the expected decrease in collagenolysis with the progression of fibrosis, he observed a trimodal (increase, decrease, unchanged) expression of collagenolysis. The explanation for this unexpected collagenolytic behavior is not yet determined.

Vallyathan and colleagues (Abstract 8–8) documented that the acute silicosis response resulted from, at least in part, the unique surface reactivity of freshly sheared silica. Using electron spin resonance, these authors determined that short-lived silicon-based radicals on the surface of mechanically sheared silica were able to effect macrophage cell membrane peroxidation leading to a respiratory burst. Finally, Sun and colleagues (Abstract 8–9) reduced the antioxidant reserve by depleting reduced glutathione levels in rodents before, during, and following an ozone challenge. Depletion of GSH led to a remodeling of lung collagen that, as yet, remains unexplained.

### New Insights Into Lung Cancer

The Randeraths (Abstract 8–10) have applied their $^{32}P$-postlabeling adduct assay to target tissues of cigarette smokers in a search for cigarette-induced DNA damage. The postlabeling adduct profile for cigarette-induced DNA damage provided a specific "fingerprint" similar to that obtained when cigarette smoke condensate is applied to mouse skin. Further, tissue DNA adduct levels for specimens of human lung, bronchus, and aryepiglottic fold correlated well with the degree of smoking exposure expressed as pack years. These data led the authors to conclude that cigarette smoking-induced DNA adduct formation is causally related to tissue damage in the target organ.

Moolgavkar and colleagues (Abstract 8–11) analyzed the Doll and Peto British doctors' data using the two-mutation, "recessive oncogenesis" model of Knudson. This model includes two rate-limiting steps that may be identified with mutations that lead to homozygous loss of antioncogene function, a concept recently validated in several solid tissue tumors. The value of this paper is the opportunity it provides to rethink the dose-response vs. duration effect of smoking on lung cancer. The age-specific risk of lung cancer among women who smoke has risen as their smoking habits have become similar to those of men (Garfinkel and Stellman, Abstract 8–12). The lung cancer standardized mortality ratio for female smokers has increased to become equivalent to that for men in the prospective studies carried out 20 years ago. Nevertheless, the recent trend toward smoking cessation has had a mitigating effect and the lung cancer rates among women (and men) aged less than 45 are beginning to fall. Higgins and Wynder (Abstract 8–13) show that the risk of lung cancer persists after smoking cessation for 20–30 years. The benefits of cessation seem to be related to cell type (with least cessation benefit for adenocarcinoma risk), but the greatest benefits for all categories accrue during the first 5 years after cessation. It is never too late to stop smoking.

The extent of environmental tobacco exposure (passive smoking) can be assessed with urinary cotinine (Haley and co-workers, Abstract 8–14). This technique is most useful for validation of self reported exposure data. However, the physiochemical properties of environmental tobacco smoke are quite different from those of inhaled mainstream smoke, and this biomarker can provide only an indirect measurement of the potential health risk associated with environmental tobacco smoke. The other major environmental lung carcinogen, environmental radon, now has been clearly characterized as hazardous, even among never-smokers. Radon-exposed never-smokers living in Sweden (Axelson and associates, Abstract 8–15) and working in Colorado uranium mines (Roscoe and associates, Abstract 8–16) both demonstrate significant excess lung cancer risk.

### Pulmonary Effects of Air Pollution

Recent reviews of the National Ambient Air Quality Standard have led to a review of the effects of particulates (Pope, Abstract 8–17). This report is one of the first to examine the association between health effects and the new NAAQS $PM_{10}$ particulate standard. Dales and co-workers (Abstract 8–18) describe the presentation of symptoms (without physiologic changes) among children, but not among adults downwind from a large point source of sulfur dioxide. Concentrations of $SO_2$ above the NAAQS standard but below the short-term exposure limit of Sweden were found by Sandström and colleagues (Abstract 8–19) to produce changes in the cellular distribution on bronchoalveolar lavage. The ultimate health consequence of $SO_2$ exposures at this level are unknown.

Oxidant responses of the murine lung to low-level concentrations of nitrogen dioxide (Parker and associates, Abstract 8–20) seem to lead to a reduction of nonspecific macrophage activation. Whether this is related to an increase in human nonfatal respiratory disease is unknown. Oxidant responses of children to ambient ozone concentrations seem to be characterized by heterogeneity (Kinney and colleagues, Abstract 8–21). Not histories of asthma, early childhood respiratory illness, nor sex were predictive of ozone "sensitivity." Two studies of responses of cells of the lung to ozone (Koren and co-workers, Abstract 8–22; Esterline and co-workers, Abstract 8–23) help clarify our understanding of acute responses to low-level ozone exposure. Of particular interst is the demonstration of an interaction between alveolar macrophages and neutrophils (Esterline). Depression of macrophage oxidant response directly by ozone is followed by a renewed respiratory burst mediated by the myeloperoxidase reactions of neutrophils summoned to the scene.

RESPIRATORY PROTECTIVE DEVICES

Wilson and Raven (Abstract 8–24) found that the 15-second maximal voluntary ventilation was the best predictor of work performance while wearing a respirator. They propose that, by measuring the 15-second MVV, calculating the potential reduction caused by respirator wear, and combining this information with the required ventilation of the work task, physicians will be able to determine each worker's ability to work while wearing a respirator, regardless of the presence of pulmonary disease. Harber and associates (Abstract 8–25) examined the effects of various types of respiratory loads characteristically imposed by respiratory protective devices, and suggested that inspiratory resistance is the dominant factor determining the ventilatory response to respiratory loading. Akkersdijk (Abstract 8–26) illustrates that wearing personal protective devices does not necessarily protect the worker. How best to validate a worker protection program must be addressed.

**Melvyn S. Tockman, M.D., Ph.D.**

## Mechanisms of Occupational Alveolitis

**Evaluation of the Causal Relationship Between Crocidolite Asbestos-Induced Lipid Peroxidation and Toxicity to Macrophages**
Goodglick LA, Pietras LA, Kane AB (Brown Univ, Providence, RI)
*Am Rev Respir Dis* 139:1265–1273, May 1989 8–1

Macrophages, through phagocytosis of asbestos fibers, are presumed to have a role in both acute and chronic reactions to asbestos. Acute cytotoxicity from crocidolite asbestos is mediated by the production of reactive oxygen metabolites, but the specific intracellular target is not clear. The role of lipid peroxidation in macrophage toxicity induced by crocidolite asbestos was studied in mouse peritoneal macrophages. Lipid peroxidation was measured by the thiobarbituric acid assay.

Exposure of murine macrophages to crocidolite asbestos led to a dose- and time-dependent rise in lipid peroxidation breakdown products. The effect paralleled cell death. Superoxide dismutase plus catalase or deferoxamine prevented both cell death and lipid peroxidation. Macrophages were not killed by crocidolite when incubated with 3-aminobenzamide, but products of lipid peroxidation were the same as in cells not so treated. Vitamin E pretreatment prevented lipid peroxidation but not cytotoxicity from crocidolite.

Lipid peroxidation takes place when macrophages are exposed in vitro to crocidolite asbestos, but that reaction is not directly responsible for irreversible injury to the cells. Nevertheless, products of lipid peroxidation may injure adjacent cells in vivo, possibly contributing to neoplasia in the lungs and mesothelium.

▶ During phagocytosis of asbestos fiber, macrophage plasma membrane lipids may be potential targets of reactive oxygen metabolites on the asbestos fiber surface. Lipid peroxidation can be initiated by free-radical abstraction of a hydrogen atom from a plasma membrane unsaturated fatty acid. Fatty acid radicals could damage adjacent lipids and lead to a chain reaction destruction of macrophage cellular membrane. Lipid peroxidation may be terminated by vitamin E and glutathione peroxidase. Exposure of mouse peritoneal macrophages to crocidolite asbestos led to a dose- and time-dependent increase in lipid peroxidation accompanied by cell death.

However, inhibition of lipid peroxidation (by vitamin E) was not sufficient to prevent crocidolite-induced cell death. Having observed that 3-aminobenzamide decreases crocidolite-induced toxicity, the authors have come to a new hypothesis about the mechanism of toxicity. 3-Aminobenzamide is known to inhibit the enzyme adenosine diphosphoribosyl transferase (ADPRT), which regulates repair of DNA single-strand breaks. It is possible that, during the repair of extensive single-strand DNA breakage, cellular NAD+ levels are depleted, leading to cell death. Depletion of NAD+ and cell suicide (from exhaustive DNA repair) could be prevented by pretreatment with the ADPRT inhibitor 3-aminobenzamide. Thus, it is not the direct lipid peroxidation of cell membrane that is responsible for the asbestos fiber cytotoxicity, but energy-depleting repair of oxidant-damaged DNA. This model also might account for the development of asbestos-related neoplasia, either from direct oxidant DNA injury or from clastogenic or mutagenic lipid oxidation products.—M.S. Tockman, M.D., Ph.D.

---

**Alveolar Macrophages From Patients With Asbestos Exposure Release Increased Levels of Leukotriene $B_4$**

Garcia JGN, Griffith DE, Cohen AB, Callahan KS (Indiana Univ, Indianapolis; Univ of Texas, Tyler)

*Am Rev Respir Dis* 139:1494–1501, June 1989 8–2

---

Current explanations of fibrosis in interstitial lung disorders postulate a central role for infiltration of inflammatory cells into the alveolar compartment. There is good evidence for asbestos-induced alveolitis. Indices of abnormalities of the lower respiratory tract detected by bronchoalveolar lavage (BAL) were investigated in 93 consecutively seen patients with occupational asbestos exposure and in 12 smoking and 10 nonsmoking controls.

The 12 patients with clinical asbestosis had increased numbers of neu-

Levels of Leukotriene $B_4$ in Cell-Free BAL Supernatants From Asbestos Workers and Controls

| Group (*n*) | $LTB_4$ (*ng/mL*) |
|---|---|
| I (8) | 2.1 ± 0.5† |
| II (15) | 2.2 ± 0.7† |
| III (10) | 0.92 ± 0.2 |
| IV (5) | 0.4 ± 0.2 |

†$P < .05$ compared with groups III and IV.
(Courtesy of Garcia JGN, Griffith DE, Cohen AB, et al: *Am Rev Respir Dis* 139:1494–1501, June 1989.)

trophils and eosinophils in BAL specimens. Greater numbers of neutrophils also were found in exposed workers without clinical disease. These abnormalities correlated with in vitro BAL alveolar macrophage production of the potent chemotaxin leukotriene $B_4$ ($LTB_4$, table).

The stimulated release of $LTB_4$ from BAL alveolar macrophages was more marked in asbestos-exposed workers with or without asbestosis. Cell-free BAL supernates from asbestos-exposed patients contained significantly more $LTB_4$ than those from controls. Both pulmonary dysfunction and abnormalities seen on radiographic study correlated well with the percentage and total numbers of neutrophils and eosinophils in BAL fluid.

In vivo production of $LTB_4$ by alveolar macrophages may be an important means by which alveolar inflammation is amplified after exposure to asbestos. The consequent infiltration of inflammatory cells into alveolar spaces may lead to both inflammatory and fibrotic responses.

▶ This paper addresses the cellular mechanisms by which asbestos exerts its cytotoxic and fibrogenic effects. In particular, emphasis is placed on the elaboration of the chemoattractant $LTB_4$ by the activated alveolar macrophage. The powerful ability of $LTB_4$ to recruit inflammatory cells has been described previously, and $LTB_4$ has been recognized by the authors as "the most potent chemotactic agent generated by arachidonic acid metabolism" (1). However, as demonstrated in the table, BAL supernatant $LTB_4$ levels are significantly greater among asbestos-exposed workers than among both smoking and nonsmoking controls, but no $LTB_4$ difference exists between those with and those without fibrosis (asbestosis) among the asbestos-exposed workers.

Further, this report focuses on the significant increase of BAL eosinophils. Like neutrophils, eosinophils can secrete proteolytic enzymes and toxic oxygen radicals that might mediate inflammatory destruction. It is important that there seems to be an emerging recognition of the role of the eosinophil in the pathogenesis of interstitial fibrosis. The authors describe the work of Peterson and associates (2), who report that only BAL eosinophil content predicted functional deterioration in a group of patients with idiopathic pulmonary fibrosis. In the present study, the increased BAL eosinophils were inversely and significantly correlated with diminished pulmonary function indices (FVC, TLC) and directly correlated with chest radiograph profusion score. Further, BAL eosinophils (percent and total BAL eosinophils) were elevated among those with fibrosis, but not among the exposed workers without asbestosis.—M.S. Tockman, M.D., Ph.D.

*References*

1. Ford-Hutchinson AW, Bray MA, Doig MV, et al: Leukotriene B, a potent chemokinetic and aggregating substance released from polymorphonuclear leukocytes. *Nature* 286:264–265, 1980.
2. Peterson MW, Monick M, Hunninghake GW: Prognostic role of eosinophils in pulmonary fibrosis. *Chest* 92:51–56, 1987.

---

**Asbestos Fibers and Silica Particles Stimulate Rat Alveolar Macrophages to Release Tumor Necrosis Factor: Autoregulatory Role of Leukotriene $B_4$**

Dubois CM, Bissonnette F, Rola-Pleszczynski M (Univ of Sherbrooke, PQ)

*Am Rev Respir Dis* 139:1257–1264, May 1989 8–3

Alveolar macrophages have a critical role in lung disease through the production of potent inflammatory and fibrogenic mediators. The role of leukotriene $B_4$ ($LTB_4$) in mediating lung disease was assessed by determining the effects of endogenous and exogenous $LTB_4$ on the release of tumor necrosis factor (TNF) by rat alveolar macrophages exposed to mineral dust.

Alveolar macrophages cultured with 1 to 100 μg/mL of silica particles or asbestos fibers produced TNF and $LTB_4$ in a concentration dependent manner (Fig 8–1). Latex beads were inactive. After 2 hours of exposure to silica or asbestos, an increase in $LTB_4$ was preceded by a rise in TNF activity. Most of the stimulatory effect was prevented by actinomycin D and cycloheximide. Lipoxygenase inhibitors lowered asbestos- and silica-stimulated TNF release. When exogenous $LTB_4$ was added to macrophages treated with lipoxygenase inhibitors, TNF production was partially restored.

There appears to be common mechanism by which asbestos and silica may modulate the production of inflammatory and fibrogenic cytokines. Inhibition of TNF activity by lipoxygenase inhibitors could be a useful approach to interrupting the processes of chronic inflammation and fibrosis.

▶ Cachectin (TNF) is a cytokine macrophage product that augments neutrophil and eosinophil activity and stimulates fibroblast growth. In this paper, the investigators evaluate the role of $LTB_4$ on the regulation of mineral-dust-induced TNF release. They found that the increase in $LTB_4$ produced by asbestos and silica-stimulated macrophages preceded the rise in TNF activity. Further, a positive correlation existed between the effects of lipoxygenase inhibitors and TNF activity. The potential mechanism for these autoregulatory effects of $LTB_4$ on

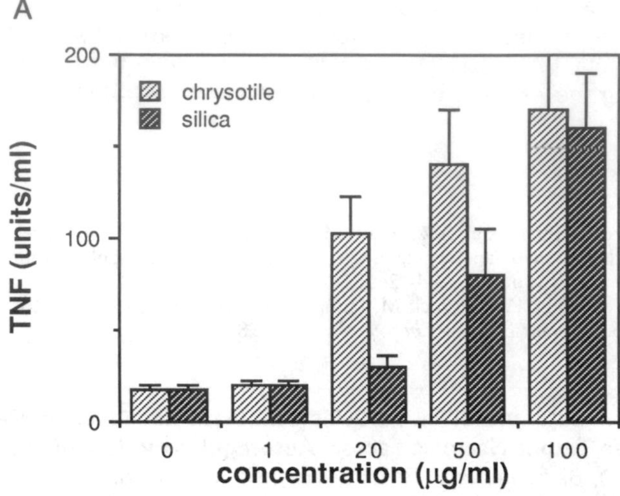


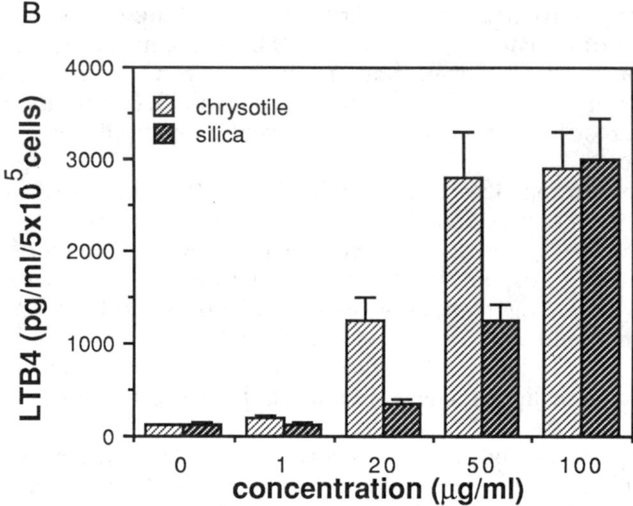


**Fig 8–1.**—Concentration-dependent stimulation of TNF (**A**) and $LTB_4$ (**B**) production by mineral dust. Data represent means ± SEM of 5 separate experiments. Confidence level is $P < .05$ for TNF generated in presence of 20 to 100 μg/mL particles and $LTB_4$ generated in presence of 20 μg/mL chrysotile A and 20 or 50 μg/mL silica; $P < .01$ for $LTB_4$ produced in presence of 50 and 100 μg/mL asbestos and 100 μg/mL silica. (Courtesy of Dubois CM, Bissonnette E, Rola-Pleszczynski M: *Am Rev Respir Dis* 139:1257–1264, May 1989.)

TNF production could be attributed to intracellular activation messengers (e.g., influx of external calcium).

If TNF is the means by which activated macrophages stimulate inflammation and fibrogenesis, then the possibility of inhibiting this destruction with lipoxygenase inhibitors of TNF activity exists. The authors report that nordihydroguaiaretic acid (NDGA), a lipoxygenase inhibitor, has been used successfully to inhibit bleomycin-induced murine fibrosis (1).—M.S. Tockman, M.D., Ph.D.

*Reference*

1. Phan SH, Kunkel S: Inhibition of bleomycin-induced pulmonary fibrosis by nordihydroguaiaretic acid. *Am J Pathol* 124:343–352, 1986.

## Monocyte-Derived Growth Factors in Asbestos-Induced Interstitial Fibrosis

Schwartz DA, Rosenstock L, Clark JG (Univ of Washington)
*Environ Res* 49:283–294, August 1989 8–4

Despite a dose-response relationship between asbestos exposure and the occurrence of interstitial fibrosis, radiographically evident fibrosis does not develop in a majority of workers exposed to even high levels of asbestos. The pathogenesis of asbestos-induced fibrosis was examined by quantifying monocyte-derived growth factor production in 5 persons with asbestosis and 5 normal exposure-matched controls. Because immunologic differences have been related to race, sex, and cigarette smoking history, only white, nonsmoking men were included in the study.

All patients with asbestosis had interstitial fibrosis established by chest radiography and a forced vital capacity of 70% of predicted or less. Monocytes from both patients with asbestosis and controls released a factor that promoted the growth of noncycling fibroblasts (table). Mitogenic activity persisted through 8 days of culture. Conditioned medium from monocytes of healthy men affected fibroblast growth more than did medium from monocytes of patients with asbestosis. Similar proliferative responses were seen with concanavalin A stimulation. After stimulation, monocyte preparations from healthy men had detectable messenger RNA for platelet-derived growth factor, whereas no expression of the gene for

Proliferative Response[a] of Swiss 3T3 Cells After Exposures to Monocyte Conditioned Medium From Subjects With Asbestosis and Exposure-Matched Controls

| Days of monocyte culture | Asbestosis Medium | Asbestosis Medium + Con A | Asbestosis *P* value | Controls Medium | Controls Medium + Con A | Controls *P* value |
|---|---|---|---|---|---|---|
| 2 | 186.3 ± 17.1[b] | 279.2 ± 93.7 | 0.05 | 424.9 ± 136.3 | 238.1 ± 33.6 | 0.02 |
| 4 | 138.8 ± 17.3 | 216.0 ± 77.6 | 0.05 | 229.7 ± 62.8 | 203.7 ± 21.7 | >0.10 |
| 6 | 94.5 ± 9.2 | 175.1 ± 73.5 | 0.05 | 100.8 ± 15.6 | 136.0 ± 19.4 | >0.10 |
| 8 | 94.2 ± 14.7 | 103.2 ± 14.0 | >0.10 | 158.4 ± 36.6 | 118.1 ± 20.6 | >0.10 |

[a]Reported as a percentage above baseline activity: [(monocyte conditioned medium − acellular incubated medium)/acellular incubated medium] × 100.
[b]Mean ± SD.
(Courtesy of Schwartz DA, Rosenstock L, Clark JG: *Environ Res* 49:283–294, August 1989.)

the B-chain of the growth factors was noted in stimulated monocyte preparations from the patients with asbestosis.

Peripheral blood monocytes from patients with asbestosis may be less mature than cells from exposure-matched persons without asbestosis. It is possible that the fibrogenic process recruits blood monocytes to the lung, leaving relatively immature cells in the circulation.

▶ This paper addresses the hypothesis that host factors—in particular, the capacity for monocytes and macrophages to produce growth factors—may be responsible for the variable fibrotic response to asbestos inhalation. The investigators theorized that interstitial fibrosis develops in patients with asbestosis because their mononuclear phagocytes produce fibroblast stimulating cytokines, whereas the macrophages of exposure-matched controls would be less likely to do so. However, analyses of mitogenic activity and platelet-derived growth factor (PDGF) and messenger RNA levels indicated that the activity of peripheral blood monocytes does not support such a theory. Peripheral blood monocytes from patients with asbestos-induced fibrosis appear to have a lesser capacity to produce monocyte-derived growth factor activity and express the B chain of PDGF gene than exposure-matched controls have.

The authors speculate on an explanation for the lack of expression of fibroblast-stimulating cytokines by peripheral blood monocytes from asbestosis patients. They suggest that potential recruitment of mononuclear cells to the asbestos-containing lungs of these patients would result in a less mature population of circulating blood monocytes. Support for this explanation would require a further study that includes concurrent testing of alveolar macrophages for cytokine release.—M.S. Tockman, M.D., Ph.D.

---

**Maintenance of Alveolitis in Patients With Chronic Beryllium Disease by Beryllium-Specific Helper T Cells**

Saltini C, Winestock K, Kirby M, Pinkston P, Crystal RG (Natl Heart, Lung, and Blood Inst, Bethesda, Md)

*N Engl J Med* 320:1103–1109, Apr 27, 1989 8–5

---

Chronic beryllium lung disease appears to be immunologically mediated. Beryllium may serve as an antigen, alone or as a hapten, that drives the T cell-mediated lung disease. The nature of the process was studied by examining T cells from peripheral blood and bronchoalveolar lavage fluid in 8 patients with chronic beryllium disease and 5 healthy controls. All the patients had noncaseating granulomas, and in vitro analysis revealed lymphocyte proliferation in response to beryllium (Fig 8–2). Lung volumes and diffusing capacity were consistently reduced, and mild hypoxemia occurred at rest.

Increased numbers of CD4+ T cells were present in lavage fluid, and these cells proliferated in response to beryllium in a dose-dependent manner proliferation of T cells was mediated by antigen-specific, class II-restricted recognition of beryllium. The response to beryllium was specific when T cells were tested with other metal salts and recall antigens.

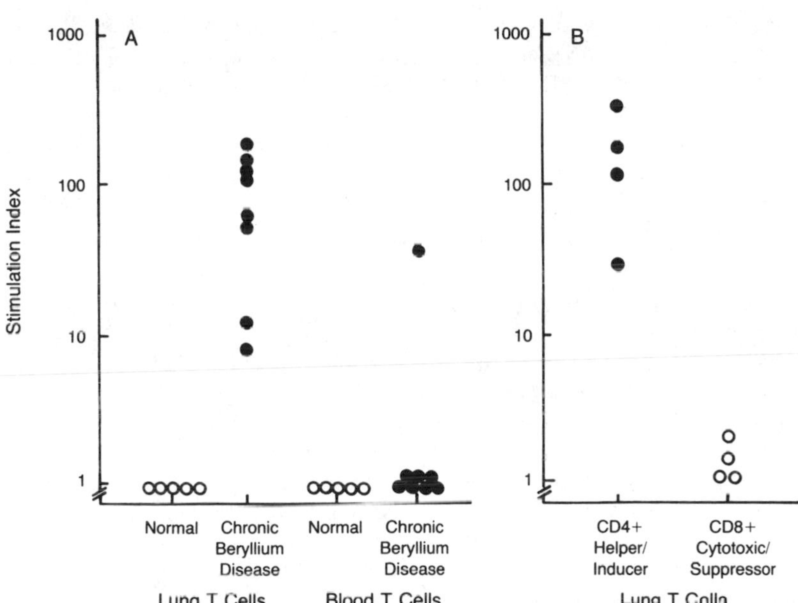


**Fig 8–2.**—In vitro proliferation of purified T Cells (**A**) and T cell subpopulations (**B**) from the lungs and blood of patients with chronic beryllium disease and controls in response to beryllium. Each symbol represents the average of 3 determinations of the stimulation index in each person. (Courtesy of Saltini C, Winestock K, Kirby M, et al. *N Engl J Med* 320:1103–1109, Apr 27, 1989.)

The alveolitis of beryllium lung disease involves a specific delayed-type hypersensitivity reaction to beryllium rather than a nonspecific mitogenic or adjuvant effect of the metal. Chronic beryllium disease is basically identical to sarcoid, except that the antigen is known. Selective activation of CD4+ T cells appears to be a central pathogenctic event in granulomatous disorders involving helper–inducer T cells.

▶ In this paper, Saltini and associates addressed whether the T cells that lead to the chronic granulomatous beryllium disease are responding to a specific beryllium antigen–hapten or to beryllium as a nonspecific mitogen similar to that seen with nickel, lithium, and zirconium. The investigators conclude that, in patients with chronic beryllium disease, the proliferation of lung T cells occurs as a specific response to beryllium antigen–hapten. This conclusion supports that the chronic beryllium alveolitis results from a specific delayed-type hypersensitivity response of T cells and macrophages.

This conclusion is based on 5 lines of evidence: (1) berylliosis-patient lung CD4+ (helper) T cells proliferate on exposure to beryllium without similar proliferation of blood T cells or lung T cells from non-beryllium-exposed controls; (2) studies using anti-class I and anti-class II antibodies demonstrated that beryllium-induced proliferation of lung CD4+ T cells was mediated by antigen-specific, class II-restricted recognition of beryllium–hapten; (3) it is possible to develop beryllium-specific T cell lines that do not respond to other metal salts, such as zirconium, lithium, and nickel; (4) the proliferative response of these derived T cell lines to beryllium is similarly class-II restricted (typical of soluble-antigen responsive CD4+ cells); and (5) beryllium-specific CD4+ T cell clones can be derived from single T cells isolated from patient lungs.

These observations indicate that chronic beryllium disease is identical to sarcoid. The essential difference is that the antigen is known in chronic beryllium disease. Similar proliferative CD4+ T cell response also is found in tuberculoid leprosy, another chronic granulomatous disorder.—M.S. Tockman, M.D., Ph.D.

## Mechanisms of Occupational Fibrosis

**Effect of Aluminum Inhalation on Alveolar Phospholipid Profiles in Experimental Silicosis**

Bégin R, Possmayer F, Ormseth MA, Martel M, Cantin A, Massé S (Univ of Western Ontario, London, Ont)

*Lung* 167:107–115, March–April 1989 8–6

Increased levels of phospholipids have been detected in a sheep tracheal lobe model of nodular silicosis. Inhalation of aluminum suppressed silica-induced alveolitis and reduced pathology. The biochemical features of lung lavage fluid in this model, with and without aluminum inhalation, were characterized in 40 sheep.

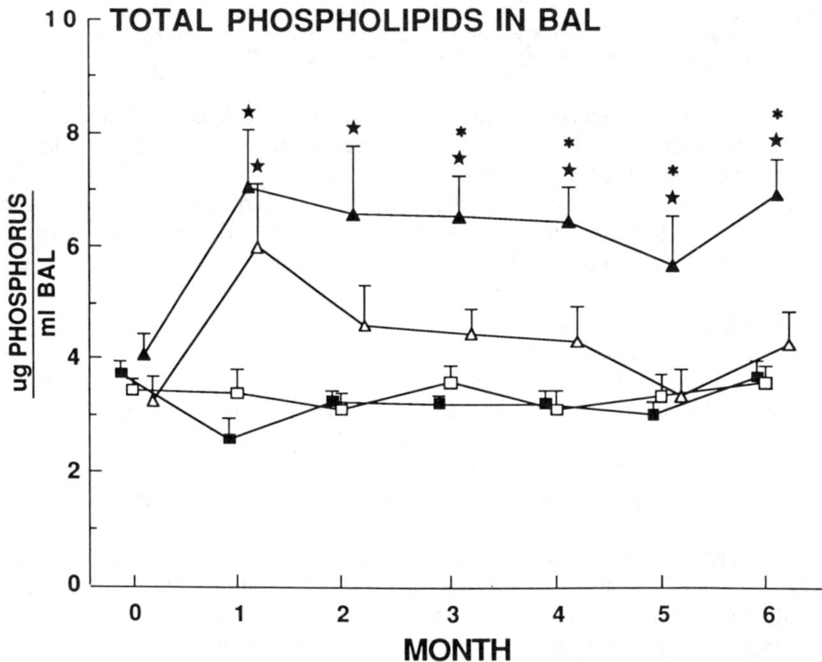


Fig 8–3.—Time course of total phospholipids in bronchoalveolar lavage fluids. *Shaded squares,* the phosphate buffered saline group; *open squares,* the phosphate buffered saline–aluminum group; *closed triangle,* the saline–phosphate buffered saline group; *open triangle,* the saline–aluminum group; *star,* $P < .05$ between *closed triangle* and *closed square;* *, $P < .05$ between *closed triangle* and *open triangle; BAL,* bronchoalveolar lavage. (Courtesy of Bégin R, Possmayer F, Ormseth MA, et al: *Lung* 167:107–115, March–April 1989.)

Lung lavage phospholipids remained constant with saline and saline–aluminum exposure but increased rapidly in the silica-buffered saline group (Fig 8–3). With silica and aluminum combined, an initial increase in phospholipids preceded baseline values within 2 months.

In the absence of lipidoproteinosis, lavage-fluid phospholipids can be altered by quartz exposure. The effect of quartz on type 2 alveolar cells is totally reversed by inhalation of aluminum lactate. Alveolar phospholipids are important because they can reduce dust toxicity, promote influx of macrophages, and regulate other cell groups in the alveolar and interstitial spaces.

▶ The authors have developed a sheep model of nodular silicosis with results of bronchoalveolar lavage similar to those found in granite workers. Using the sheep model, the investigators found that aluminum inhalation 1 month after exposure significantly suppressed the silica-induced alveolitis, reduced the phospholipid production, and decreased the parenchymal retention of quartz. This study characterizes the phospholipids produced in response to silica exposure.

Silica exposure induced a 200% increase in total phospholipid levels and in each of the lipid components, particularly in phosphatidylglycerol, phosphatidylethanolamine, and phosphatidylinositol. This increase in the production and release of alveolar phospholipids was suppressed by inhalation of aluminum lactate. These alveolar phospholipids are of interest because such molecules may reduce dust toxicity and may have a chemotactic effect on macrophages and other inflammatory effector cells.—M.S. Tockman, M.D., Ph.D.

---

**Collagen Metabolism in Experimental Lung Silicosis: A Trimodal Behavior of Collagenolysis**

Ramos C, Montaño M, González G, Vadillo F, Selman M (Natl Inst of Respiratory Illnesses; Natl Inst of Perinatalogy, Mexico City)

*Lung* 166:347–353, 1988 8–7

---

The pathogenesis of silicosis remains uncertain despite the many studies that focus on the role of inflammatory cells, chiefly macrophages, and the effects of their products on fibroblasts. The content, synthesis, and degradation of collagen were examined in a rat model of silicosis. Intratracheal instillation of silica was carried out at age 8 to 9 weeks, and the animals were studied 7, 15, 30, 45, and 60 days after instillation.

Collagen content and synthesis increased significantly from day 15 onward. Some animals had increased collagenolysis, others had decreased collagen degradation, and a third group had values for collagenolytic activity similar to those of controls. More animals had decreased collagen degradation in the latter part of the course.

Increased collagen in silicotic lungs appears to result from increased biosynthesis and in at least some instances from decreased degradation.

▶ Rather than focus solely on the model of macrophage activation, mediator production, and collagen synthesis, these investigators also examined the contribution of collagen degradation in a rat silicosis model.

Silica instillation produced the expected morphological changes, including peribronchial and perivascular granulomas. Silicotic lung then showed a progressive increment in collagen content. Almost all the experimental animals had increases in collagen synthesis. The authors then expected, from their experience with idiopathic pulmonary fibrosis patients, that diminished collagen degradation would play an important role in the maintenance and progression of fibrosis. Instead, collagenolysis showed a trimodal behavior; some animals had an increased degradation, others had values similar to those of the controls, and others had a decrease of collagenolytic activity. As fibrosis in granulomas progressed, collagen degradation decreased simultaneously in an increasing number of animals. These results suggest that the collagen increase in silicotic lungs results from both a rise in biosynthesis and, at least in some animals, a decrease in degradation. The mechanisms underlying these observations and the reasons for the different rates of collagenolysis have not yet been determined.—M.S. Tockman, M.D., Ph.D.

---

**Generation of Free Radicals From Freshly Fractured Silica Dust: Potential Role in Acute Silica-Induced Lung Injury**

Vallyathan V, Shi X, Dalal NS, Irr W, Castranova V (Natl Inst for Occupational Safety and Health; West Virginia Univ, Morgantown)

*Am Rev Respir Dis* 138:1213–1219, November 1988 8–8

---

Acute silicosis is characterized by the rapid accumulation of granular lipoprotein exudate in the air spaces and the occurrence of respiratory disability within a few years. Is freshly ground silica more surface-reactive or cytotoxic than aged silica? The generation of short-lived silicon-based radicals on freshly ground silica and the release of radical oxygen species were studied via the electron spin resonance approach. Alveolar macrophages were exposed to freshly ground and aged silica, and those

Effect of Grinding Crystalline Silica on the Rate of Lipid Peroxidation and Time-Dependent Loss of Lipid Peroxidation Potential on Storage in Air

| Silica (*mg/ml*) | Malondialdehyde Formation (*μ mol*) Time After Grinding 0–5 min | 24 h | 48 h | 96 h |
|---|---|---|---|---|
| 1.25 | 5.71 ± 0.70 | 4.72 ± 0.55 ($p < 0.03$) | 1.95 ± 0.45 ($p < 0.01$) | 2.03 ± 0.49 ($p < 0.01$) |
| 2.5 | 6.48 ± 0.11 | 4.58 ± 0.36 ($p < 0.01$) | 1.66 ± 0.26 ($p < 0.01$) | 1.43 ± 0.14 ($p < 0.01$) |
| 5.0 | 7.50 ± 0.63 | 4.34 ± 0.32 ($p < 0.01$) | 1.96 ± 0.26 ($p < 0.01$) | 1.54 ± 0.36 ($p < 0.01$) |

*Note:* Data presented are means ± SD of a minimum of 4 sets of experiments in duplicate. *P* values given are for differences compared with values of 0–5 minutes after grinding silica. Each experimental set used the same stock of freshly ground silica at various times after grinding.

(Courtesy of Vallyathan V, Shi X, Dalal NS, et al: *Am Rev Respir Dis* 138:1213–1219, November 1988.)

agents were compared for their effects on release of lactic dehydrogenase by alveolar macrophages and on lipid peroxidation.

Grinding of silica produced silicon-based radicals that interacted with aqueous media to form hydroxyl radicals. The ability of silica to generate hydroxyl radicals in solution declined with a half-life of about 20 hours. Freshly ground silica activated a greater respiratory burst in alveolar macrophages than did aged silica. It also had a greater cytotoxic effect on cell membrane, as exemplified by release of lactic dehydrogenase from macrophages, increased hemolytic activity, and enhanced lipid peroxidation (table).

Freshly ground silica of respirable size contains silicon-based radicals that react in an aqueous environment to produce hydroxyl radicals. Those radicals may have a significant role in damaging cell membranes through initiating lipid peroxidation, which results in acute silicosis. Fresh silica is inhaled in sandblasting, rock drilling, tunneling, and silica flour mill operations.

▶ In contrast to chronic silicosis, little is known about the development of acute silicosis. The authors hypothesized that the qualitatively different acute silicosis response was, at least in part, caused by some unique feature of the inhaled dust. They focused on the unique surface reactivity of freshly sheared silica.

Using electron spin resonance, the authors determined that the fresh grinding of silica generated short-lived silicon-based radicals. The silicon-based radicals react with aqueous media to produce hydroxyl radicals. The concentration of silicon-based radicals in silica decreases with aging in air; the half-life is 30 hours. Upon storage in aqueous media, the ability to generate hydroxyl radicals decreases significantly within minutes. Thus, freshly ground silica is more reactive than aged silica. This was demonstrated by the induction of a greater respiratory burst in alveolar macrophages, leading to lipid peroxidation and the production of superoxide and hydrogen peroxide. Occupations in which freshly fractured crystalline silica of respirable size is generated may produce acute silicosis by such a mechanism.—M.S. Tockman, M.D., Ph.D.

---

**Effects of Buthionine Sulfoximine on the Development of Ozone-Induced Pulmonary Fibrosis**

Sun JD, Pickrell JA, Harkema JR, McLaughlin SI, Hahn FF, Henderson RF (Inhalation Toxicology Research Inst, Albuquerque)

*Exp Mol Pathol* 49:254–266, October 1988 8–9

---

Pulmonary fibrosis may occur when damaged epithelium fails to heal and fibroblasts proliferate through the normally intact epithelium and produce tissue scarring. Reduced glutathione (GSH) may act to neutralize the active oxygen species that damage epithelial cells, and its depletion could delay healing and allow fibrosis to develop. That hypothesis was examined in mice exposed to as much as 1 ppm ozone 23 hours a day for 2 weeks. Subgroups of exposed mice received L-buthionine-*S,R*-sulfoximine (BSO) in drinking water to reduce GSH levels.

The administration of BSO to unexposed mice lowered blood glutamylcysteine synthetase, a regulatory enzyme for GSH biosynthesis, and also lung levels of nonprotein sulfhydryl. Ozone exposure increased blood glutamylcysteine synthetase activity and lung levels of nonprotein sulfhydryl in a concentration-dependent manner. The increases were less marked in BSO-treated mice. Ozone produced an inflammatory response, but no signs of developing fibrosis were evident. Modest evidence of fibrosis was present 90 days later in mice exposed to 1 ppm ozone and not given BSO. Treatment with BSO after ozone exposure enhanced pulmonary fibrosis.

Suppression of GSH biosynthesis worsens pulmonary fibrosis in mice exposed to ozone for 2 weeks. Further work is needed to determine specifically how GSH can protect the lungs from fibrosis.

▶ This paper represents an interesting manipulation of reduced glutathione levels in rodents exposed to an ozone challenge. By exposing mice with an inhibited ability to synthesize GSH in response to ozone, the investigators observed an increased degree of pulmonary fibrosis compared with nontreated, ozone-challenged controls.

Buthionine-*S,R,*-sulfoximine (BSO) inhibits glutamylcysteine synthetase, the regulatory enzyme for GSH biosynthesis. The authors had demonstrated previously that the addition of BSO to the drinking water of mice results in a reduction of lung tissue GSH by 50%. As might be expected, at the end of the 1-ppm ozone exposure, BSO-treated mice had lungs with evidence of an acute inflammatory response. Bronchiolar walls were thickened from edema, an influx of neutrophils and a moderate accumulation of macrophages. Continued BSO treatment, however, caused progression to fibrosis. The absence of evidence for increased collagen content in the fibrotic lungs led to the conclusion that a remodeling of lung collagen had occurred. The mechanism by which GSH depletion might have led to a collagen remodeling is unclear.—M.S. Tockman, M.D., Ph.D.

## New Insights Into Lung Cancer

### Covalent DNA Damage in Tissues of Cigarette Smokers as Determined by $^{32}$P-Postlabeling Assay

Randerath E, Miller RH, Mittal D, Avitts TA, Dunsford HA, Randerath K (Baylor College of Medicine, Houston; Tulane Univ, New Orleans; Univ of Texas Med Branch, Galveston)

*J Natl Cancer Inst* 81:341–347, March 1, 1989 8–10

The DNA addition products, or DNA adducts, formed during DNA damage associated with the covalent binding of carcinogens to cellular DNA may provide insight into the mechanisms of action of genotoxicants. A highly sensitive phosphorus 32-postlabeling assay was used for DNA adduct analysis to study the damage done by cigarette smoke in tissues of smokers. Nontumorous tissues were taken from areas near lung

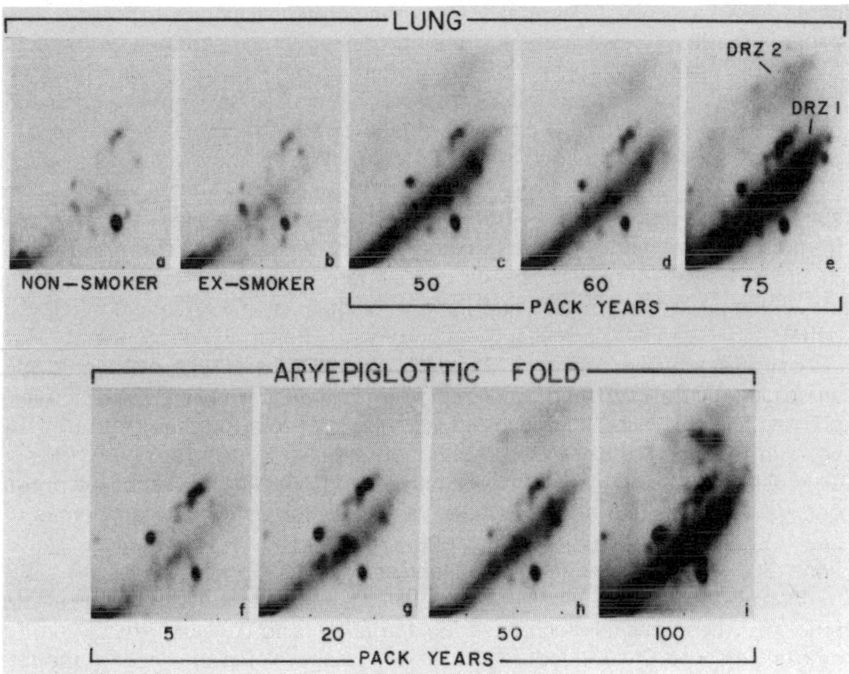


**Fig 8–4.**—Autoradiographic profiles of covalent DNA lesions in smokers' lungs and larynges, as determined with $^{32}$P-postlabeling. DNA (10 μg) from nontumorous surgical specimens of patients with cancer of the lung or larynx was analyzed. Labeled adducts were separated by anion-exchange thin-layer chromatography on polyethyleneimine-cellulose layers in 2 directions in solvent I (from bottom to top) and solvent II (from left to right) and located by screen-enhanced autoradiography. A nonsmoker control sample (**a**) had background spots that were also present in the smokers' samples. Diagonal radioactive zones DRZ 1 and DRZ 2 (**e**) were detected in all smokers' specimens. Low levels of DRZ 2 adducts not seen in panels **b** and **f** were detected on > 18-hr film exposure (not shown). (Courtesy of Randerath E, Miller RH, Mittal D, et al: *J Natl Cancer Inst* 81:341–347, March 1, 1989.)

and laryngeal tumors during cancer surgery in 18 patients. Three autopsies were included in the study.

Multiple DNA adducts occurred in a dose- and time-dependent manner in the lung, bronchus, and larynx of smokers with cancer of those organs (Fig 8–4). Levels of adducts declined only slowly after cessation of smoking, and low levels persisted for up to 14 years in the lungs of ex-smokers with a history of high exposure. In autopsy samples, smoking-associated DNA lesions were found in the lungs and heart and to a lesser extent in the kidneys, bladder, esophagus, aorta, and liver.

Epidemiologic data indicating that lung cancer risk increases with the duration and intensity of smoking and declines only slowly after smoking ceases were corroborated. Smoking-induced DNA damage probably contributes to smoking-related degenerative changes in the lungs and heart.

▶ Deoxyribonucleic acid addition products (DNA adducts) formed by the covalent binding of carcinogens or their metabolites to cellular DNA have been evaluated as a molecular dosimeter for environmental carcinogen exposure. This paper is the first to evaluate actual genetic damage in smokers' target organs. Cigarette smoke is a complex mixture of more than 3,800 chemicals. The postlabeling assay is well suited to look for smoking-induced covalent DNA damage because it does not require prior knowledge of the specific DNA-reactive carcinogens or their metabolites.

The postlabeling adduct profile for cigarette-induced DNA damage provided a specific "fingerprint." The smoking-associated adduct profiles were distinct from those detected in the white blood cells of foundry workers or in experimental animals treated with specific carcinogens, but were qualitatively similar for all human tissues investigated (lung, bronchus, larynx) and were similar to patterns in mice after dermal application of cigarette smoke condensate.

Tissue DNA adduct levels for 21 surgical specimens of lung, bronchus, and aryepiglottic fold correlated well with the degree of smoking exposure expressed as pack years. Low levels of adducts appeared to persist for up to 14 years in the lungs of ex-smokers with high previous exposures. Deoxyribonucleic acid adduction is known to be associated with the activation of proto-oncogenes (Ki-ras activation has been described for lung adenocarcinomas of heavy smokers). In addition to oncogene activation, smoking-induced mutations also may be involved in the inactivation of the cancer-suppressing RB (retinoblastoma) gene in small-cell lung cancer, known to be related to cigarette smoking. These observations have led the authors to conclude that cigarette smoking-induced DNA adduct formation is causally related to cancer in the target organs.—M.S. Tockman, M.D., Ph.D.

---

**Cigarette Smoking and Lung Cancer: Reanalysis of the British Doctors' Data**

Moolgavkar SH, Dewanji A, Luebeck G (Fred Hutchinson Cancer Research Ctr, Seattle)

*J Natl Cancer Inst* 81:415–420, March 15, 1989 8–11

---

The British doctors' study is a relatively precise and complete prospective study of smoking-related disease. A mathematical formulation of the recessive oncogenesis model, which posits that inactivation of both alleles of specific genes leads to cancer, was fitted to lung cancer incidence data from the British doctors' study. The model described the data well. Data were analyzed for men aged 40–79 years who either were nonsmokers or regularly smoked up to 40 cigarettes a day.

The chief questions in tobacco carcinogenesis deal with the issue of dose-response (Fig 8–5). For a given level of smoking, the incidence rate of lung cancer at age 60 depends to a substantial degree on the age at which smoking began. Age is independent of the duration of smoking in determining the lung cancer risk in smokers. The predicted risk for ex-smokers continues to increase.

The 2-stage model that fits these data best is one in which the effect of cigarette smoke on the kinetics of growth of intermediate cells is negligi-

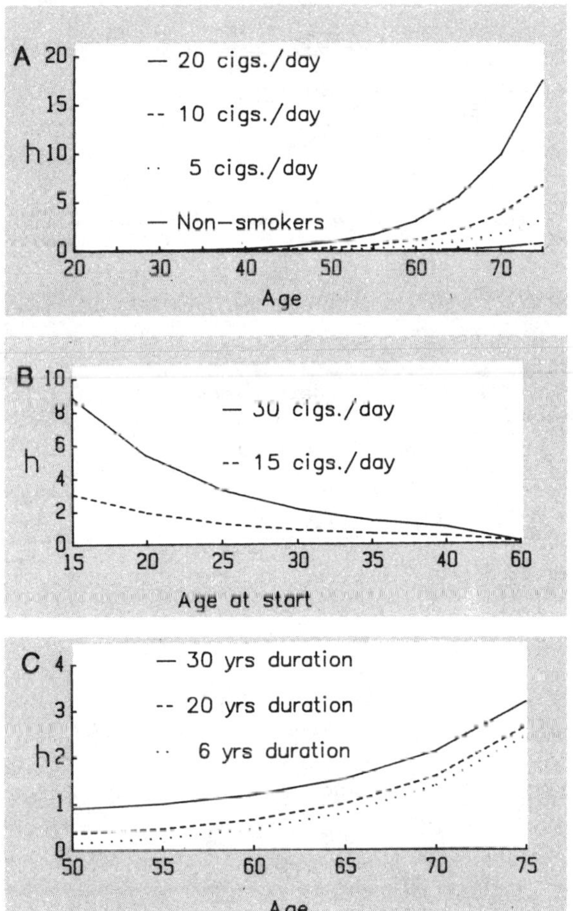


**Fig 8–5.—A,** plot of age-specific incidence rates of lung cancer among nonsmokers and smokers as predicted by the model. **B–E,** different perspectives on dose-response. *(Continued on p 332.)*

ble. A better idea of the importance of mutation rates and the rate of intermediate cell growth would be gained by simultaneously analyzing data for ex-smokers.

▶ Doll and Peto (1) reported from their British doctor's study that lung cancer risk was proportional to the fourth or fifth power of (t − 22.5), where t is age measured in years, and the second power of the number of cigarettes smoked per day. This observation has led to the conclusion that the duration of smoking is more important than the number of cigarettes smoked per day (daily dose of cigarettes). The authors of the present report analyzed the British doctors' data within the framework of the 2-mutation, "recessive oncogenesis" model of Knudson (2). From this reanalysis, they concluded that age has a large influence on lung cancer risk among smokers even after smoking duration is con-

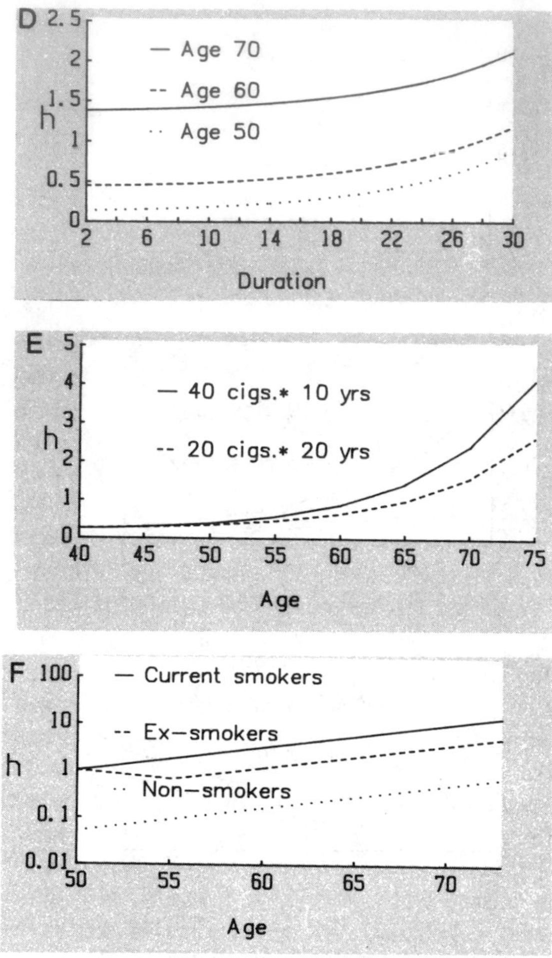


**Fig 8–5, cont.—F,** semilogarithmic plot of predicted age-specific incidence among nonsmokers, continuing smokers (20 cigarettes/day), and smokers quitting at age 50. *h,* lung cancer incidence/1,000 persons. (Courtesy of Moolgavkar SH, Dewanji A, Luebeck G: *J Natl Cancer Inst* 81:415–420, March 15, 1989.)

sidered, and that daily dose of smoking is as important to lung cancer risk as smoking duration.

The 2-mutation model incorporates 2 features: (1) transition of target stem cells into cancer cells via an intermediate stage in 2 rate-limiting mutations of the genome, and (2) growth and differentiation of normal target and intermediate cells. The 2 rate-limiting steps may be identified with mutations that lead to homozygous loss of antioncogene function. The association of allele loss with chromosome regions harboring recessive oncogenes has been demonstrated for retinoblastoma, Wilms' tumor, colorectal carcinoma, and most recently, lung cancer as well (3).

The value of this paper is the opportunity it provides to rethink the dose-response vs. duration effect of smoking on lung cancer. Determination of which of several possible models is correct must await analysis of the lung cancer incidence rates in ex-smokers.—M.S. Tockman, M.D., Ph.D.

*References*


1. Doll R, Peto R: Cigarette smoking and bronchial carcinoma: Dose and time relationships among regular smokers and life-long nonsmokers. *J Epidemiol Community Health* 32:303–313, 1978.
2. Knudson AG Jr: Mutation and cancer: Statistical study of retinoblastoma. *Proc Natl Acad Sci USA* 68:820–823, 1971.
3. Takahashi T, Nau MM, Chiba I, et al: p53: A frequent target for genetic abnormalities in lung cancer. *Science* 246:491–494, 1989.


**Smoking and Lung Cancer in Women: Findings in a Prospective Study**

Garfinkel L, Stellman SD (American Cancer Society, New York)

*Cancer Res* 48:6951–6955, Dec 1, 1988 8–12

Although past studies of lung cancer showed much lower relative risk ratios for women than for men, smoking patterns of women have changed and women—especially those aged more than 50 years—now are exposed much more than in the past. Lung cancer rates in relation to smoking habits were reviewed in a cohort of 619,225 women followed up from 1982 to 1986. There were 1,006 lung cancer deaths in this population.

Standardized mortality ratios (SMRs) were 12.7 for current smokers

Observed and Expected Lung Cancer Deaths and SMRs Among Women With No History of Chronic Illness, According to Number of Cigarettes/Day Currently Smoked and Number of Years of Smoking Habit

| Duration of smoking habit (yr) | No. of cigarettes/day, current smokers | | | | |
|---|---|---|---|---|---|
| | 1–10 | 11–19 | 20 | 21–30 | 31+ |
| 21–30 | | | | | |
| O[a] | 3 | 3 | 16 | 9 | 7 |
| E | 1.0 | 0.4 | 1.2 | 0.5 | 0.4 |
| SMR | 2.9 | 6.7 | 13.6 | 18.4 | 18.9 |
| 31–40 | | | | | |
| O | 18 | 22 | 59 | 36 | 27 |
| E | 2.3 | 1.1 | 3.1 | 1.4 | 1.1 |
| SMR | 7.9 | 19.2 | 19.2 | 26.5 | 25.3 |
| 41–70 | | | | | |
| O | 29 | 23 | 83 | 36 | 30 |
| E | 2.9 | 1.4 | 3.3 | 1.0 | 0.8 |
| SMR | 10.0 | 17.0 | 25.1 | 34.3 | 38.8 |

[a]O, observed; *E*, expected (based on age-specific rates in nonsmoking women).
(Courtesy of Garfinkel L, Stellman SD: *Cancer Res* 48:6951–6955, Dec 1, 1988.)

and 4.8 for ex-smokers. Current smokers without a history of chronic disease had SMRs of 17.6. Mortality ratios increased with the number of cigarettes smoked each day and with the depth of inhalation, independent of the number of cigarettes smoked. Mortality ratios also increased with the duration of smoking (table) and declined after smoking stopped.

More lung cancer deaths are occurring as women begin smoking earlier in life, smoke more, and inhale more deeply. Current SMRs for women are similar in magnitude to those seen for men in the past. Nevertheless, a fall in rates is starting to appear in younger women, as in men, and it is hoped that lung cancer rates will decline markedly as more smokers quit.

▶ Studies of lung cancer in the 1960s and 1970s showed that smoking was associated with a much lower risk in women than in men. The major reason for the sex difference in the risk of smoking was a lower lifetime exposure to cigarettes among women. Women in those studies started smoking later in life, smoked fewer cigarettes per day, and inhaled less deeply than men.

Over the 26 years since the first studies, the age-standardized lung cancer rate in female nonsmokers has remained the same. However, the lung cancer standardized mortality ratio for female smokers has increased to become equivalent to those of men in the prospective studies carried out in the 1960s and 1970s. The age at which women began smoking decreased 8–10 years, the proportion of 1-pack-per-day smokers rose 20% and the index of inhalation was higher at each age. The observed increases in lung cancer risk related to these dosage factors clearly outweighed the much smaller beneficial effect of reduced tar and nicotine yield in cigarettes over the same period.

The optimistic side of the data is that a sufficiently large number of younger women have quit so that the lung cancer rates for women aged less than 45 years are beginning to fall and there is a leveling off of rates for women aged 45 to 54 years. This effect also has been seen for younger men.—M.S. Tockman, M.D., Ph.D.

---

**Reduction in Risk of Lung Cancer Among Ex-Smokers With Particular Reference to Histologic Type**

Higgins IT, Wynder EL (American Health Found, New York)

*Cancer* 62:2397–2401, Dec 1, 1988 8–13

---

The risk of lung cancer declines when smoking stops, but how does the risk reduction depend on the duration of cessation and the amount of smoking that took place? Data from patients with histologic diagnoses of lung cancer at 26 hospitals in 6 cities in the United States were reviewed. Controls were matched with the patients for age, sex, race, time of diagnosis, and hospital. There were 534 ex-smokers among 2,085 male lung cancer patients and 1,106 ex-smokers among 3,948 controls. For women, there were 195 ex-smokers among 1,012 patients and 394 among 1,819 controls.

The lung cancer risk declined with the number of years of cessation for both men and women. Among women the risk was higher for those who had quit for 30 years compared with those stopping for a shorter time, but this might have been the result of small numbers. Among men, the decline in risk with an increasing time of cessation was consistent within each category of smoking, with certain exceptions. The risk for those quitting for only 1 to 4 years was similar to that for continuing smokers or even slightly greater. The cancer risk was greater for those with Kreyberg I than those with Kreyberg II cancers, and the risk decline with time of cessation was more consistent for the former type. Women had a higher proportion of Kreyberg II to Kreyberg I tumors.

Those who stop smoking retain a lung cancer risk appreciably greater than that for persons who have never smoked, even after 20 to 30 years of cessation. It is never too late to stop, however; even the heaviest smokers will have a lower risk of lung cancer after having stopped.

▶ Cases of lung cancer have been classified into 2 histologic types: Kreyberg I includes primarily squamous cell, small cell and large cell types; Kreyberg II consists primarily of the adenocarcinomas. This paper reports the common observation of a more frequent occurrence of Kreyberg II (adenocarcinoma) lung cancer in women. Analysis by histologic type showed that, for both sexes, cigarette smoking was associated with a greater risk for Kreyberg I types of lung cancer. The decline in risk with number of years of smoking cessation was more consistent for Kreyberg I lung cancer. The authors conclude that the weaker relationship between Kreyberg II cancers and cigarette smoking plus the greater frequency of Kreyberg II cancers among women are likely to be responsible for the less consistent association of decline in lung cancer risk with years of smoking cessation observed in women than in men.

Unfortunately, the risk of lung cancer persists longer than previously thought, with a twofold to fourfold excess lung cancer risk persisting 20–30 years after cessation. Nevertheless, the greatest improvement occurs after the first 5 years of cessation even in the heaviest smoking categories. It is never too late to stop smoking.—M.S. Tockman, M.D., Ph.D.

---

**Biochemical Validation of Self-Reported Exposure to Environmental Tobacco Smoke**

Haley NJ, Colosimo SG, Axelrad CM, Harris R, Sepkovic DW (American Health Found, Valhalla, NY, and New York)

*Environ Res* 49:127–135, June 1989 8–14

---

The correlation between self-reported exposure to environmental tobacco smoke and urinary cotinine levels was studied in 148 men and 112 women with respective mean ages of 39 and 35 years. Questions were asked about smoke exposure at home, at work, in social circumstances, and during transportation.

Both men and women who reported being exposed to smoke on social occasions had higher urinary cotinine levels than those who responded negatively. Levels also were increased in those reporting that they lived with a smoker. Smoke exposure at home was the most prominent factor in increased cotinine levels for both men and women. For those exposed at work only, the reported degree of exposure correlated well with urinary cotinine values.

Validation of exposure status using a biologic maker is necessary for reliable epidemiologic studies of passive smoking. Studies correlating urinary cotinine levels with perceived smoke exposure before and after worksite restrictions are implemented will help in assessing those measures.

▶ Cotinine, a major metabolite of nicotine, currently is thought to be the best marker of tobacco exposure through active inhalation (1). It is of great interest that, among nonsmokers, urinary cotinine is also an effective biologic marker for the modest levels of environmental tobacco smoke encountered by passive smokers. The results of this study show that people who work or reside with smokers have significantly higher levels of urinary cotinine than those who do not work or live with smokers. Thus, it seems reasonable to agree that urinary cotinine can be used as a direct assessment of environmental exposure to tobacco smoke and can validate self-reported exposure data. If a quantitative estimate of tobacco smoke exposure is desired, normalization against creatinine is necessary. However, creatinine normalization does not remove sex differences. Overall, the women in this study had significantly higher levels of cotinine in urine than did the men after urinary creatinine normalization. Therefore, comparisons of environmental tobacco smoke exposures that depend on urinary cotinine must be sex-specific.

The author clearly points out, however, that this biomarker measures only indirectly the potential health risk associated with environmental tobacco smoke. The physicochemical properties of environmental tobacco smoke are quite different from those of inhaled mainstream smoke. It would be inappropriate to extrapolate either lung cancer or cardiovascular risk based on urinary cotinine estimates of tobacco smoke exposure.—M.S. Tockman, M.D., Ph.D.

*Reference*

1. Haley NJ, Axelrad CM, Tilton KA: Validation of self-reported smoking behavior: Biochemical analyses of cotinine and thiocyanate. *Am J Public Health* 93:1204–1207, 1983.

---

**Indoor Radon Exposure and Active and Passive Smoking in Relation to the Occurrence of Lung Cancer**

Axelson O, Andersson K, Desai G, Fagerlund I, Jansson B, Karlsson C, Wingren G (Univ Hosp, Linköping, Sweden; Örebro Med Ctr Hosp, Örebro, Sweden; County Council of Skaraborg, Skövde, Sweden)

*Scand J Work Environ Health* 14:286–292, October 1988 8–15

---

Concern that exposure to indoor radon and radon daughters may cause lung cancer is supported by several trials. However, most have rel-

Lung Cancer Patients and Referents According to Exposure Categories and Sex, 1960–1981

| Sex | Exposure category[a] | | | |
|---|---|---|---|---|
| | 0 | 1 | 2 | 1+2 |
| Male | | | | |
| Cases | 27 | 46 | 52 | 98 |
| Referents | 120 | 131 | 128 | 259 |
| Female | | | | |
| Cases | 16 | 16 | 20 | 36 |
| Referents | 113 | 93 | 88 | 181 |
| Total | | | | |
| Cases | 43 | 62 | 72 | 134 |
| Referents | 233 | 224 | 216 | 440 |
| Crude rate ratio | 1.0 | 1.5 | 1.8 | 1.7 |
| Mantel-Haenszel rate ratio | 1.0 | 1.4 | 1.7 | 1.6 |
| 90 % confidence interval | | 1.0—2.1 | 1.2—2.5 | 1.1—2.2 |

Mantel extension chi-square: 6.33

[a]Category 0, reference, i.e., wooden houses without a basement on normal ground; 1, all types of houses not classed as 0 or 2; 2, wooden houses with basements on radiation ground or stone, brick, and plaster houses with basements on any ground, alternatively without a basement on radiation ground.

(Courtesy of Axelson O, Andersson K, Desai G, et al: *Scand J Work Environ Health* 14:286–292, October 1988.)

atively small numbers of participants or are weak in their assessment of exposure. A trial without these methodologic weaknesses was done to evaluate the risk of indoor radon and radon daughter exposure in 177 patients with lung cancer and 677 without cancer. The particpants were all deceased, and all had 30 years or more of residency in the same house in an area with radon-leaking alum shale deposits in the central part of southern Sweden. Exposure categories were defined by building material, type of house, and ground conditions, and measurements of the indoor radon daughter concentration were obtained for 142 patients and 264 referents. Active and passive smoking behaviors were determined through questionnaires sent to next-of-kin.

Overall, the lung cancer risk was about twofold greater for the persons in categories of assumed radon daughter exposure in the rural sector of the population but not for the same categories of the urban sector, possibly because of less precise exposure evaluation and influence from other factors (table). Both occasional and passive smokers and passive smokers alone had a higher risk of lung cancer associated with the increased exposure categories.

These data and findings from other trials suggest that the risk of lung cancer may double because of an elevation above the unavoidable background of indoor radon daughter levels. Indoor radon daughter exposure at unavoidable levels might have some role in the cause of lung cancer. Further tests are needed to help define the risk of lung cancer from indoor radon.

▶ Approximately a twofold risk of lung cancer was found for those with radon daughter exposure in a rural region of Sweden. Similar exposure categories of the urban population did not show a similar level of risk, perhaps because of less precise exposure estimates or the effects of other covariates, primarily smoking. The primary problem with such studies is accurate estimation of radon dose. This study actually made measurements of radon exposure in 80% of the lung cancer case homes and 38% of controls.—M.S. Tockman, M.D., Ph.D.

---

**Lung Cancer Mortality Among Nonsmoking Uranium Miners Exposed to Radon Daughters**

Roscoe RJ, Steenland K, Halperin WE, Beaumont JJ, Waxweiler RJ (Natl Inst for Occupational Safety and Health, Cincinnati; Ctrs for Disease Control, Atlanta; Harvard School of Public Health, Boston; Univ of California, Davis)
*JAMA* 262:629–633, Aug 4, 1989 8–16

---

Exposure to radon daughters is associated with lung cancer, but the cancer risk from such exposure in the absence of cigarette smoking has proved difficult to assess. Risk estimates were made for 516 white men from the U.S. Public Health Service cohort of Colorado Plateau uranium miners, followed up from 1950 through 1984, who had never smoked cigarettes, cigars, or pipes. Mortality data from nonsmoking U.S. veterans were used for comparison.

Fourteen men died of lung cancer among the nonsmoking miners, with 1.1 deaths expected. The standardized mortality ratio was 12.7 with 95% confidence limits of 8.0 and 20.1. Also, 8 men died as a result of nonmalignant respiratory diseases, with 0.68 expected. Three of those deaths were caused by silicosis; 3, by chronic obstructive lung disease; and 1 each by pulmonary fibrosis and emphysema.

Nonsmoking uranium miners have a substantially increased risk of dying of lung cancer. Exposure to radon daughters is itself a potent carcinogen that must be strictly controlled.

▶ An overall lung cancer standardized mortality ratio of 12.7 (95% confidence interval, 8.0–20.1) is reported for white, male, lifetime nonsmoking uranium miners. The observation is striking because the magnitude of risk encountered by these miners after a median exposure of 296 working level months (WLM; mean, 720 WLM) is comparable to that experienced by smokers of 1 pack of cigarettes per day. Essentially all of this risk seems to be encountered at exposure levels greater than 465 WLM. However, the small number of deaths (14 observed, 1.1 expected) and small denominator (7,861 person-years) gave only a small power (12%) to detect lung cancer risks as low as 2.0.—M.S. Tockman, M.D., Ph.D.

## Pulmonary Effects of Air Pollution

**Respiratory Disease Associated With Community Air Pollution and a Steel Mill, Utah Valley**

Pope CA III (Brigham Young Univ, Provo, Utah)

*Am J Public Health* 79:623–628, May 1989 8–17

In 1984, the Environmental Protection Agency proposed that total suspended particulates be replaced by a new indicator of particulate pollution including only those particulates having an aerodynamic diameter of 10 μm or less ($PM_{10}$). In 1987 the total suspended particulate standards were replaced by a 24-hour $PM_{10}$ standard of 150 $\mu g/m^3$ with no more than 1 measurement in excess expected per year and an annual $PM_{10}$ standard of an expected arithmetic mean of 50 $\mu g/m^3$.

Hospital admissions were correlated with $PM_{10}$ in Utah Valley during a 3-year period when a local steel mill was closed and reopened. The mill was the chief industrial source of fine particulate pollution in the area. Elevated $PM_{10}$ levels were associated with hospital admissions for pneumonia, pleurisy, bronchitis, and asthma (table). Admissions of children nearly tripled in months when the 24-hour $PM_{10}$ exceeded 150$\mu g/m^3$. Particulate levels when the mill was open were nearly double those found when the mill was closed. On regression analysis, $PM_{10}$ levels correlated most closely with admissions of children and with admissions for bronchitis and asthma.

Hospital admissions for respiratory illness correlated closely with $PM_{10}$ levels. The close association is partly because $PM_{10}$ is a better indicator of particulate pollution than previous indicators. In addition, when relatively few persons in the population being studied smoke, particulate pollution is a relatively large contributor to respiratory disease.

▶ "Particulates" may include a variety of chemically and physically diverse substances that exist in the atmosphere as discrete particles. As noted by the *Indoor Air Quality Environmental Information Handbook: Combustion Sources*, "Particulates present a risk to health out of proportion to their concentration in the atmosphere because they deliver a high-concentration package of potentially harmful substances" (U.S. Dept of Energy, 1985; DOE/EV10450-1, National Technical Information Service, U.S. Dept. of Commerce, Springfield, Va). Particulate effect is determined by both particle size, which affects location and magnitude of deposition in the respiratory tract, and chemical composition, which determines health effects of the deposited particles.

The *Indoor Air Quality Environmental Information Handbook* summarizes the major effects of concern attributed to particle exposure as (1) impairment of respiratory mechanics; (2) aggravation of existing respiratory and cardiovascular disease; (3) reduction in particle clearance and other host defense mechanisms; (4) morphological alterations; (5) carcinogenesis; and (6) mortality from respiratory infections, cancer, or heart failure.

This report by Pope is one of the first examinations of the association be-

Comparisons of Hospital Impatient Admissions for Utah Valley Regional Medical Center and American Fork Hospital Across Time Periods With Geneva Steel Mill Open and Closed

| Year | Steel Mill Open? | Mean $PM_{10}$ Level for Months Included | Mean High $PM_{10}$ Level for Months Included | Bronchitis and Asthma Ages 0–17 | Bronchitis and Asthma Age 18+ | Simple Pneumonia and Pleurisy Ages 0–17 | Simple Pneumonia and Pleurisy Age 18+ | Subtotal Ages 0–17 | Subtotal Age 18+ | TOTAL |
|---|---|---|---|---|---|---|---|---|---|---|
| Winter Months (December–February) | | | | | | | | | | |
| 1985/86 | yes | 90 | 235 | 78 | 75 | 76 | 73 | 154 | 148 | 302 |
| 1986/87 | no | 51 | 96 | 23 | 67 | 32 | 83 | 55 | 150 | 205 |
| 1987/88 | yes | 84 | 177 | 78 | 65 | 71 | 126 | 149 | 191 | 340 |
| Fall Months (September–November) | | | | | | | | | | |
| 1985 | yes | 35 | 63 | 49 | 46 | 20 | 51 | 69 | 97 | 166 |
| 1986 | no | 31 | 47 | 23 | 48 | 25 | 60 | 48 | 108 | 156 |
| 1987 | yes | 47 | 83 | 55 | 46 | 24 | 66 | 79 | 112 | 191 |
| Fall and Winter (September–February) | | | | | | | | | | |
| 1985/86 | yes | 63 | 149 | 127 | 121 | 96 | 124 | 223 | 245 | 468 |
| 1986/87 | no | 41 | 71 | 46 | 115 | 57 | 143 | 103 | 258 | 361 |
| 1987/88 | yes | 66 | 130 | 133 | 111 | 95 | 192 | 228 | 303 | 531 |

(Courtesy of Pope CA III: *Am J Public Health* 79:623–628, May 1989.)

tween health effects and the new National Ambient Air Quality Standard (NAAQS) for particulate pollution. Pope demonstrated a convincing association between elevation of fine particulate pollution (particulates with an aerodynamic diameter ≤10 micrometers, $PM_{10}$) and hospital admissions for pneumonia, pleurisy, bronchitis, and asthma, especially among children. The author suggests that the strength of this association may be explained (at least, in part) because $PM_{10}$ is a better indicator of particulate pollution as it relates to respiratory health than previously used indicators. However, insofar as the health effects of particulates depend primarily on their chemical nature, the absence of information regarding either the nature of the pollutant compound or its acidity are critical limitations of this study. The degree to which sulfates or other acid aerosols may have been present to condense on the fine particulates for transport deep into the parenchyma is unknown. It is unlikely, for example, that the observed health effects would have resulted from inhalation of similar quantities of respirable inert dust.—M.S. Tockman, M.D., Ph.D.

---

**Respiratory Health of a Population Living Downwind From Natural Gas Refineries**

Dales RE, Spitzer WO, Suissa S, Schechter MT, Tousignant P, Steinmetz N (McGill Univ, Montreal; Univ of Ottawa; Univ of British Columbia, Vancouver)
*Am Rev Respir Dis* 139:595–600, March 1989 8–18

---

Natural gas refineries in Alberta release mainly sulfur dioxide but also hydrogen sulfide into the atmosphere. Since the late 1950s excessive illness has been perceived in a rural Canadian population living downwind of 2 such refineries. A health survey undertaken in 1985 included 2,157 persons in the exposed population and 839 reference subjects.

More respiratory symptoms were reported by exposed persons in the

---

Probability of Respiratory Symptom Reporting and Physiologic Impairment as a Function of Total Sulfation Levels in the Index Area

| | Children | | | Adults | | |
|---|---|---|---|---|---|---|
| | Odds Ratio* | 95% CI | p Value | Odds Ratio | 95% CI | p Value |
| Symptom | | | | | | |
| Persistent cough | 1.31 | 1.14–1.51 | 0.000 | 1.00 | 0.88–1.14 | 0.987 |
| Persistent phlegm | 1.31 | 1.13–1.52 | 0.000 | 0.97 | 0.86–1.10 | 0.662 |
| Dyspnea | 1.10 | 0.82–1.48 | 0.523 | 0.89 | 0.74–1.08 | 0.244 |
| Wheeze | 1.18 | 1.03–1.35 | 0.019 | 0.98 | 0.89–1.08 | 0.667 |
| Wheeze with dyspnea | 1.10 | 0.96–1.27 | 0.172 | 1.00 | 0.90–1.10 | 0.991 |
| Lower 10th centile of function | | | | | | |
| $FEV_1$ | 1.03 | 0.82–1.30 | 0.454 | 0.97 | 0.84–1.13 | 0.694 |
| FVC | 0.65 | 0.38–1.19 | 0.075 | 0.93 | 0.80–1.09 | 0.380 |
| MMEFR | 1.18 | 0.97–1.43 | 0.837 | 0.93 | 0.79–1.10 | 0.408 |

*Abbreviations: $FEV_1$*, forced expiratory volume in 1 second; *FVC*, forced vital capacity; *MMEFR*, maximal midexpiratory flow rate.

*For every 10 mg/100 $cm^2$/day × 1,000 increase in total sulfation, there was a relative increase in the adjusted odds (indicated in column) of reporting the symptom or being in the lower 10th centile of function (indicated in rows).

(Courtesy of Dales RE, Spitzer WO, Suissa S, et al: *Am Rev Respir Dis* 139:595–600, March 1989.)

age range 5 to 13 years and among never-smokers aged 14 and older. Lung function values were similar for the 2 populations. In the area of exposure there tended to be more respiratory symptoms in younger than in older persons. Logistic regression analysis confirmed a lack of significant correlation between respiratory symptoms and reduced lung function (table).

Long-term exposure to emissions of gas refineries has effects similar to those of other sulfur-containing forms of pollution. Future studies of environmental pollution should include, in addition to objective measures of respiratory disease, methods of assessing those psychological factors that might influence symptom reporting.

▶ The *Indoor Air Quality* (IAQ) *Environmental Information Handbook* describes sulfur dioxide ($SO_2$) as an irritant that is known to cause significant bronchoconstriction in exercising asthmatic persons at concentrations of about 0.25 to 0.50 ppm. Otherwise, $SO_2$ has no direct health effects on healthy persons at concentrations currently encountered in the United States. Sulfur dioxide, however, dissolves rapidly in water to form sulfurous acid, which oxidizes to sulfuric acid, which in turn reacts with many substances to form particulate sulfates. Roughly 20% of atmospheric particles, 5 μm or less in diameter, are sulfates (U.S. Dept of Energy, 1985; DOE/EV10450-1, National Technical Information Service, U.S. Dept. of Commerce, Springfield, Va).

Toxicity of $SO_2$ and particulate sulfates have been described in the *IAQ Environmental Information Handbook* as airway inflammation primarily due to (1) direct acidic trauma to the airways; (2) acid-related increased permeability of the upper airway lining mucosa leading to increase toxic gas absorption; and (3) direct toxicity of cations in the sulfates. There is no national ambient air quality standard (NAAQS) for acid aerosols; however, the particles of concern within the aerosol are subject to regulation under the $PM_{10}$ NAAQS.

Elevations of ambient $SO_2$ most often are caused by large point sources that burn fossil fuels. The present study by Dales and colleagues describes a survey of health effects downwind from 2 natural gas refineries emitting primarily $SO_2$. Unfortunately, the reported measures of total sulfation (deposition of sulfur-containing products) cannot be converted directly to atmospheric levels, making difficult any generalization of the response to this level of exposure. Nevertheless, the observations of symptoms among children, but not among adults, without physiologic changes are consistent with the authors' hypothesis that exposure to gas refinery emissions has mild physiologic effects similar to other sulfur-containing pollution.—M.S. Tockman, M.D., Ph.D.

---

**Cell Response in Bronchoalveolar Lavage Fluid After Sulfur Dioxide Exposure**

Sandström T, Stjernberg N, Andersson M-C, Kolmodin-Hedman B, Lindström K, Rosenhall L (Univ Hosp, Umeå; Natl Inst of Occupational Health, Umeå, Sweden)

*Scand J Work Environ Health* 15:142–146, 1989 8–19

---

The dose-response relationship between brief exposure to sulfur dioxide and inflammatory response in the lungs was examined in 22 healthy nonsmoking men aged 22–37 years. The men were exposed to $SO_2$ levels of 10 to 30 $mg/m^3$ (4 to 11 ppm) for 20 minutes. Bronchoalveolar lavage was done at least 2 weeks before exposure and was repeated 24 hours afterward.

Mast cells, lymphocytes, and macrophages all were increased significantly after $SO_2$ exposure, as was the subset of lysozyme-positive macrophages. A dose-dependent increase in cellular response was noted after exposure to 10 to 20 $mg/m^3$, but no greater response was seen after 30 $mg/m^3$. Small, insignificant reductions in forced expiratory volume in 1 second followed exposure to $SO_2$; respiratory symptoms were not significant.

An inflammatory response takes place in the lungs at levels of $SO_2$ exposure that occur in indoor industrial environments worldwide. Inflammation occurs with levels below the short-term exposure limit prevailing in Sweden and many other countries (13 $mg/m^3$). Repeated exposure to $SO_2$ may be an important factor in the increased morbidity from chronic lung disease in exposed workers.

▶ In this report, the authors have found enhanced concentrations of inflammatory cells (alveolar macrophages, mast cells, and lymphocytes) in the bronchoalveolar lavage fluid of healthy, nonsmoking volunteers exposed to $SO_2$ at concentrations as low as 10 $mg/m^3$. This concentration is approximately 30 times greater than the National Ambient Air Quality Standard, but it is below the 13 $mg/m^3$ accepted as the short-term exposure limit in Sweden and several other countries. Although a 10-year study of paper workers in New Hampshire showed no increase in mortality from either respiratory or other diseases (1), Sandstrom and co-workers in the present study question the safety of the short-term exposure limit for $SO_2$.—M.S. Tockman, M.D., Ph.D.

*Reference*

1. Ferris BG Jr et al: *Br J Ind Med* 36:127, 1979.

**Short-Term Exposure to Nitrogen Dioxide Enhances Susceptibility to Murine Respiratory Mycoplasmosis and Decreases Intrapulmonary Killing of *Mycoplasma pulmonis***

Parker RF, Davis JK, Cassell GH, White H, Dziedzic D, Blalock DK, Thorp RB, Simecka JW (Univ of Alabama, Birmingham)

*Am Rev Respir Dis* 140:502–512, August 1989 8–20

Circumstantial epidemiologic data indicate that inhaled pollutants—especially oxidants such as $NO_2$—enhance the development of respiratory diseases caused by infectious agents. The effects of $NO_2$ on susceptibility to murine respiratory mycoplasmosis (MRM) was studied in strains of mice that are relatively resistant to MRM and those susceptible

Effect of Nitrogen Dioxide Exposure on Mortality in Mice Caused by Murine Respiratory Mycoplasmosis

| Strain of Mouse | $NO_2$ Exposure (*ppm*) | *M. pulmonis* in Nebulizer (*cfu/ml*) | Incidence of Death at 7 Days | Incidence of Death at 21 Days |
|---|---|---|---|---|
| C57BL/6N | 0 | $5.01 \times 10^{10}$ | 1/12 (8%) | 1/12 (8%) |
| | 10 | $5.01 \times 10^{10}$ | 5/12 (42%) | 9/12 (75%)* |
| | 15 | $5.01 \times 10^{10}$ | 8/13 (62%)* | 11/13 (85%)* |
| C3H/HeN | 0 | $5.01 \times 10^{9}$ | 0/12 (0%) | 3/12 (25%) |
| | 10 | $5.01 \times 10^{9}$ | 0/12 (0%) | 0/13 (0%) |
| | 15 | $5.01 \times 10^{9}$ | 2/12 (17%) | 7/14 (50%) |

*Group significantly different from group exposed to 0 ppm of $NO_2$ at $P \leq .05$.
(Courtesy of Parker RF, Davis JK, Cassell GH, et al: *Am Rev Respir Dis* 140:502–512, August 1989.)

to MRM. Mice were exposed to $NO_2$ for 4 hours before receiving aerosols of *Mycoplasma pulmonis.*

In the relatively resistant mice, $NO_2$ exposure increased mortality and the incidence of gross and microscopic lung lesions but not the incidence of lung infection (table). More *Mycoplasma* organisms occurred in the lungs of mice of both strains exposed to $NO_2$. Exposure to $NO_2$ lowered the clearance of organisms from the lungs but did not alter the rate of physical removal of organisms from the lungs. Reduced clearance was the result of impaired intrapulmonary killing of the organisms.

Reduced clearance of organisms after $NO_2$ exposure is related to more severe disease. It is hoped that further studies will reveal which host mechanisms are affected by $NO_2$ exposure and are responsible for impaired killing of *M. pulmonis* in the lungs.

▶ The effects of oxidizing agents, particularly nitrogen dioxide ($NO_2$) and ozone ($O_3$) on human health have been sumarized by the *IAQ Environmental Information Handbook* (U.S. Dept of Energy, 1985; DOE/EV10450-1, National Technical Information Service, U.S. Dept. of Commerce, Springfield, Va) as follows: (1) an immediate short-term increase in airway reactivity (sensitivity); (2) increased incidence of acute respiratory infections, especially in infants and children; (3) impairment of lung function in children; (4) production of methemoglobin, reducing the oxygen carrying capacity of the blood.

Heightened reactivity can make airways more vulnerable to nonspecific, irritant stimuli, such as other pollutants and cold or dry air. Persons with preexisting hyperreactive airways from asthma or acute respiratory infections (current or recent) are likely to be most susceptible. An increase in acute childhood respiratory infections increases the probability that chronic lung disease will develop in adolescence and adulthood or that lung growth and development will be retarded, or both.

In the study by Parker and associates, an animal model is described to help understand the mechanism underlying the oxidant-related increase in nonfatal respiratory disease. The authors have observed a reduction in intrapulmonary killing of the *Mycoplasma* organisms, which, they suggest, may result from a reduction of nonspecific macrophage activation. The failure of intrapulmonary mycoplasma killing then results in a heightened neutrophil influx and increased neutrophil lung destruction.—M.S. Tockman, M.D., Ph.D.

**Short-Term Pulmonary Function Change in Association With Ozone Levels**

Kinney PL, Ware JH, Spengler JD, Dockery DW, Speizer FE, Ferris BG Jr (Harvard Univ; Brigham and Women's Hosp, Boston)

*Am Rev Respir Dis* 139:56–61, January 1989 8–21

Mounting evidence indicates that short-term, reversible pulmonary dysfunction occurs in response to relatively low levels of ozone exposure. Short-term changes in lung function in schoolchildren living in Kingston and Harriman, Tennessee, were examined as part of a larger study of respiratory health in the United States. Function was evaluated weekly in 154 children for a 2-month period in 1981. Ambient ozone, sulfate, and fine particle concentrations were measured at the same time.

The peak hourly ozone concentration during the period was 78 parts per billion (ppb). Levels of ozone, but not of particulates, were associated

Summary of Basic Regression Results: Kingston Acute Study

| Pollution Variable | Lung Function Variable | Mean Slope | Standard Error |
|---|---|---|---|
| $O_3$max, ppb | FVC, ml | −0.92* | 0.36 |
| | $FEV_{75}$, ml | −0.99† | 0.36 |
| | MMEF, ml/s | −1.9* | 0.88 |
| | $\dot{V}max_{75}$, ml/s | −2.4† | 0.78 |
| FP, μg/m³ | FVC, ml | 0.85 | 1.2 |
| | $FEV_{75}$, ml | 2.3 | 1.2 |
| | MMEF, ml/s | 6.5* | 2.7 |
| | $\dot{V}max_{75}$, ml/s | 3.4 | 2.9 |
| $FSO_4$, μg/m³ | FVC, ml | 0.2 | 1.7 |
| | $FEV_{75}$, ml | −1.0 | 1.5 |
| | MMEF, ml/s | 5.8 | 4.3 |
| | $\dot{V}max_{75}$, ml/s | −1.6 | 3.4 |
| Temp, °F | FVC, ml | −0.92† | 0.33 |
| | $FEV_{75}$, ml | −0.64 | 0.39 |
| | MMEF, ml/s | −1.7* | 0.85 |
| | $\dot{V}max_{75}$, ml/s | −2.7† | 0.71 |

*Abbreviations: $O_3max$,* maximal hourly $O_3$ in the 24 hours before pulmonary function testing; *FP,* fine particle concentration; *$FSO_4$,* fine sulfate; *temp,* temperature; *FVC,* forced vital capacity; *$FEV_{75}$,* forced expiratory volume in 75 seconds; *MMEF,* maximal mid-expiratory flow rate; *$Vmax_{75}$,* flow rate at 75% of expired FVC.

*$P < .05$.

†$P < .01$.

(Courtesy of Kinney PL, Ware JH, Spengler JD, et al: *Am Rev Respir Dis* 139:56–61, January 1989.)

with declines in forced vital capacity, forced expiratory volume, and maximal mid-expiratory flow rates (table). Individual responses to ozone could not be related to sex, respiratory illness early in life, or asthma.

Exposure to environmental ozone at levels well below the National Ambient Air Quality Standard of 120 ppb are associated with transient reductions in pulmonary function in schoolchildren. Whether these effects will lead to clinically significant changes remains to be determined.

▶ In ambient air, ozone is derived from the photochemical action of the sun on a mixture of hydrocarbon vapor and nitrogen oxides. The oxidant damage producing the health effects of ozone are similar to those of the nitrogen oxides summarized in the preceding section. The study by Kinney and colleagues joins several others described in the YEAR BOOKS OF PULMONARY DISEASE for 1988 and 1989 demonstrating a reversible physiologic effect on pulmonary function in children at ozone levels below the NAAQS of 120 ppb. However, the health significance of these changes is not yet clear. The investigators suggest that 2 factors are important in resolving this issue: the magnitude of the function decrements and their relationship to longer-term effects.

On average, the ozone response is small (1-mL loss of forced vital capacity per part per billion of $O_3$). However, this and other studies of childhood ozone responsiveness have shown substantial heterogeneity. These investigators assessed whether "sensitivity," as measured by the child-specific slopes of ozone response, could be predicted by available individual characteristics. Not histories of asthma, early childhood respiratory illness, nor sex was predictive of ozone "sensitivity" in this study.—M.S. Tockman, M.D., Ph.D.

**Ozone-Induced Inflammation in the Lower Airways of Human Subjects**

Koren HS, Devlin RB, Graham DE, Mann R, McGee MP, Horstman DH, Kozumbo WJ, Becker S, House DE, McDonnell WF, Bromberg PA (US Environmental Protection Agency, Research Triangle Park, NC; Univ of North Carolina, Chapel Hill; Wake Forest Univ, Winston-Salem; Environmental Monitoring and Services, Inc, Chapel Hill, NC)

*Am Rev Respir Dis* 139:407–415, February 1989 8–22

Ozone exposure leads to acute, reversible changes in pulmonary function and also to inflammation and temporary airway hyperresponsiveness to bronchoconstrictor drugs. The cellular and biochemical sequelae of ozone exposure were examined in 11 healthy nonsmoking men aged 18–35 years, who were exposed to 0.4 ppm ozone for 2 hours with intermittent exercise; bronchoalveolar lavage was carried out 18 hours later. Control exposures were to filtered air.

The percentage of polymorphs in bronchoalveolar lavage specimens increased eightfold after exposure to ozone. Macrophages declined to a significant degree. Immunoreactive neutrophil elastase rose fourfold in lavage fluid and more than 20-fold in lavaged cells (Fig 8–6). Protein, albumin, and immunoglobulin G levels approximately doubled, suggesting increased vascular permeability of the lung. Levels of prostaglandin $E_2$ and

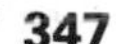

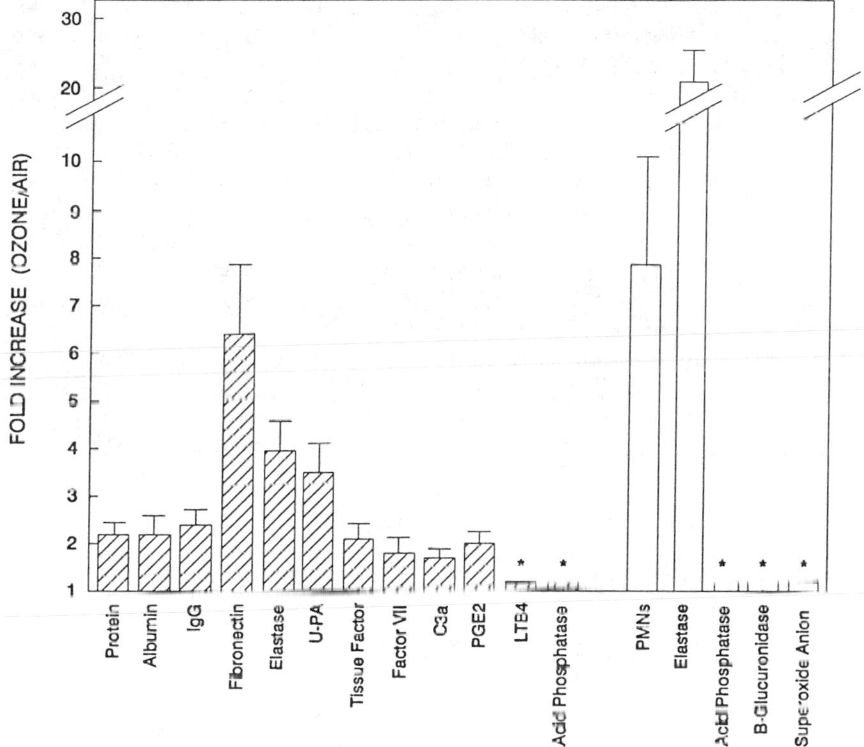


**Fig 8–6.**—Cellular and biochemical changes in bronchoalveolar lavage specimens of subjects exposed to ozone and air. *Bars* represent mean ratios (fold increase) of measurements in lavage fluid *(shaded bars)* and on assayed cells *(open bars)* determined after ozone and air exposures. *No detectable changes (ozone vs. air) were observed. (Courtesy of Koren HS, Devlin RB, Graham DE, et al: *Am Rev Respir Dis* 139:407–415, February 1989.)

$C_{3a}$ increased after ozone exposure. Lysosomal enzymes and NADPH-oxidase were not increased. Fibronectin was increased sixfold in lavage fluid. Urokinase plasminogen activator, which has fibrinolytic activity, increased more than threefold.

Acute ozone exposure associated with moderate exercise leads to a relatively prolonged inflammatory response in the lower airways. The response presumably is transient, but recurrent inhalation of ozone may entail a significant risk.

▶ This study measured a range of ozone effects on the airway, focusing on enzymes, proteins, and mediators with relevance to inflammation, chronic lung disease, and host defense. The investigators have grouped their studies to evaluate (1) molecules associated with chemotaxis (complement component $C_{3a}$ and arachidonic acid metabolite prostaglandin $E_2$ were increased approximately twofold, but no elevation of leukotriene $B_4$ was detected); (2) enzymes associated with tissue damage and microorganism defense (NADPH oxidase and the lysosomal enzymes acid phosphatase and β-glucuronidase were not increased); and (3) proteins involved in fibrotic and fibrinolytic processes (fibronectin was elevated 6.4-fold; a fibrinolytic protease, urokinase plasminogen activator, was increased 3.6-fold).

That ozone inflames both upper and lower airways of animals and human beings has been previously demonstrated. This paper quantitates the human acute (18-hour) cellular and biochemical response to a 2-hour inhalation of 0.4 ppm ozone detectable via bronchoalveolar lavage. The paper thus represnts an intermediate step in our understanding of the inflammatory potential of acute, moderate-dose ozone exposure to human airways. Knowledge of the cellular and biochemical consequences of long-term human ozone exposure, or of ozone exposures at levels more typical of ambient concentrations, must await further study. Furthermore, the surprising absence of an expected $LTB_4$ elevation is discussed by the authors; it, too, requires further study because this lipoxygenase metabolite, a powerful neutrophil and eosinophil chemotactic factor and lymphocyte immunoregulator, has been found in ozone-exposed animals and asbestos-exposed humans (1).—M.S. Tockman, M.D., Ph.D.

*Reference*

1. Garcia JGN et al: *Am Rev Respir Dis* 139:1494–1501, June 1989.

---

**Characterization of the Oxidant Generation by Inflammatory Cells Lavaged From Rat Lungs Following Acute Exposure to Ozone**

Esterline RL, Bassett DJP, Trush MA (Johns Hopkins Univ School of Hygiene and Public Health)

*Toxicol Appl Pharmacol* 99:229–239, June 1989 8–23

---

Exposure to irritant gases, such as ozone, is a health hazard to human beings, partly because of an influx of inflammatory cells that generate molecular oxygen-derived oxidants. Those oxidants have been implicated in damage to lung cells and in the activation of xenobiotics. An attempt was made to characterize the oxidant-generating capacity of inflammatory cells after acute exposure of adult rats to ozone in an inhalation chamber.

After the rat's exposure to 2 ppm ozone for 4 hours, superoxide production stimulated by 12-O-tetradecanoylphorbol-13-acetate or opsonized zymosan was maximally inhibited at 24 hours. In contrast, luminol-amplified chemoluminescence was increased after ozone exposure, paralleling an increase in the percentage of neutrophils and myeloperoxidase in the inflammatory cells. Chemoluminescence was inhibited by azide but not by superoxide dismutase. The cells generated taurine chloramines, a myeloperoxidase-dependent function that was not present before ozone exposure. Addition of myeloperoxidase to control alveolar macrophages enhanced chemoluminescence and taurine chloramine generation.

Acute exposure of rats to ozone depresses the ability of alveolar macrophages to produce superoxide and enhances myeloperoxidase-mediated reactions. Human polymorphs have even greater oxidant-generating capacity than do rat cells, suggesting that human beings may be at particular risk for the deleterious effects of inflammatory cell-mediated reactions.

▶ This paper contributes to our understanding of the effects of the interaction of polymorphonuclear leukocytes (PMNs) and macrophages on the oxidant moieties produced by inflammatory cells within the lung after exposure to ozone.

The investigators demonstrate that, immediately after acute exposure of rats to ozone (2 ppm), superoxide generation by the inflammatory cell population (primarily alveolar macrophages) was depressed. Yet, after a large influx of neutrophils into the lung that peaked at 24 hours, the spectrum of oxidant-dependent reactions changed. The newly recruited PMNs were not exposed directly to ozone and retain their capacity to produce superoxide as well as the hydrogen peroxide necessary for myeloperoxidase activity. In the presence of exogenous (PMN-derived) myeloperoxidase, possibly ingested as leukocyte debris by macrophages, the macrophages then contribute to myeloperoxidase-mediated pathologic reactions.

The advent of peroxidase activity, associated with neutrophil influx, is potentially important also as a mechanism of procarcinogen activation. The authors raise the possibility that ozone exposure may increase the carcinogenic risk of xenobiotics (e.g., benzo[a]-pyrene), which are substrates for peroxidases in the lung. This point is further discussed by Witschi (1).—M.S. Tockman, M.D., Ph.D.

*Reference*

1. Witschi H: Ozone, nitrogen dioxide, and lung cancer: A review of some recent issues and problems. *Toxicology* 48:1–20, 1988.

## Respiratory Protective Devices

### Clinical Pulmonary Function Tests as Predictors of Work Performance During Respirator Wear

Wilson JR, Raven PB (Texas College of Osteopathic Medicine, Fort Worth)
*Am Ind Hyg Assoc J* 50:51–57, January 1989 8–24

Physicians have available little information on how to assess workers' ability to use a respirator safely. To predict the capability of workers to wear respirator during work, a heterogeneous population of 38 men and women, including 19 firefighters, underwent clinical pulmonary function testing with or without a full-face-piece respiratory mask (MSA Ultravue). The pressure-demand respiratory was used in the demand mode to assess pulmonary function at work and at rest.

Most pulmonary measures were reduced significantly from 7% to 15% with respiratory wear. The forced vital capacity (FVC) declined significantly by 12%, and the ratio of forced expiratory volume in 1 second to FVC fell significantly by 5%. Peak expired flow declined significantly from 8.4 L/sec without 7.1 L/sec with the respirator. Flow at 50% vital capacity was not affected significantly, whereas flow at 25% vital capacity was increased significantly with respirator use. The average maximal voluntary ventilation in 15 seconds ($MVV_{.25}$) fell 7.4% with respirator use. Participants worked at 11% more of their reserve capacity with the respirator. The only predictor of maximal work performance was the $MVV_{.25}$ test with the respirator; the only predictor of endurance exercise time with the respirator was the change in peak inspiratory flow with and without respirator use. The $MVV_{.25}$ scores with and without the respirator mask were well correlated, and the higher the $MVV_{.25}$ without the respirator, the greater the decrease caused by wearing the respirator.

To evaluate worker capability for respirator wear, a physician must know both a worker's functional lung capacity and the demands of the work. Otherwise indiscriminate assignment of workers to tasks requiring respirators may produce physical distress.

▶ These authors report the results of their search to find a simple clinical test that can be used to screen industrial workers for their capability to wear a respirator. Justification for a single-item screening test of pulmonary function lies in several of the standard pulmonary function measures being highly correlated with each other. Results of the stepwise linear regression incorporating clinical pulmonary function tests to predict work performance indicated the best predictor of work performance during maximal exercise was the 15-second MVV with the respirator.

The authors found that greater lung impairment, or smaller lung capacities, resulted in lesser reduction in the 15-second MVV. They propose that, by measuring the 15-second MVV, calculating the potential reduction caused by respirator wear, and combining this information with the required ventilation of the work task, a physician will be able to determine each worker's ability to work while wearing a respirator, regardless of the presence of pulmonary disease.— M.S. Tockman, M.D., Ph.D.

---

**Effects of Respirator Dead Space, Inspiratory Resistance, and Expiratory Resistance Ventilatory Loads**

Harber P, Shimozaki S, Barrett T, Losides P, Fine G (Univ of California, Los Angeles; Univ of California Southern Occupational Health Ctr, Los Angeles)
*Am J Ind Med* 16:189–198, 1989 8–25

---

The physiologic effects of respiratory protective devices remain incompletely understood, partly because many combinations of inspiratory resistance (IR), expiratory resistance (ER), and dead space are incorporated into respirator designs. The effects of varying those parameters were examined in 11 healthy persons during both moderate steady-stage and rapidly incremented exercise.

The physiologic effects of IR predominated. They included increasing inspiratory time and several measures of ventilatory work. The effects of dead space appeared to be related to increased minute ventilation; they included an increased flow rate and greater ventilatory work. The effect of dead space was relatively less at higher levels of rapidly incremented exercise. Expiratory resistance had the effect of compressing expiratory time.

These observations of healthy persons suggest that dead space may be physiologically less significant than inspiratory resistance. If a respirator simulation test is used in the course of medical certification testing, an IR generally should be used. Expiratory resistance may be relatively unimportant, and adding expiratory bypass valves to lower expiratory flow resistance may not greatly promote tolerance of a respirator. Inspiratory resistance should be minimized in designing respirators, even at the expense of increasing dead space to some degree.

► This paper examines the effects of various types of respiratory loads characteristically imposed by respiratory protective devices: inspiratory flow resistance, expiratory flow resistance, and dead space. The experimental model described by the investigators could impose these loads individually and in combination. All loads were measured at steady state and during rapidly incremented exercise.

It has long been known that individuals adjust their respiratory patterns to minimize inspiratory effort (1). Subjects adjusted their respiratory patterns to compensate for the respiratory loads. Additional inspiratory resistance led to lengthening of the inspiratory time and lower peak inspiratory flows. Additional expiratory resistance prolonged the expiratory phase. Increasing the dead space lengthened the inspiratory time but increased the flow rate, so that no change in respiratory frequency was observed. The authors suggest that inspiratory resistance is the dominant factor determining the ventilatory response to increasing respiratory loading.—M.S. Tockman, M.D., Ph.D.

*Reference*

1. Mead J: Control of respiratory frequency. *J Appl Physiol* 15:325–336, 1960.

---

**Effect of Respiratory Protective Equipment on Exposure to Asbestos Fibers During Removal of Asbestos Insulation**

Akkersdijk H, Bremmer CF, Schliszka C, Spee T (Ministry of Social Affairs and Employment, Voorburg, The Netherlands)

*Ann Occup Hyg* 33:113–116, 1989 8–26

---

Adequate protective gear is important for workers who remove sprayed asbestos. Asbestos concentrations were measured within powered respirators that were used by workers in removing asbestos-containing insulation. Fiber concentrations within the protective equipment exceeded the Dutch threshold limit for crocidolite, 0.2 fibers/$cm^3$.

After daily rather than weekly replacement of filters, thorough cleaning and inspection of protective overalls after each shift, and cleaning of the changing facility every week, fiber concentrations in the breathing zone fell significantly to about 0.08 fibers/$cm^3$. The fiber concentration outside the helmet was 28 fibers/$cm^3$ yielding a protection factor of about 350.

▶ This study points out the importance of monitoring workplace exposures via personal air sampling. Mandated worker protection procedures were being followed, so it was only investigator concern and personal air sampling that determined that actual worker exposures exceeded the threshold limit value. Unfortunately, this study does not provide criteria for deciding when to undertake personal air sampling so as to assure the efficacy of mandated protective procedures.—M.S. Tockman, M.D., Ph.D.

# Subject Index

## A

## B

# C

## F



## G

## H



## I

## K



## L

## M

## S

## T

## U



## V

## W

# Author Index

## A



## B



## C

## D



## E



## F



## G

## H



## I



## J



## K

## L



## M

## R



## S

## T



## U



## V



## W



## Y



## Z

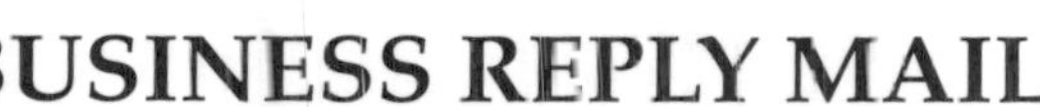

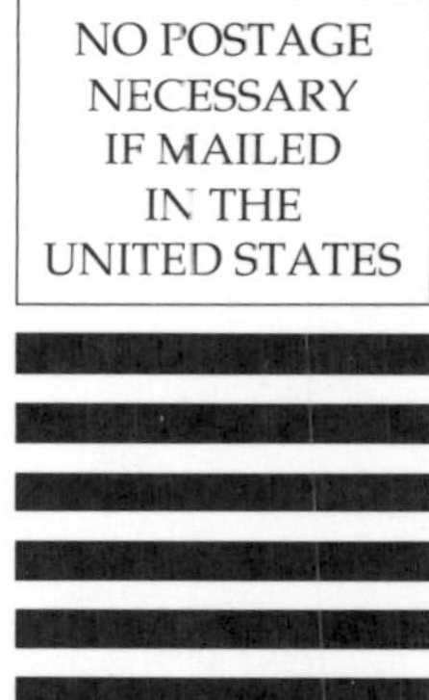



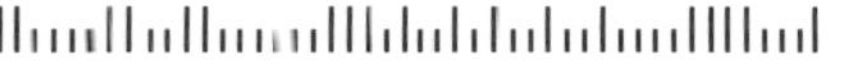

# *YEAR BOOK READY-ACCESS CARD!*

[✗] Yes! I'd like to keep current. Please send me a *free* 30-day examination copy of the Year Book(s) checked below:

| | |
|---|---|
| [ ] *Year Book of Anesthesia*® (AN) | $54.95 |
| [ ] *Year Book of Cardiology*® (CV) | $54.95 |
| [ ] *Year Book of Critical Care Medicine*® (16) | $51.95 |
| [ ] *Year Book of Dermatology*® (10) | $51.95 |
| [ ] *Year Book of Diagnostic Radiology*® (9) | $54.95 |
| [ ] *Year Book of Digestive Diseases*® (13) | $51.95 |
| [ ] *Year Book of Drug Therapy*® (6) | $54.95 |
| [ ] *Year Book of Emergency Medicine*® (15) | $51.95 |
| [ ] *Year Book of Endocrinology*® (EM) | $54.95 |
| [ ] *Year Book of Family Practice*® (FY) | $51.95 |
| [ ] *Year Book of Geriatrics and Gerontology* (GE) | $51.95 |
| [ ] *Year Book of Hand Surgery*® (17) | $54.95 |
| [ ] *Year Book of Hematology*® (24) | $51.95 |
| [ ] *Year Book of Infectious Diseases*® (19) | $51.95 |
| [ ] *Year Book of Infertility* (IN) | $51.95 |
| [ ] *Year Book of Medicine*® (1) | $51.95 |
| [ ] *Year Book of Neonatal-Perinatal Medicine* (23) | $51.95 |
| [ ] *Year Book of Neurology and Neurosurgery*® (8) | $54.95 |
| [ ] *Year Book of Nuclear Medicine*® (NM) | $54.95 |
| [ ] *Year Book of Obstetrics and Gynecology*® (5) | $51.95 |
| [ ] *Year Book of Oncology* (CA) | $54.95 |
| [ ] *Year Book of Ophthalmology*® (EY) | $51.95 |
| [ ] *Year Book of Orthopedics*® (OR) | $54.95 |
| [ ] *Year Book of Otolaryngology – Head and Neck Surgery*® (3) | $54.95 |
| [ ] *Year Book of Pathology and Clinical Pathology*® (PI) | $54.95 |
| [ ] *Year Book of Pediatrics*® (4) | $51.95 |
| [ ] *Year Book of Plastic and Reconstructive Surgery*® (12) | $54.95 |
| [ ] *Year Book of Psychiatry and Applied Mental Health*® (11) | $49.95 |
| [ ] *Year Book of Pulmonary Disease*® (21) | $51.95 |
| [ ] *Year Book of Sports Medicine*® (SM) | $51.95 |
| [ ] *Year Book of Surgery*® (2) | $54.95 |
| [ ] *Year Book of Urology*® (7) | $54.95 |
| [ ] *Year Book of Vascular Surgery*® (20) | $54.95 |

*All Year Books are published annually. For the convenience of its customers, Year Book enters each purchaser as a subscriber to future volumes and sends annual announcements of each volume approximately 2 months before publication. The new volume will be shipped upon publication unless you complete and return the cancellation notice attached to the announcement and it is received by Year Book within the time indicated (approximately 20 days after your receipt of the announcement). You may cancel your subscription at any time. The new volume may be examined on approval for 30 days, may be returned for full credit, and if returned Year Book will then remove your name as a subscriber. Return postage is guaranteed by Year Book to the Postal Service.

NAME/ACCT. NO.

ADDRESS

CITY/STATE/ZIP CODE: EBF1

Prepaid orders are shipped postage free; add $3.50 per order to cover handling. Other orders will be billed a shipping and handling charge. IL, MA, TN residents are billed appropriate sales tax. Prices quoted in U.S. dollars. Canadian orders will be billed in Canadian funds at the current exchange rate. All prices subject to change without notice.

**Mosby-Year Book, Inc. • 200 North LaSalle Street • Chicago, Illinois 60601**